VIROLOGY RESEARCH PROGRESS

EPSTEIN-BARR VIRUS (EBV)

TRANSMISSION, DIAGNOSIS AND ROLE IN THE DEVELOPMENT OF CANCERS

VIROLOGY RESEARCH PROGRESS

Additional books in this series can be found on Nova's website under the Series tab.

Additional e-books in this series can be found on Nova's website under the e-book tab.

VIROLOGY RESEARCH PROGRESS

EPSTEIN-BARR VIRUS (EBV)

TRANSMISSION, DIAGNOSIS AND ROLE IN THE DEVELOPMENT OF CANCERS

JAN STYCZYNSKI
EDITOR

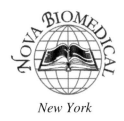

New York

Copyright © 2014 by Nova Science Publishers, Inc.

All rights reserved. No part of this book may be reproduced, stored in a retrieval system or transmitted in any form or by any means: electronic, electrostatic, magnetic, tape, mechanical photocopying, recording or otherwise without the written permission of the Publisher.

For permission to use material from this book please contact us:
Telephone 631-231-7269; Fax 631-231-8175
Web Site: http://www.novapublishers.com

NOTICE TO THE READER

The Publisher has taken reasonable care in the preparation of this book, but makes no expressed or implied warranty of any kind and assumes no responsibility for any errors or omissions. No liability is assumed for incidental or consequential damages in connection with or arising out of information contained in this book. The Publisher shall not be liable for any special, consequential, or exemplary damages resulting, in whole or in part, from the readers' use of, or reliance upon, this material. Any parts of this book based on government reports are so indicated and copyright is claimed for those parts to the extent applicable to compilations of such works.

Independent verification should be sought for any data, advice or recommendations contained in this book. In addition, no responsibility is assumed by the publisher for any injury and/or damage to persons or property arising from any methods, products, instructions, ideas or otherwise contained in this publication.

This publication is designed to provide accurate and authoritative information with regard to the subject matter covered herein. It is sold with the clear understanding that the Publisher is not engaged in rendering legal or any other professional services. If legal or any other expert assistance is required, the services of a competent person should be sought. FROM A DECLARATION OF PARTICIPANTS JOINTLY ADOPTED BY A COMMITTEE OF THE AMERICAN BAR ASSOCIATION AND A COMMITTEE OF PUBLISHERS.

Additional color graphics may be available in the e-book version of this book.

Library of Congress Cataloging-in-Publication Data

ISBN: 978-1-63117-476-6

Library of Congress Control Number: 2014933507

Published by Nova Science Publishers, Inc. † New York

Contents

Preface		vii
Chapter I	Epstein-Barr Virus: Clinical and Laboratory Characteristics of Infectious Mononucleosis *Napoleón González Saldaña, Eduardo Liquidano Pérez and Hugo Juárez Olguín*	1
Chapter II	The Role of Epstein-Barr Virus in the Management of Undifferentiated Nasopharyngeal Carcinoma *Thian-Sze Wong, Yu-Wai Chan and Wei Gao*	29
Chapter III	Epstein-Barr Virus (EBV) –Associated B-Cell Lymphoma *Prakash Vishnu and David M. Aboulafia*	41
Chapter IV	The Role of the Epstein-Barr Virus in the Pathogenesis of Post-Transplant Lymphoproliferative Disorders *Julie Morscio and Thomas Tousseyn*	73
Chapter V	EBV-Related Post-Transplant Lymphoproliferative Disorders (PTLD): Background, Diagnosis and Treatment *Ghaith Abu-Zeinah and Mustafa Al-Kawaaz*	153
Chapter VI	Differences between EBV-Associated Post-Transplant Lymphoproliferative Disorders after Hematopoietic Stem Cell Transplantation and Solid Organ Transplantation *Jan Styczynski*	175
Chapter VII	T-Cell Lymphoproliferative Disorders: The Role of the Epstein-Barr Virus *Jan Styczynski*	207
Chapter VIII	Results of Therapy of EBV-Associated Post-Transplant Lymphoproliferative Disorder in Children and Adults with Anti-CD20 Antibodies after Hematopoietic Stem Cell Transplantation *Jan Styczynski*	239
Index		269

Preface

The Epstein-Barr Virus (EBV), also known as Human Herpes Virus 4, has been identified and described as the etiological agent of infectious mononucleosis. It is the first human virus found to be implicated in oncogenesis. EBV is associated with a number of biologically diverse cancers, mainly lymphoproliferations of B-cell origin. With the development of basic research and clinical medicine, new ideas related to the pathogenesis and clinical aspects of EBV-associated diseases have arisen recently.

A significant progress in the number of hematopoietic stem cell and solid organ transplantations performed worldwide, involving high-risk patients, has contributed to an increase in the development of EBV-associated malignant post-transplant lymphoproliferative disorders. In the stem cell transplant setting, a post-transplant lymphoproliferative disorder has in most cases the nature of a secondary cancer. Apart from post-transplant lymphoproliferative disorders, other types of lymphoproliferative disorders are recognized and presented in this book.

The main aim of this book is to provide readers with an overview of the impact of EBV on parameters that contribute to the development of malignancy in immunocompromised patients, particularly in recipients of a solid organ or hematopoietic stem cell transplant. Also, current concepts and practices in the diagnosis, management and prevention of EBV-associated malignancies are highlighted, with special emphasis on transplant patients.

The book is organized in two sections. The first section describes the oncogenic potential of the Epstein-Barr Virus along with a thorough appraisal of its role in nasopharyngeal carcinoma and B-cell lymphoma. This part is essential for situating EBV in the field of oncogenesis, and presenting the pivotal role of EBV in contemporary oncology and transplantology. This is followed by the second section, which answers some of the questions related to post-transplant lymphoproliferative disorders.

The book is a comprehensive collection of papers that describe the active processes induced by EBV in oncogenesis. As we live in the world where transplantation science is making rapid progress, the book is focused mostly on post-transplant lymphoproliferative disorders, as this topic is developing considerably.

The issue of post-transplant lymphoproliferative disorder is of great interest to scientists and clinicians due to significant changes in its epidemiology, diagnostics and therapy over the last decade. The epidemiology of post-transplant lymphoproliferative disorders has been influenced by a tremendous increase in mismatched and unrelated donor transplants. Current diagnostics of EBV-associated diseases is based on modern pathology, quantitative viremia and the use of positron emission tomography. A significant progress has been achieved in the therapy of post-transplant lymphoproliferative disorders with the use of rituximab and EBV-specific cytotoxic T lymphocytes.

The content of the book was critically reviewed by Dr Lidia Gil from Department of Hematology, Poznan Medical University. I wish to thank her for excellent guest service.

This book seeks a more comprehensive application of the knowledge on EBV and its role in the development of cancer. The publication is not a purely academic monograph as it contains a number of novel insights, concepts and hypotheses. We are presenting a book related to both basic and clinical research, and whose main audience is the healthcare community.

Jan Styczynski, MD, PhD
Department of Pediatric Hematology and Oncology,
Collegium Medicum, Nicolaus Copernicus University,
Bydgoszcz, Poland
jstyczynski@cm.umk.pl

Note from the Reviewer

Epstein-Barr virus, with its oncogenic abilities, is known to be involved in a development of a wide range of nonmalignant or malignant diseases, especially among immunocompromised patients. Substantial progress in medicine with new drugs and methods resulting in prolonged survival but interfering with immune system, is related to a growing risk for EBV-related complications.

The importance of EBV-related complications, including malignancies, far exceeds their frequency, as with the application of recent advances in cellular and molecular biology to the understanding of their pathogenesis, diagnosis and treatment, have become a model approach of relevance to different forms of cancer.

The book, including 8 chapters, does approach the subject of EBV-related hematological, non-hematological and infectious complications from a basis scientific standpoint and will be of value to both clinicians and scientists working in the field. Presented management (diagnosis, prevention, treatment) of neoplastic complications in different settings, based not only on case reports, but also on designed studies is of great value, especially as it is in line with international recommendations. Most of texts dealing with EBV-related lymphoma are dedicated to B-lymphoproliferations, however interesting is also part concerning rare entity, EBV-related T/NK-lymphomas. Careful analysis of the chapters related to lymphomas, confirms the differences between patient populations, i.e., PTLD after HSCT versus PTLD after SOT, with respect to clinical presentation, prognosis, prevention and treatment.

I was honored to review papers prepared by acknowledged experts in their field, thus providing a multidisciplinary and international perspective.

Lidia Gil, MD, PhD
Department of Hematology,
Medical University, Poznan, Poland

In: Epstein-Barr Virus (EBV)
Editor: Jan Styczynski

ISBN: 978-1-63117-476-6
© 2014 Nova Science Publishers, Inc.

Chapter I

Epstein-Barr Virus: Clinical and Laboratory Characteristics of Infectious Mononucleosis

Napoleón González Saldaña[1], Eduardo Liquidano Pérez[2] and Hugo Juárez Olguín[2,3],*

[1]Servicio de Infectología, Instituto Nacional de Pediatría (INP), Mexico City, Mexico
[2]Laboratorio de Farmacología, INP, Mexico City, Mexico
[3]Departamento de Farmacología, Facultad de Medicina, Universidad Nacional Autónoma de México, Mexico City, Mexico

Abstract

Epstein Barr virus (EBV) belongs to the group of herpes virus. The virus is regarded as the etiology of infectious mononucleosis (IM). Its genome consists of a double chain DNA that exclusively infects lymphoreticular system, thereby giving rise to lymphoproliferative diseases. There are two types of EBV: "A and B", also designated as 1 and 2, a classification which is principally based on their allelic differences that define their development in B lymphocytes. The infection has a universal distribution although, in developing countries, the presentation is seen more in early ages of life. The principal means of transmission is through the saliva, a means which gives rise to its denomination as "kissing disease", with its first site of budding being the oropharyngeal epithelium. Invasion of EBV in B lymphocytes induces cellular response with the participation of NK lymphocytes, cytotoxic cells, and T lymphocytes all of which function as mediators of the clinical symptoms of the disease in acute phase. The symptoms of the infection depend on age. In little children, it is generally asymptomatic while in adolescents and

---

* Corresponding author: Hugo Juarez Olguin, Laboratorio de Farmacología, Instituto Nacional de Pediatria, Av. Iman #1, 3er piso, Col Cuicuilco, CP 04530, Mexico City, Mexico. Tel/ fax: 5255 1084 3883. E-mail: juarezol@yahoo.com.

adults, it is symptomatic with the principal presentation being fever, pharyngitis and adenopathies.

In general, IM has a benign prognosis for being a self-limited disease, normally resolved in 1 to 3 weeks. The incidence of complications in general population is low. EBV is the first human virus that was associated with malignant neoplasm due to the presence of its genome in different neoplasmic tissues which leads to the confirmation of its contribution in development of the same. The infection can range from self-limited benign disease, such as IM, to non aggressive malignants as hemophagocytic syndrome or completely malignants as nasopharyngeal carcinoma, Burkitt lymphoma, or Hodgkin disease. Diagnostic tests include blood test, Paul-Bunnell test, and detection of specific antibodies as well as the use of end markers, and polymerase chain reaction (PCR). Currently, there are studies that focused on the development of recombinant vaccine with protein Gp350 of the virus for its prevention. The treatment of the acute form of the virus is mainly symptomatic with the principal objectives being to mellow down such symptoms as fever and inflammatory process. Usually, increasing liquid intake and adequate diet are recommended as part of this treatment. Although assays with acyclovir *in vitro* have shown positive results by inhibition of viral multiplication, clinically favorable results have not been reported. In the present chapter, the concepts referent to the transmission, diagnosis of EBV, and its relation with cancer development are analyzed in detailed and updated form.

Keywords: Epstein-Barr virus, oncogenesis, infectious mononucleosis, Paul-Bunnell test

Introduction

The herpetic family virus is very numerous and ranges from benign to malignant viruses and from viruses with immediate action to those with slow participation in human pathology. Within these groups is Epstein-Barr virus (EBV), a type 4 herpes virus, with two sub-classes – EBV-1 and EBV-2, and the causal agent of infectious mononucleosis (IM), Burkitt lymphoma, and nasopharyngeal carcinoma. EBVs can be reproduced *in vitro* in lymphocytes. They are considered as responsible for IM and with affinity for B lymphocytes. The EBVs are also associated with Burkitt lymphoma and nasopharyngeal carcinoma [1, 2].

History

Epstein-Barr virus (EBV) was discovered as a result of pioneering work in the 1950s, by Denis Burkitt. Burkitt identified a previously unrecognized form of cancer in the jaws of young African children, and made a crucial insight that the distribution of this common tumor (now known as Burkitt's lymphoma) appeared to be influenced by climatic factors, notably temperature and elevation.

His work was followed by Tony Epstein, an English pathologist. Epstein with his graduate student Yvonne Barr identified by electron microscopy a novel herpes virus in lymphoma cell cultures. This virus was named Epstein-Barr virus (EBV) with an ability to confer unlimited growth on peripheral blood B lymphocytes in tissue culture (called immortalization).

In 1968, the virus was described as an etiological agent of IM while in 1979, the DNA was detected in tissues of patients with nasopharyngeal carcinoma. Later, it was found in tissues of other tumors like T cell lymphomas and Hodgkin disease [3-5].

Epidemiology, Prevalence and Geographical Distribution

EBV infection has a universal distribution. In developing countries, the infection is found in early ages of life and often asymptomatic or with unspecific symptoms while in developed countries or in socially privileged zones, the infection is seen in older ages such as school age or young people [6]. The virus has a cosmopolitan distribution, but the majority of the primary infections are found in subclinical form. The transmission is by oropharyngeal secretions but as well, could be transmitted by sexual activity since it has been isolated in vaginal and cervical secretions [7, 8].

Two distinct types of EBV, type 1 and 2 (also denominated as type A and B) have been characterized with type 1 being the most frequent in the world. Type 2 is more common in Africa than in America and Europe. EBV-1 has been found to provoke B lymphocyte growth transformation with more efficacy than EBV-2 *in vitro*. However, pathological manifestations or specific clinical differences between the two have not been identified [9]. IM epidemiology is related to the age of acquisition of EBV infection, a virus that affects more than 95% of world population. The transmission is by penetrated sexual relationships or by contact with oral secretions through kisses and exchange of saliva among children in nursery centers. Non intimate contact and enviromental sources do not contribute in the dissemination of the virus [10, 11].

In developing countries and less privileged socioeconomic groups in developed countries, EBV infection usually occurs during lactation and preschool period. In Central Africa, almost all children are affected at 3 years of age. The first infection by EBV in childhood is usually asymptomatic and indistinguishable from other infections in children. The clinical syndrome of IM is almost completely unknown in underdeveloped regions of the world. In the richest populations of industrialized countries of the world, the infection is also common however, with less frequency, perhaps due to a better level of hygiene with about one-third of the cases occurring in adolescents and the first part of adult life [9]. The incidence of infectious mononucleosis varies in each country in such a way that in US, 500 cases per 100,000 inhabitants are reported every year with a higher incidence in the age group from 15 to 24 years. Ebell reported a higher incidence of infectious mononucleosis in people from 10 to 19 years old (6 to 8 cases per 1,000 per year), and a lower incidence in children less than 10 years old (1 case per 1,000 people per year) and a milder clinical manifestations which is frequently underdiagnosed [6]. The prevalence of serological indices of having suffered from an EBV infection increases with age. Almost all adult in United States of America are seropositive [9, 12].

In a study carried out in Mexico in 1973, in a town close to Mexico City, it was found that at two years of age, 88.8% of the children had antibodies against EBV (anti-EBV) and that at the age 18 years, 93.5% were positive suggesting that in this place, the virus is acquired in younger age than in others. Gonzalez and collaborators, in a study carried out 22 years later, in a group of low socioeconomic level in Mexico City, found that 49% had anti-EBV at 4 years of age and 73% at 15 years old [6]. A similar event was described in other countries of Latin America. For instance, in Sao Pablo, 80% of the population was found to be positive for anti-EBV while a seroprevalence study carried out in Chile showed that 50% of 663 healthy children in low and medium socioeconomic levels had had the infection at 2 years of age while in high socioeconomic level, only 5.9% of children less than 2 years old were seroconverted.

However, at 20 years of age, 90% of the population in this age had specific antibodies against the virus. Another study carried out in Great Britain concluded that between 30% and 40% of the children acquired the infection at 5 years of age while in US, from 50 to 70% of the infections by EBV are present in adolescents [6]. In developing countries, EBV infection occurs early in life. Nearly the entire population of a developing country becomes infected before adolescence. Thus, symptomatic infectious mononucleosis is uncommon in such countries. In areas with high standards of hygiene, such as the United States and Western Europe, where EBV infection may be delayed until adulthood, infectious mononucleosis is more prevalent. The increase in the incidence of infectious mononucleosis with improved sanitary conditions may explain why this disease was not described until the latter half of the nineteenth century [13]. Because primary EBV infections occur early in life in Asia and developing countries, asymptomatic primary infections are common in these areas, whereas acute MI is fairly common in the United States and Western Europe, where a primary infection often occurs during adolescence [14].

Virological Characteristics of EBV

EBV is a member of herpes virus family, belonging to gammaherpesvirus sub-family and a prototype of lymphocryptovirus genus. The viral genome is located in a nucleocapsid surrounded by a viral envelope, before the virus penetrates into B lymphocytes. The glycoprotein of its membrane, gp 350, is united to the viral receptor (CD 21 molecule). Two major types of EBV, EBV-1 and EBV-2 (also known as types A and B), have been detected in humans. These two types differ in the sequence of the genes that code for the EBV nuclear antigens (EBNA-2, EBNA-3A/3, EBNA-3B/4, and EBNA-3C/6) [13, 15, 16].

Structure of the Virion

Like other herpes viruses, EBV is a DNA virus with a toroid-shaped protein core that is wrapped with DNA, a nucleocapsid with 162 capsomers, a protein tegument between the nucleocapsid and the envelope, and an outer envelope with external virus-encoded glycoprotein spikes [13, 17-19].

Structure of the Viral Genome

EBV genome is a linear, double-stranded, ~172-kb DNA molecule that encodes >85 genes. The genome is a double stranded DNA molecule of approximately 172,000 base pairs. As in other herpes viruses, the molecule is divided into unique, internal repeat, and terminal repeat domains [20-24]. The genome encodes approximately 80 proteins. The function of many of the genes involved in viral replication has been inferred from their homology to herpes simplex virus genes; however, genes expressed during latent infection of B cells do not have recognized counterparts in other human herpes viruses.

Two strains or types of EBV infect the humans [26, 27]. These strains differ in sequences of genes expressed during latent infection and in their ability to transform B lymphocytes (Table 1).

Although earlier studies suggested that type A (or EBV-1) virus infection was more prevalent in North America and Europe and that type B (or EBV-2) virus infection was more prevalent in Africa, more recent studies suggest that both strains are prevalent in the United States and that people can be co-infected with both strains. Epstein-Barr virus infects epithelial cells of the oropharynx and of the cervix and resting B lymphocytes. The receptor for the virus on epithelial cells and B lymphocytes is CD21 molecule, formerly called CR2, which is also the receptor for C3d component of complement [13, 25, 28].

Pathogenesis

The infection in humans is by contact with oral secretions and therefore, the infection begins with viral inversion of the pharynge. The transmission is principally through exposure to infected saliva and as such the denomination "kissing disease" [6, 29]. Viral replication takes place once it is found in epithelial cells of oropharynge from where it spreads to B lymphocytes when the later get in contact with these cells.

The B lymphocytes with latent memory constitute the permanent site of EBV in the organism. The virus, now in the cells of the epithelium and B lymphocytes begins to replicate and to produce cellular lysis.

Table 1. EBV latency and associated malignancies

EBV latency pattern and associated malignancies		
Latency type	Viral products expressed	Associated malignancies
Latency I	EBN-1 EBERs BARF0	Burkitt lymphoma Gastric carcinoma[b]
Latency II	EBN-1 EBERs LMP-1 LMP-2A BARF0	Hodgkin disease Nasopharyngeal carcinoma Peripheral T/NK lymphoma
Latency III	All EBNAs[a] EBERs LMP-1 LMP-2A BARF0	Post-transplant lymphoproliferative disorders AIDS-associated lymphomas

[a]EBNAs include EBNA-1, EBNA-2, EBNA3A(EBNA-4), EBNA-3C (EBNA-6), EBNA-LP (EBNA-5 or EBNA-4).

[b]Gastric carcinoma have been shown to express an intermediate latency I/II pattern including expression of EBNA-1, EBERs, LMP-2[a], BARF0 and some lytic infection proteins such as BARF-1, ENRF-1.

About 100 genes are expressed during the replication, but only 10 are expressed in period of latency with these being the limiting factors in genetic expression of viral proteins which impedes their recognition by cytotoxic T cells [3, 30-32].

If the first infection occurs in the first years of life, the infection is usually subclinic, but if the infection develops in the second decade of life, acute signs and symptoms such as fever, sore throat, ganglionary growth, general body pain, headache, splenomegaly, and the presence of atypic lymphocytes in blood are observed. The reason is that the virus could continue to be excreted in constant or intermittent form for a period of 18 months or more after the onset of the sickness. In small children, there could be other unknown mechanisms of transmission [33]. IM scarcely occurs by intimate contact of a patient with the disease with another person due to high level of immunity among these contacts. The incubation period of IM is from 30 to 50 days after exposition, but if the exposition is by blood transmission, which is usually rare, the incubation period is shorter [34, 35]. The transmission of EBV through blood derivatives has been described with clinical data similar to IM, but its frequency is very low in comparison with that of cytomegalovirus (CMV).

Immune Response

As commented, EBV is transmitted through the saliva and has its first site of entrance in oropharyngeal epithelium. The viral glycoprotein gH intervenes in the union with epithelial cell receptors that are independent of CD21, and in this way, the lymphoid tissue of Waldeyer chain is infected. Later, it invades the blood where a selective infection of B lymphocytes, accounting with specific surface receptors for EBV, occurs. The entrance into B lymphocytes is through the interaction of CD21 receptor cell with gp350/220 glycoprotein of the virus [36-39]. The infection of the lymphocytes leads to its destruction and shedding of viral particles in the blood which trigger the formation of antibodies. In the acute phase of IM, about 15,000 millions of lymphocytes are infected but various months later, the number declines to between 1 and 10 million lymphocytes. After IM, the virus remains for life in the infected lymphocytes [6, 40].

The latent permanence of the virus in B lymphocytes induces cellular immune response consisting in attraction of NK lymphocytes, cytotoxic cells, T lymphocytes, and activation of polyclonal B lymphocytes. It is believed that the activation of T lymphocytes and NK cells is brought into effect by the atypic lymphocytes in the peripheral blood and that these activated cells probably function as mediators of clinical symptoms in acute stage of the infection. As consequence of immune response, a drastic and notable reduction in the number of B lymphocytes occurs which gives rise to the establishment of an equilibrium in an indefinite form with the persistence in the peripheral blood of cellular immune response to the specific virus all the life, and dissemination of infected B lymphocytes in all the mononucleic phagocytic system [41-43].

The B cells with latent memory are the site of permanence of EBV in the organism. The infection by EBV generates cellular and humoral responses at the same time with cellular response being the most important for the control of the infection. The natural suppressor cells and cytotoxic T cells: CD4+ and CD8+ together with cytotoxic T cells control the proliferation of infected B cells in a primary infection by this virus.

In reality, the capacity of the virus to persist in the organism in spite of the strong immune response has been seen. This indicates that the virus coins up strategies to elude the defensive response of the organism.

The latent state of B lymphocytes in peripheral blood and possibly in other sites prolongs continuous replication of the virus, and thereby its lytic cycle in oropharyngeal epithelium. This latent state is characterized by expression of new EBV codified proteins: nuclear antigens determined by EBV such as EBNA-1, EBN-2, EBN-3A, EBN-3B, and EBN-3C; header protein; latent membrane proteins as LMP-1, LMP-2^a, and LMP-2B; and EBV codified RNA found in latency in all infected cells. EBNA-1 is essential in maintaining EBV genome like a circular extra-chromosomic episome while EBNA-2, EBNA-3A, EBNA-3C, and LMP-1 are necessary to maintain the immortalization of B lymphocytes [6, 46, 47].

Clinical Manifestations

Infectious Mononucleosis: Infectious mononucleosis (IM) or Mononucleosis syndrome is caused by an acute infection of Epstein-Barr virus (EBV). It has been reported that about 90% of the cases is caused by EBV. The natural infection by EBV occurs only in humans and the result is a life-long infection. In industrialized countries, there is greater possibility of developing mononucleosis if EBV infection occurs in the second decade of life. Seroepidemiological studies have shown that about 91% of all adults worldwide have had first-time infection by EBV. In developing countries, first-time infection by EBV is more frequent in the first decade of life [6, 48-53].

The classic syndrome of mononucleosis is defined as a clinical triad of fever, pharyngitis, and adenopathy, although many other symptoms and signs such as tonsillitis, pharyngo-laryngitis, hepatosplenomegaly, puffy eyelids, and skin eruptions can also occur. Skin rashes are most frequently induced by the administration of ampicillin, amoxicillin, and β-lactamic antibiotics. In most patients with acute IM, the illness is caused by a primary EBV infection, but similar symptoms may occur in an acute cytomegalovirus infection, and in drug-induced hypersensitivity syndrome caused by sulphates, anticonvulsants, allopurinol, and other drugs. The complications of IM include neutropenia, thrombocytopenia, splenic rupture, airway obstruction by tonsillar hypertrophy, central nervous system involvements, and fulminant hepatitis observed in developed countries [6].

The diagnosis of acute EBV infectious mononucleosis is based on clinical presentation and supportive laboratory findings, including an absolute lymphocytosis in which more than 15% of cells are atypical [13, 54].

The laboratory findings reported by Gonzalez et al in 2012 were: lymphocytosis (41.7%), atypic lymphocytes (24.5%), and increased transaminases (30.9%), there were no rupture of the spleen and no deaths among the 163 cases (Table 2) [6, 55-58].

Gonzalez and collaborators gave a general description of the clinical spectra and classified them as follows:

1 Asymptomatic
2 Unspecific respiratory manifestations
3 Classic or typical expression

4. Atypic clinical expression
5. Associated to syndromes
6. Recurring mononucleosis
7. Chronic mononucleosis
8. Congenital infection by EBV.
9. Associated to myeloproliferative diseases
10. Associated to neoplasm.

1. Asymptomatic: Babies and small children do not usually manifest any symptoms and factible diagnosis could only be by means of seroepidemiology.

2. Unspecific airway manifestations: Unspecific manifestations such as membrane-linked or non-membrane-linked pharyngitis, fever or adenopathy, and generally without the rest of the clinical spectra are usually observed in small children. Therefore, it is very difficult to carry out the clinical diagnosis and it is common to be diagnosed as pharyngitis or upper airway infection.

3. Classical or typical clinical expression: The classic triad consists in fever, pharyngitis, and adenopathy. However, the clinical spectra could also include other data as lymphadenopathy as well as some signs and symptoms as hepatosplenomegaly, skin eruption or rash, and puffy eyelid with a higher frequency in children of less than four years old in comparison with older ones were evident while red spots or papulovesicular occur with lesser frequency. Lymphadenopathy is generalized and usually important and could produce unsuppurative, hard and painful ganglions with variable sizes which could persist from 2 to 4 weeks until a maximum of 3 months. Pharyngitis is one of the most constant signs which at onset is characterized by oropharyngeal pain, reddening and growth of adenoid tissue.

Table 2. Comparison of the clinical and laboratory in different studies of patients with infectious mononucleosis secondary to Epstein–Barr virus

Clinical and laboratory data	Authors				
	Balfour 2005(%)	Grotto 2003(%)	Rea 2001(%)	Gao 2011(%)	Gonzalez et al. 2012 (%)
Lymphadenopathy	95	88.9	57	95	89.5
Fever	30	79	45	92.3	79.7
General body pain	NR	NR	77	NR	69.3
Pharyngitis	100	95	73	83.5	55.2
Hepatomegaly	25	36.7	7	58.1	47.2
Splenomegaly	35	53.3	8	47.4	36.8
Exanthema	17	16.7	15	14.8	16.5
Jaundice	NR	16.7	<10	0	9.8
Myalgia	50	32.4	0	0	0
Palpebral edema	10	NR	0	115	0.61
Atypic Lymphocytosis	NA	59.2	85.7	51.9	24.5
Transaminasemia	NA	57.9	31	48.6	30.9
Hyperbilirubinemia	NA	14.9	6	NR	42.1

NR: Not reported. NA: Not analyzed. Balfour [55], Grotto [56], Rea [57], Gao [58] From Gonzalez S. et al. [6].

In 2 to 4 days, it transforms into a whitish membrane which bleeds on detachment, a very painful process, which could leave behind red spots at the beginning that changes to brown color within 24 to 48 hours.

There could be mild or moderate fever with variable duration from some days to one week or even more but never more than three weeks. It is normal to find it present in variable form and reports have it that it occurs in up to 98% of the cases. Another sign that is usually found is the enlargement of the spleen which is observed after the appearance of pharyngitis. Although, both could simultaneously occur, this data should be investigated with caution when the sickness is suspected to avoid spleen rapture.

4. Atypic clinical expression: Mononucleosis could present with atypic clinical manifestations, just one of these like an important unique cervical adenopathy of 8 to 10 cm which appears suddenly and could last from two to three weeks. Moreover, other clinical manifestations of diverse form like facial paralysis, hepatitis, meningoencephalitis, transverse myelitis, thrombocytopenic purpura, and pneumonitis among others. At National Institute of Pediatrics, Mexico City, there was a case of infectious mononucleosis with hemophagocytic syndrome together with pericardial discharge, provoked by EBV, which is totally a rare case.

5. Associated to syndromes: EBV has been associated with different syndromes. Some of the symptomatic complexes which occur, apart from elevation of heterophilic antibodies and EBV specific antibodies are as follows: Gianotti-Crosti syndrome, Guillain-Barre syndrome, Alicia syndrome in the wonderland, post-perfusion syndrome, Reye syndrome, recurrent parotiditis, acute cerebral syndrome, chronic fatigue syndrome, and hemophagocytic syndrome, as reported Gonzalez Saldaña et al in 15 cases of his study [59].

6. Recurrent mononucleosis: Report of clinical manifestation characterized by repetitive pharyngitis together with fever, oropharyngeal pain, and body pain has been made in children. On physical exploration, reddened pharynx and cervical adenopathy which in some occasions are accompanied by puffy eyelids, artralgia and myalgia of 3 to 10 days duration meriting or no of antibiotics. The majority of the cases reported had negative pharyngeal aspiration and mild elevation of atypic lymphocytes in blood count, all of which occurs in the presence of heterophilic antibodies and possibility of abnormalities in liver function with increases in the number of EBV antibodies as an indication of early infection which ceases on conclusion of the acute manifestation.

7. Chronic mononucleosis: In world bibliography, acute and atypic manifestations related to different syndromes have been reported, however there are others in which following the resolution of the primary infection, recurrent and chronic manifestations occur. These manifestations are cataloged as chronic fatigue syndrome which is a sickness whose origin is uncertain for the fact that even if EBV is involved, there are other agents which are associated with the syndrome.

8. Congenital infection by EBV: Even when in developing countries, mononucleosis affects babies and school children, the appearance of the primary infection during pregnancy is an exceptional fact. In few cases registered in developed countries, abnormalities have been observed, in which the pregnancy was monitored until birth of the baby. However, in a retrospective studies, it has been confirmed that the disease could provoke congenital malformations such as micrognathia, cryptorchidism, and cataracts. Moreover, other data like hypotonia, persistent monocytosis, proteinuria, metaphysitis, and hearing impairment could be seen.

9. Associated to myeloproliferative diseases: The principal defense against EBV are the specific cytotoxic T lymphocytes for EBV. This is the reason why any alteration in cellular immune response affecting the activities of T cells would modify the repressive influence that these cells have in the face of lymphoproliferation. If this occurs, lymphoproliferative manifestations which go from simple monoclonal or polyclonal response to lymphoma development which may occur, above all, in primary immunodeficiency where cellular response is greatly affected (ataxia-telangiectasia, Wiskott-Aldrich syndrome, Chediak-Higashi syndrome, common variable immunodeficiency). However, X-linked lymphoproliferative disease is what has been described in general as capable of manifesting like mortal mononucleosis, hemophagocytic syndrome, fulminant hepatitis as well as malignant lymphoma.

10. Associated to neoplasm: The pathogenic inherence of EBV in development of different neoplasms is still questionable since there is no precision of its causal participation. However, the latency of EBV as well as the observation of its genome in different neoplasmic tissues suggests its possible contribution principally in the pathogenic development of neoplasms such as Burkitt lymphoma and nasopharyngeal carcinoma. However, there are other entities, although controversial, in which the etiological function of EBV infection could co-participate. Such entities are Hodgkin lymphoma, non-Hodgkin lymphomas (B cell phenotype, T cells, and NK cells), gastric carcinoma, hepatic cell cancers, breast cancer, parotid carcinoma, salivary gland lymph epithelial carcinoma, amygdale carcinoma, and thymoma. Other neoplasms like cervico-uterine cancer, bladder cancer, cutaneous tumors, and laryngeal tumors have not been associated to EBV yet, since it has not been found in the genome of their tissues [37, 59].

Studies have begun to clarify the molecular properties of several EBV-associated lymphoproliferative and neoplasmic diseases, as well as the role of the virus in their development. Burkitt lymphoma is a monoexpression of EBNA-1, the EBERs, and occasionally LMP-1 (in 40% to 70% of cases). Although expression of LMP-1 provides a target for immune destruction, the growth-transforming advantage afforded by LMP-1 may result in a selective advantage for some of these tumors. The B-cell lymphoproliferative disorders arise in congenitally immunosuppressed infants and children, as well as in immunosuppressed organ or bone marrow transplant recipients. These disorders can evolve during acute EBV infection, but most often they result from previous infection with the virus. The lesions may exhibit B-cell hyperplasia or lymphoma; regardless of the pathologic findings, the chromosomal translocations characteristic of Burkitt lymphoma are usually not present. Tissues from immunocompromised patients with B-cell lymphoproliferation contain EBV genomes and usually express the full complement of latent gene products. The marked degree of immunosuppression may allow EBV-infected B cells to express all the latency proteins and still expand without selective pressure from cytotoxic T cells. About one third of B-cell lymphomas in patients with AIDS contain EBV genomes.

Unlike the tumors seen in congenitally or iatrogenically immunosuppressed patients, these tumors show a Burkitt or Burkitt-like histology and contain chromosomal translocations similar to those seen in Burkitt lymphoma in patients without AIDS. Most of these tumors in patients with AIDS also express the full repertoire of latent genes. Patients with Hodgkin disease often have elevated levels of antibody to EBV antigens before or at the time of presentation of lymphoma; this condition was long presumed to reflect evolving impairment in cellular immunity.

Recently, however, tissues from 20% to 40% of patients with Hodgkin disease were found to contain EBV genomes, usually within the Reed-Sternberg cells. Most cases associated with EBV are of more aggressive, nodular sclerosing or mixed cellularity subtypes of Hodgkin disease. Tumors that contain EBV, the DNA show expression of LMP-1 but not of EBNA-2. Unlike the EBV-associated tumors discussed above, oral hairy leukoplakia represents a nonmalignant infection of epithelial cells, with extensive replication of EBV. Lesions contain EBV, the DNA in the upper epithelial layers, and herpesvirus-like particles have been seen on electron microscopy; EBV-DNA is not present in the lower layers. Thus, EBV may not be latent in the lower layers of the epithelium, and infection may be sustained by continuous infection of maturing cells in the upper layers. EBV replicative genes (such as ZEBRA, VCA, gp350) and LMP-1 are expressed, but the EBERs are not natural history of infections by EBV, preferentially infects human B cells, epithelial cells, T cells, natural killer cells, and smooth muscle cells. Latent EBV infection occurs in the oropharyngeal epithelium, where EBV virions are replicated and released from the epithelial cells to saliva [14, 60].

The EBV-infected cells express a different array of EBV-associated antigens depending on lytic or latent infection, and these viral antigens are targeted by EBV-specific cytotoxic T lymphocytes (CTLs). The CTL responses to EBV infections induce a variety of inflammatory systemic and cutaneous symptoms, while the lack of CTLs allows EBV-infected cells to survive and proliferate. The primary infection may cause infectious mononucleosis, and, less frequently, induce Gianotti-Crosti syndrome and virus-associated hemophagocytic syndrome. Latent EBV infection is associated with various types of neoplasms and hematological disorders including X-linked lymphoproliferative disorder (Duncan disease), malignant lymphomas arising in patients with acquired immunodeficiency syndrome (AIDS) and the recipients of organ transplantations, gastric cancer, and pyothorax associated lymphoma [14, 61].

Non-Hodgkin Lymphoma

EBV is seen in benign-like nodule biopsies in HIV patients who later presented non-Hodgkin lymphomas. About 50% of these tumors contain EBV-DNA with immunoblastic lymphoma constituting the majority of these tumors seen in patients in advanced stage of AIDS. In this kind of patients with severe immunocompromise or with Burkitt lymphoma (CNS lymphoma), the CD4 count is very low and are generally immunoblastics [3].

EBV-Related Tumors

EBV was the first human virus associated to malignant tumors. The infection can give rise to a spectrum of proliferative disorders ranging from benign self-limited diseases as IM to aggressive non-malignant proliferations as EBV-linked hemophagocytic syndrome and to lymphoid and epithelial malignant neoplasms. EBV benign neoformations consist of oral villi leucoplasts which appear, above all, in adults with AIDS, and lymphoid interstitial pneumonitis [62, 63]. In children with AIDS, EBV-linked malignant neoplasms could be nasopharyngeal tumor, Burkitt lymphoma, Hodgkin disease, lymphoproliferative disorders, and leiomyosarcoma in immunodeficiency state like AIDS [9, 64-66].

The Epstein Barr virus (EBV) is a ubiquitous human herpes virus infecting over 90% of the world population. After the acute infection, the virus establishes a life-long latency that is clinically asymptomatic. However, the clinical and biological evidence indicates that EBV may disrupt this latency and become causally linked to several tumors, especially those of lymphoid and epithelial origin [67].

EBV is associated with almost all cases of undifferentiated carcinoma of nasopharyngeal type (UCNT WHO type 3) and endemic Burkitt's lymphoma (BL), whereas in squamous cell carcinoma (WHO type 1), non-keratinizing carcinoma (WHO type 2), NK/T cell lymphoma, Hodgkin's disease (HD) and lymphoproliferative disorders of the immunocompromised host, EBV-association is variable, ranging from 10 to 100% of the cases. The EBV genome consists of approximately 100 genes, present in neoplasmic cells of EBV-related tumors in an episomal form, and replicated during cellular division by host cell machinery. Of these 100 genes, only 10 are expressed in infected B cells during latency. LMP-1, LMP-2, EBNA-1, EBNA-2 and EBNA-3, are the most important genes expressed during latency. In particular, LMP-1 and LMP-2 genes are important in the process of neoplasmic transformation by acting as oncogenes [67, 68].

This carcinoma predominates in south of China, North Africa, and Alaska. About 99% of anaplasic or poorly differentiated carcinomas contain EBV genome. This genome is found in transformed epithelial cells. The patients could present elevated IgA titration against viral structural protein with this being used in some western countries for the detection of early nasopharyngeal carcinoma and for treatment response assessment basically for the fact that increase in these titration is highly related to poor prognosis [3, 69-71].

Burkitt lymphoma is frequently found in the jaws (mandibles) and constitutes the most common child cancer in equatorial zone of West Africa and New Guinea, the endemic zone of *Plasmodium falciparum*, with a history of presentation of EBV infections at a very early age. The median age of onset in this region is 5 years [72, 73]. The constant exposition to malaria acts as a mitogen for B lymphocytes, which contributes to polyclonal proliferation of B lymphocytes with EBV infection, thus, prejudicing the control of T lymphocytes of EBV infected B lymphocytes, and in this way, increase the risk of development of Burkitt lymphoma [9]. Malaria infection reduces the T cells which control the proliferation EBV infected B cells. This lymphoma contains a chromosomic translocation of 8, 14, and 22 chromosomes which epidemiological studies cited as the causal agent of Burkitt lymphoma. Children with high titration of antibodies presented a high risk of suffering Burkitt lymphoma with the presence of EBV DNA in the lymphoma tissue as well as in EBV genome which indicates that the tumor comes from EBV infected cell [3, 74].

Hodgkin Disease

The incidence of Hodgkin disease reaches maximum level in childhood in developing countries and in the first part of adult life in developed countries. The systemic levels of antibodies against EBV are elevated before the development of Hodgkin disease. Only a small number of the patients are EBV seronegatives. The infection by the virus seems to increase the risk of development of Hodgkin disease [9].

EBV DNA is detected in 40%-60% of the patients suffering from this disease in US. EBV genome is present in Reed-Sternberg cells in which they are found to be monoclonals.

The virus is found in tumors of mixed or subtype cellularity with more frequent lymphocyte depletion than in other subtypes of tumors.

EBV Associated NK/T Cell Lymphomas

EBV is involved in the majority of LPD arising in patients with congenital and acquired immunodeficiencies, and methotrexate-associated lymphoproliferative disorders. Most EBV-associated LPDs are of B cell lineage, but T cell neoplasms and Hodgkin lymphoma may occur [75]. Latent EBV infection plays a pivotal role in the occurrence of African Burkitt lymphoma, pyothorax-associated lymphomas (PAL), Hodgkin lymphoma, primary effusion lymphoma (PEL) induced by HHV-8 co-infection, and various types of B cell lymphomas. The association of latent EBV infection with NK/T cell lymphomas is less common than B cell lymphomas, but their clinical and histological features are characteristic enough to predict the presence of EBV infection. Extranodal NK/T cell lymphoma, nasal type (according to WHO classification), is a prototype of EBV-associated NK/T cell lymphomas preferentially arising in nasal cavity, which often affects the nasopharynx, palates, skin, soft tissues, gastrointestinal tract, and testis. Neoplasmic cells in most cases appear to be of NK cell lineage, but rare cases show a cytotoxic T cell phenotype. It is, therefore, designated as NK/T (NK or T) cell lymphoma. Cases involving the nasal cavity are identical to the former categories, including nasal lymphoma, angiocentric T cell lymphoma (according to REAL classification), and lethal midline granuloma. EBV associated NK/T cell lymphoma is more prevalent in Asia, Mexico, and Central and South America. Angiocentric or angiodestructive infiltration is a hallmark of NK/T cell lymphoma, and prominent ulceration or tissue necrosis is often seen. The neoplasmic cells of typical cases express CD2, cytoplasmic CD3ε, CD 56, and cytotoxic molecules such as TIA-1 and granzyme B, without surface CD3. EBV is usually present in neoplasmic cells in a clonal episomal form [76-78].

Apart from the prototypic nasal NK/T cell lymphoma, EBV-associated cutaneous lymphomas often show characteristic clinical features of HV-like lymphoma in children or young adults, puffy eyelid swelling with intramuscular infiltration, masquerading dermatomyositis, and panniculitis-like plaque associated with high fever, pancytopenia, and beanbag cells, mimicking cytophagic histiocytic panniculitis. Other clinical phenotypes associated with EBV infections include aggressive NK/T cell lymphoma, and chronic NK/T cell leukemia. NK/T cell lymphoma occurs most often in adults, but children who have suffered from chronic active EBV infection (CAEBV) and HMB often progress to EBV-associated NK/T cell lymphomas. We believe that EBV-associated NK/T cell lymphomas can be separated into 2 groups: de novo, adult-onset EBV-associated NK/T cell lymphomas, and those arising in children or young adults, preceded by various EBV-related complications.

Overt EBV-associated lymphomas are usually resistant to conventional chemotherapy, including adriamycin, probably because of multidrug resistant (MDR) gene expression, and frequently complicate to a fatal hemophagocytic syndrome. No treatment protocol has been established at present time. Recent advances have made it possible to apply the adoptive immune transfer of EBV-specific cytotoxic T cells for EBV-associated lymphomas arising in patients with bone marrow transplantation or severe CAEBV [79]. This procedure might be applicable for patients with latency II or III infection, in which some EBV antigens for CTLs are expressed by neoplasmic cells.

The infusion of donor leukocytes or gene-modified virus-specific T cells has been successfully used to control EBV-associated lymphoproliferative disorders after allogenic bone marrow transplantation. Because EBV-specific T cells are selectively proliferating in this system, graft versus host disease (GVHD) caused by alloreactive CTL clones are absent or minimal [80, 81].

Nasopharyngeal Carcinoma

Nasopharyngeal carcinoma occurs worldwide, but it is 10 times more common in South of China where it represents the most frequent malignant tumor among male adults. Also, it is frequent in white people of North Africa and in the Eskimos of North America. The patients usually present cervical lymphadenopathy, Eustachian tube blockage, and epistemic nasal obstruction.

All undifferentiated nasopharyngeal malignant carcinoma cells contain a high number of copies of EBV episomes.

The people with partially undifferentiated non-keratinized nasopharyngeal carcinoma have a very high titration of anti-EBV which is very useful diagnostic and prognostic tool.

In asymptomatic people, high levels of IgA antibodies against EA and VCA antigens can be detected and this can be used to monitor antitumoral treatment response. Well-differentiated keratinized nasopharyngeal carcinoma cells contain little or no copies of EBV genome. These people show serologic patterns similar to the general population [82-84].

Computed tomography and magnetic resonance imaging are very useful diagnostic tools to identify and define the presence of mass in head and neck while definitive diagnosis is established by biopsy of mass or of a suspicious cervical lymphatic ganglion.

For their staging as well as diagnosis, the surgery plays a vital role. The management is usually radiotherapy which has shown to be very efficient in controlling primary tumors and regional ganglionary metastasis.

Also, the therapeutic approach using chemotherapy has shown that 5-fluorouracil, cisplatin, and methotrexate are efficient but not curative. Prognosis is usually good when the tumor is localized [9, 85-87].

EBV is also related to saliva-gland carcinoma. Other possible related EBV tumors are some T lymphomas such as lethal midline granuloma.

In lymphadenopathy-angioimmunoblastic-like lymphomas, thymomas, supraglotic laryngeal carcinomas, respiratory tract lymphoepithelial tumors, gastrointestinal lympho-epithelial tumors, and gastric adenocarcinoma, the exact contribution of EBV is not defined (Table 3) [9, 88-90].

EBV and HIV

HIV patients are more vulnerable to EBV infection. 10 to 20% of these patients have more EBV-infected B cells in circulation than in healthy individuals. The T cells of HIV patients are less effective in suppressing the infected cells. The infections described in these patients are oral leukoplakia, lymphoid interstitial pneumonia, and non-Hodgkin lymphoma [91-93].

Table 3. Principal diseases associated with EBV

Principal disease associations of Epstein-Barr virus	
Disease	Comments
1. Infectious mononucleosis	1. Primary infection, self-limiting. Occurs in 50% of primary infections of adolescents and young adults.
2. Burkitt´s lymphoma (BL)	2. EBV found as latent infection in 97% endemic, 15-85% sporadic and 30-40% AIDS BL cases.
3. Hodgkin´s disease	3. Sporadic lymphoma; latent EBV found in aprox. 50% of cases.
4. B-lymphoproliferative disease	4. Lymphoproliferative disease/lymphomas, almost exclusively in the immunocompromised host, especially post-transplant (as a result of immunosuppressive drug therapy) and in AIDS. Might occur in primary infection or persistent infection.
5. X-linked lympho-proliferative syndrome	5. Rare genetic immune dysfunction results in fatal primary infection.
6. Nasopharyngeal carcinoma	6. Malignant squamous epithelial tumor of the nasopharynx; cells contain latent virus.
7. Oral hairy leukoplakia	7. Viral replication in the superficial layers of tongue epithelium results in a benign lesion, almost exclusively in HIV-positive individuals.

Diagnosis

The most useful laboratory studies for the diagnosis of IM, suggested by Gonzalez and collaborators, are blood test, Paul-Bunnell test, and detection of EBV specific antibodies. The diagnosis is basically clinical and serologic through a search of heterophilic agglutinins by immunofluorescence, Paul-Bunnell test, and monotest. The virus can be isolated and cultured when there is mucous necrotizing lesion. Microscopic observation of the material obtained from the lesions revealed infected cells with inclusion bodies.

Blood count: This study would permit the finding of leukocytes with 40-50% of lymphocytosis and detect atypic lymphocytes of Downey cells which are big-sized leukocytes with basophilic vacuolated cytoplasm and irregular, dense nucleic chromatin nucleus. Only in exceptional cases can nucleoli be observed.

Leukocytosis and also lymphocytosis usually appear in the second week of the disease. So, in the first week, the profiles appear normal or leukopenic after which high levels are seen which continues for 2 to 3 weeks and in some occasions more time.

However, it has to be reiterated that these data are not pathognomic of mononucleosis for the fact that such data are seen in many viral infections such as measles, chicken-pox, and hepatitis.

Paul-Bunnell test: Consists of detection of antibodies (heterophils) that reacts with antibodies of other species (erythrocytes of ram) in patients with mononucleosis. They are not specific in this entity because they can be found in serum disease, hepatitis, syphilis, measles, and others.

For this reason, it is necessary to carry out absorption with horse antigen (Forssman antigen) which suppresses the antibodies of other sicknesses but not that of mononucleosis in such a way that the titration continued to be high without reduction to more than two dilution tubes. On the other part, heterophilic antibodies of mononucleosis are absorbed by antibodies of ox but not that of other diseases, in such a way that heterophilic antibody titration of 1:56 which does not reduce more than two dilutions with Forssman antibodies and which is suppressed by erythrocytes of ox is considered positive. It appears starting from the second week and continues to be high till six months or more. However, in children less than five years of age, they can be negative all the time. Many techniques of fast diagnosis like Monospot, Monosticon, and Monotest that use erythrocytes of horse or ram as antigen (with a gutter of problem serum) have been developed with the aim of looking for agglutination effect.

EBV specific antibodies: The diagnosis of EBV acute infection is founded in one or more of the following serologic criteria: elevation of IgM antibody, elevation of IgG antibodies against capsid (anti-VCA), elevation of IgG antibodies against early antigen of diffuse component (anti-D). The elevation of antibodies against the nucleus (anti-EBNA) is observed in long time acquired infection.

Serology in relation with infection state: Today, many specific serological tests for the detection of antibodies against EBV are available in different virology laboratories. The most common test is the detection of antibodies against viral capsid antigen (VCA) for the fact that VCA antibodies of IgG quickly elevates in one week with high titration. For this reason, once the infection started, it is not necessary to obtain a paired sample of anti-VCA in order to define the infection. The detection of IgM antibodies against VCA and of antibodies against early antigen is employed in the diagnosis of recent infections. Antibodies against Epstein Barr nuclear antigen (anti-EBNA) are not present until many weeks or months after the onset of infection. The presence of anti-EBNA excludes recent infection.

EBV Prevention

For specific prevention, a recombinant vaccine containing EBV Gp350 protein is under investigation. Vaccination against EBV could be effective in seronegatives patients. Presently, studies in high risk pediatric populations viral vaccine using Gp350 protein is under way. Also, a test involving vaccination with EBV peptides which activate cellular and humoral immunity in humans is being carried out [3].

Treatment

In acute forms of infectious mononucleosis, the treatment is fundamentally symptomatic focusing on fever and inflammatory processes with increase in liquid intake and adequate diet. Antiviral treatment has been tried with acyclovir which although inhibits viral replication in vitro but without observed improvement in the clinical manifestations and until date, there is no specific treatment [59].

The existing symptoms constitute the basis of better control in children. In the same way, it is convenient to reduce physical activities and to be on rest. In severe cases involving central nervous system, obstruction of airways, and severe hematologic alterations (autoimmune hemolytic anemia, neutropenia, and thrombocytopenia associated with bleeding) steroids (prednisone) 1-2 mg/kg have been used with favorable response. Even when we can favorably argue on its use, such medication should never be administered in mild cases or systemically. Other treatments like intravenous gammaglobulins and metisazone in convalescent subjects have been used however, with unsatisfactory results. Recent reports showed the efficacy of metronidazole but this could be explained by the fact that in EBV pharyngitis, there could be associated anaerobic microorganisms that are the target action of metronidazole. Nevertheless, there is no specific antiviral treatment, since no therapeutic scheme has been demonstrated to either ameliorate the symptoms or reduce the complications. Generally, the prognosis is good in terms of complete recovery if there are no complications in the acute phase. The aforementioned principal symptoms usually last from 2 - 4 weeks. Prolonged tiredness and weakness, the sensation of general body pain, and certain level of incapacity could be variable during many weeks or until six months.

Conclusion

The infection by EBV is regarded as the etiology of infectious mononucleosis (IM) and has a universal distribution although, in developing countries, the presentation is seen more in early ages of life. The principal means of transmission is through the saliva and the treatment of the acute form of the virus is mainly symptomatic with the principal objectives being to mellow down such symptoms as fever and inflammatory process. Usually, increasing liquid intake and adequate diet are recommended as part of this treatment. For specific prevention, a recombinant vaccine containing EBV Gp350 protein is under investigation. Also, a test involving vaccination with EBV peptides which activate cellular and humoral immunity in humans is being carried out. Although assays with acyclovir *in vitro* have shown positive results by inhibition of viral multiplication, clinically favorable results have not been reported.

Glossary

Alice in Wonderland syndrome
Includes an array of symptoms involving altered perception of shape (meta-morphopsia) of objects or persons who appear to be smaller (micropsia) or larger (macropsia) than normal, of impaired sense of passage of time, of zooming of the environment.

Ataxia-telangiectasia (A-T)
Also called Louis-Bar syndrome, it is a rare, genetic neurological disorder of childhood that progressively destroys part of the motor control area of the brain, leading to a lack of balance and coordination. A-T also affects the immune system and increases the risk of leukemia and lymphoma in affected individuals.

Burkitt lymphoma

It is a type of non-Hodgkin lymphoma (NHL) that most often occurs in young people between the ages of 12 and 30, accounting for 40% to 50% of childhood NHL. The disease usually causes a rapidly growing tumor in the abdomen. Up to 90% of these tumors are in the abdomen.

Other sites of involvement include the testis, sinuses, bone, lymph nodes, skin, bone marrow, and central nervous system.

Chédiak–Higashi syndrome

It is a rare autosomal recessive disorder that arises from a microtubule polymerization defect which leads to a decrease in phagocytosis. The decrease in phagocytosis results in recurrent pyogenic infections, partial albinism and peripheral neuropathy.

Chronic fatigue syndrome (CFS)

It is a common name for a group of significantly debilitating medical conditions characterized by persistent fatigue and other specific symptoms that lasts for a minimum of six months in adults (and 3 months in children or adolescents).

The fatigue is not due to exertion, not significantly relieved by rest, and is not caused by other medical conditions. CFS may also be referred to as myalgic encephalomyelitis (ME), post-viral fatigue syndrome (PVFS), chronic fatigue immune dysfunction syndrome (CFIDS), or by several other terms. Biological, genetic, infectious and psychological mechanisms have been proposed, but the etiology of CFS is not understood and it may have multiple causes

Duncan's disease (X-linked lymphoproliferative syndrome)

It is a rare X-linked immunodeficiency in which there is a normal response to childhood infection but infection with Epstein-Barr produces a fatal lymphoproliferative disorder. Most patients die of acute infection. Others develop hypogammaglobulinemia, B-cell lymphoma, aplastic anemia, or agranulocytosis.

Gianotti-Crosti syndrome (GCS)

It is a distinct infectious exanthem with associated lymphadenopathy and acute anicteric hepatitis. Gianotti and Crosti initially described GCS as associated with a hepatitis B virus exanthem, which they termed popular acrodermatitis of childhood.

A similar constellation of characteristics was later found to be associated with several infectious agents and immunizations that were called papulovesicular acrolocated syndromes.

Subsequent retrospective studies have shown that these 2 entities are indistinguishable from one another, and they are now consolidated under the unifying title of GCS.

Guillain-Barré syndrome (GBS)

It is a rare neurological disorder that occurs when the body's immune system attacks the peripheral nerves in the body.

A temporary inflammation of the nerves, causing pain, weakness, and paralysis in the extremities and often progressing to the chest and face. It typically occurs after recovery from a viral infection or, in rare cases, following immunization for influenza.

Hemophagocytic syndrome

Also called as hemophagocytic lymphohistiocytosis (HLH). Represent a severe hyperinflammatory condition with the cardinal symptoms prolonged fever, cytopenias, hepatosplenomegaly, and hemophagocytosis by activated, morphologically benign macrophages. Biochemical markers include elevated ferritin and triglycerides, and low fibrinogen.

Frequent triggers are infectious agents, mostly viruses of the herpes group. Malignant lymphomas, especially in adults, may be associated with HLH. A special form of HLH in rheumatic diseases is called macrophage-activation syndrome. Initially HLH may masquerade as a normal infection since all symptoms, even though less pronounced, may also be found in immune competent patients.

Infectious mononucleosis

Frequently called "mono" or the "kissing disease," is a contagious illness caused by the Epstein-Barr virus (EBV) found in saliva and mucus; that can affect the liver, lymph nodes, and oral cavity. The virus affects a type of white blood cell called the B lymphocyte producing characteristic atypical lymphocytes that may be useful in the diagnosis of the disease. While mononucleosis is not usually a serious disease, its primary symptoms of fatigue and lack of energy can linger for several months.

Paul Bunnell test

Called also *Paul-Bunnell reaction is* a test for infectious mononucleosis based on increased agglutination of sheep red blood cells resulting from heterophil antibodies in the serum. The test is considered positive if dilution of serum of 1:80 or higher agglutinates the sheep cells. Elevated agglutinin titers are more likely to be found during the second or third week of the disease, but the serum may not become positive until 7 weeks have elapsed.

Postperfusion syndrome

Also known as "*pumphead*" is a constellation of neurocognitive impairments attributed to cardiopulmonary bypass (CPB) during cardiac surgery. Symptoms of postperfusion syndrome are subtle and include defects associated with attention, concentration, short term memory, fine motor function, and speed of mental and motor responses. Studies have shown a high incidence of neurocognitive deficit soon after surgery, but the deficits are often transient with no permanent neurological impairment. Occurs after recovery from a viral infection or, in rare cases, following immunization for influenza.

Reye's syndrome

It is a potentially fatal disease that has numerous detrimental effects to many organs, especially the brain and liver, as well as causing a lower than usual level of blood sugar (hypoglycemia).

The classic features are a rash, vomiting, and liver damage. The exact cause is unknown and, while it has been associated with aspirin consumption by children with viral illness, it also occurs in the absence of aspirin use.

The disease causes fatty liver with minimal inflammation and severe encephalopathy (with swelling of the brain). The liver may become slightly enlarged and firm, and there is a change in the appearance of the kidneys.

Waldeyer's tonsillar ring

It is an anatomical term collectively describing the annular arrangement of lymphoid tissue in the pharynx. Waldeyer's ring circumscribes the naso- and/or pharynx, with some of its tonsillar tissue located above and some below the soft palate (and to the back of the oral cavity); formed by the two palatine tonsils, the pharyngeal tonsil, the lingual tonsil, and intervening lymphoid tissue.

Wiskott-Aldrich syndrome
A hereditary sex-linked recessive disorder characterized by chronic eczema, recurring infections, and a decrease in the number of white blood cells and platelets.

Summary Points List

- Epstein Barr virus (EBV) is regarded as the etiology of infectious mononucleosis (IM).
- It exclusively infects lymphoreticular system giving rise to lymphoproliferative diseases.
- There are two types of EBV, based on their allelic differences.
- In developing countries is seen more in early ages of life.
- The principal means of transmission is through the saliva, its first site of budding being the oropharyngeal epithelium.
- The symptoms of the infection depend on age, in little children it is generally asymptomatic.
- In adolescents and adults, symptoms are fever, pharyngitis and adenopathies
- IM has a benign prognosis; normally is resolved in 1 to 3 weeks.
- The incidence of complications in general population is low.

Future Issue List

- The transmission could be transmitted by sexual activity since it has been isolated in vaginal and cervical secretions.
- In small children there could be other unknown mechanisms of transmission.
- Neoplasms like cervico-uterine cancer, bladder cancer, cutaneous tumors, and laryngeal tumors have not been associated to EBV yet, since it has not been found in the genome of their tissues.
- Currently there are studies focused on the development of recombinant vaccine for its prevention.
- Although assays with antiviral *in vitro* have shown positive results by inhibition of viral multiplication, clinically favorable results have not been reported.

Acknowledgment

We thank Dr. Cyril Ndidi Nwoye, an expert translator and a native English speaker for reviewing and correcting the chapter.

References

[1] Robinson, M., Suh, Y., Paleri, V., Devlin, D., Ayaz, B., Pertl, L., Thavaraj, S.: Oncogenic human papillomavirus associated nasopharyngeal carcinoma: an observational study of correlation with ethnicity, histological subtype and outcome in a UK population. *Infect. Agent Cancer* 2013, 8:30.
[2] Wai-Ming, L. R., Hung-Man, T. J., Ka-Fai, T.: Emerging roles of small Epstein-Barr virus derived non-coding RNAs in epithelial malignancy. *Int. J. Mol. Sci.* 2013,14: 17378-17409.
[3] Cohen, J. I.: Infeccion por el virus de Epstein Barr (VEB). *N. Engl. J. Med.* 2000, 343: 481-492.
[4] Bhat, R. A., Thimmappaya, B.: Two small RNAs encoded by Epstein-Barr virus can functionally substitute for the virus-associated RNAs in the lytic growth of adenovirus 5. *Proc. Natl. Acad. Sci. US* 1983, 80:4789–4793.
[5] Wang, Y., Xue, S. A., Hallden, G., Francis, J., Yuan, M., Griffin, B. E., Lemoine, N. R.: Virus-associated RNA I-deleted adenovirus, a potential oncolytic agent targeting EBV-associated tumors. *Cancer Res.* 2005, 65:1523–1531.
[6] Gonzalez, S., Monroy, C., Piña, R., Juarez, O.: Clinical and laboratory characteristics of infectious mononucleosis by Epstein-Barr virus in Mexican children. *BMC Res. Notes* 2012, 5:361-365.
[7] Lima, M.: Aggressive mature natural killer cell neoplasms: from epidemiology to diagnosis, *Orphanet J. Rare Dis.* 2013, 8:95.
[8] Burke, A. P., Yen, T. S., Shekitka, K. M., Sobin, L. H.: Lymphoepithelial carcinoma of the stomach with Epstein-Barr virus demonstrated by polymerase chain reaction. *Mod. Pathol.* 1990, 3:377–380.
[9] Kliegman, R. M., Behrman, R. E., Jenson, H. B., Stanton, B. F.: *Nelson Tratado de Pediatria* 18ª edición, 2008.
[10] Kutok, J. L., Wang, F.: Spectrum of Epstein-Barr virus-associated diseases. *Annu. Rev. Pathol.* 2006, 1:375–404.
[11] Timms, J. M., Bell, A., Flavell, J. R., Murray, P. G., Rickinson, A. B., Traverse-Glehen, A., Berger, F., Delecluse, H. J.: Target cells of Epstein-Barr-virus (EBV)-positive post-transplant lymphoproliferative disease: Similarities to EBV-positive Hodgkin's lymphoma. *Lancet* 2003, 361:217–223.
[12] Lung, R. W., Tong, J. H., Sung, Y. M., Leung, P. S., Ng, D. C., Chau, S. L., Chan, A. W., Ng, E. K., Lo, K. W., To, K. F.: Modulation of LMP2A expression by a newly identified Epstein-Barr virus-encoded microRNA miR-BART22. *Neoplasia* 2009, 11: 1174–1184.
[13] Straus, S. E., Cohen, J. I., Tosato, G., Meier, J.: Epstein Barr virus infections: biology, pathogenesis, and management. *Arch. Inter. Med.* 1993, 118:45-58.

[14] Iwatsuki, K., Yamamoto, T., Tsuji, K., Suzuki, D., Fujii, Matsuura H., Oono, T.: A spectrum of clinical manifestations caused by host immune responses against Epstein Barr virus infections. *Acta Med.* 2004, 58:169-180.

[15] Fok, V., Friend, K., Steitz, J. A.: Epstein-Barr virus noncoding RNAs are confined to the nucleus, whereas their partner, the human La protein, undergoes nucleocytoplasmic shuttling. *J. Cell Biol.* 2006, 173:319–325.

[16] Moss, W. N., Steitz, J. A.: Genome-wide analyses of Epstein Barr virus reveal conserved RNA structures and novel stable intronic sequence RNA. *BMC Genimics* 2013, 14:543.

[17] Zur Hausen, H., Schulte-Holthausen, H.: Presence of EB virus nucleic acid homology in a "virus-free" line of Burkitt tumour cells. *Nature* 1970, 227:245–248.

[18] Schwemmle, M., Clemens, M. J., Hilse, K., Pfeifer, K., Troster, H., Muller, W. E., Bachmann, M.: Localization of Epstein-Barr virus-encoded RNAs EBER-1 and EBER-2 in interphase and mitotic Burkitt lymphoma cells. *Proc. Natl. Acad. Sci. US 1992*, 89: 10292–10296.

[19] Toczyski, D. P., Steitz, J. A.: EAP, a highly conserved cellular protein associated with Epstein-Barr virus small RNAs (EBERs). *EMBO J.* 1991, 10:459–466.

[20] Kai, Y., Yuk-Lap, K., Ka-Yan, C., Tin-Yun, G., Lee, S., Cheung, S., Ka-Fai, T., Kwok-Wai, L.: Complete genomic sequence of Epstein-Barr virus in nasopharyngeal carcinoma cell line C666-1. *Infectious Agents and Cancer* 2013, 8:29.

[21] Xiao-yan, Y., Wang, M., Xiao-yan, W., Chang, A., Jie, L.: Non-detection of Eptein-Barr virus and human Papillomavirus in a region of high gastric cancer risk indicates a lack of a role for these viruses in gastric carcinomas. *Gen. Mol. Biol.* 2013, 36:183-184.

[22] Sample, J., Kieff, E.: Transcription of the Epstein-Barr virus genome during latency in growth-transformed lymphocytes. *J. Virol.* 1990, 64:1667–1674.

[23] Howe, J. G., Shu, M. D.: Epstein-Barr virus small RNA (EBER) genes: Unique transcription units that combine RNA polymerase II and III promoter elements. *Cell* 1989, 57:825–834.

[24] Toczyski, D. P., Matera, A. G., Ward, D. C., Steitz, J. A.: The Epstein-Barr virus (EBV) small RNA EBER1 binds and relocalizes ribosomal protein L22 in EBV-infected human B lymphocytes. *Proc. Natl. Acad. Sci. US* 1994, 91:3463–3467.

[25] Young, L. S., Rickinson, A. B.: Epstein-Barr virus: 40 years on. *Nat. Rev. Cancer* 2004, 4:757–768.

[26] Ishtiaq, S., Hassan, U., Mushtaq, Akhtar N.: Determination of frequency of Epstein Barr virus in Non-Hodgkin lymphomas using EBV latent membrane protein 1 (EBV-LMP1) immunohistochemical staining. *Asian Pacific J. Cancer Prev.* 2013, 14:3963-3967.

[27] Friis, A., Akerlund, B., Christensson, B., Gyllensten, K., Aleman, A., Zou, J., Emberg, I.: Epstein Barr virus DNA analysis in blood predicts disease progression in a rare case of plasmablastic lymphoma with effusion. *Agents and Cancer* 2013, 8:28.

[28] Babcock, G. J., Decker, L. L., Volk, M., Thorley-Lawson, D. A.: EBV persistence in memory B cells in vivo. *Immunity* 1998, 9:395–404.

[29] Raab-Traub, N.: Epstein-Barr virus in the pathogenesis of NPC. *Semin. Cancer Biol.* 2002, 12:431–441.

[30] Rosa, M. D., Gottlieb, E., Lerner, M. R., Steitz, J. A.: Striking similarities are exhibited by two small Epstein-Barr virus-encoded ribonucleic acids and the adenovirus-associated ribonucleic acids VAI and VAII. *Mol. Cell. Biol.* 1981, 1:785–796.

[31] Iwakiri, D., Eizuru, Y., Tokunaga, M., Takada, K. Autocrine growth of Epstein-Barr virus-positive gastric carcinoma cells mediated by an Epstein-Barr virus-encoded small RNA. *Cancer Res.* 2003, 63, 7062–7067.

[32] Glickman, J. N., Howe, J. G., Steitz, J. A. Structural analyses of EBER1 and EBER2ribonucleoprotein particles present in Epstein-Barr virus-infected cells. *J. Virol.* 1988, 62, 902–911.

[33] Sitki-Green, D. L., Edwards, R. H., Covington, M. M., Raab-Traub, N.: Biology of Epstein-Barr virus during infectious mononucleosis. *J. Infect. Dis.* 2004, 189:483–492.

[34] Lo, K. W., To, K. F., Huang, D. P.: Focus on nasopharyngeal carcinoma. *Cancer Cell* 2004, 5:423–428.

[35] Gottschalk, S., Heslop, H. E., Rooney, C. M.: Adoptive immunotherapy for EBV-associated malignancies. *Leuk. Lymphoma* 2005, 46:1–10.

[36] Sano, M., Kato, Y., Taira, K.: Sequence-specific interference by small RNAs derived from adenovirus VAI RNA. *FEBS Lett.* 2006, 580:1553–1564.

[37] Aparicio, O., Razquin, N., Zaratiegui, M., Narvaiza, I., Fortes, P.: Adenovirus virus-associated RNA is processed to functional interfering RNAs involved in virus production. *J. Virol.* 2006, 80:1376–1384.

[38] Fok, V., Mitton-Fry, R. M., Grech, A., Steitz, J. A.: Multiple domains of EBER 1, an Epstein-Barr virus noncoding RNA, recruit human ribosomal protein L22. *RNA* 2006, 12:872–882.

[39] Gilligan, K., Sato, H., Rajadurai, P., Busson, P., Young, L., Rickinson, A., Tursz, T., Raab-Traub, N.: Novel transcription from the Epstein-Barr virus terminal EcoRI fragment, DIJhet, in a nasopharyngeal carcinoma. *J. Virol.* 1990, 64:4948–4956.

[40] Imai, S., Nishikawa, J., Takada, K.: Cell-to-cell contact as an efficient mode of Epstein-Barr virus infection of diverse human epithelial cells. *J. Virol.* 1998, 72:4371–4378.

[41] Brooks, L., Yao, Q. Y., Rickinson, A. B., Young, L. S.: Epstein-Barr virus latent gene transcription in nasopharyngeal carcinoma cells: Coexpression of EBNA1, LMP1, and LMP2 transcripts. *J. Virol.* 1992, 66:2689–2697.

[42] Shaknovich, R., Basso, K., Bhagat, G., Mansukhani, M., Hatzivassiliou, G., Murty, V. V., Buettner, M., Niedobitek, G., Alobeid, B., Cattoretti, G.: Identification of rare Epstein-Barr virus infected memory B cells and plasma cells in non-monomorphic post-transplant lymphoproliferative disorders and the signature of viral signaling. *Haematologica* 2006, 91:1313–1320.

[43] Kieff, E., Johannsen, E., Calderwood, M. A.: *Epstein-Barr virus: latency and transformation.* Robertson, E. S. Ed. Caister Academic Press: Norfolk, UK, 2010; pp. 1–24.

[44] Faulkner, G., Krajewski, A., Crawford, D.: *The ins and outs of EBV infection.* Elsevier 2000, Vol. 8 No. 4.

[45] Yang, X., Wada, T., Imadome, K., Nishida, N., Mukai, T., Fujiwara, M., Kawashima, H., Kato, H., Shigeyoshi, F., Akihiro, Y., Xiaodong, Z., Toshio, M., Kanegane, H.: Characterization of Epstein-Barr virus (EBV)-infected cells in EBV-associated hemophagocytic lymphohistiocytosis in two patients with X-linked lymphoproliferative syndrome type 1 and type 2. *Herpesviridae* 2012, 10:3.

[46] Rowe, D. T.: Epstein-Barr virus latent gene expression in uncultured peripheral blood lymphocytes. *J. Virol.* 1992, 66:3715–3724.
[47] Clarke, P. A., Schwemmle, M., Schickinger, J., Hilse, K., Clemens, M. J.: Binding of Epstein-Barr virus small RNA EBER-1 to the double-stranded RNA-activated protein kinase DAI. *Nucleic Acids Res.* 1991, 19:243–248.
[48] Smith, P. R., de Jesus, O., Turner, D., Hollyoake, M., Karstegl, C. E., Griffin, B. E., Karran, L., Wang, Y., Hayward, S. D., Farrell, P. J.: Structure and coding content of CST (BART) family RNAs of Epstein-Barr virus. *J. Virol.* 2000, 74:3082–3092.
[49] Pfeffer, S., Zavolan, M., Grasser, F. A., Chien, M., Russo, J. J., Ju, J., John, B., Enright, A. J., Marks, D., Sander, C.: Identification of virus-encoded microRNAs. *Science* 2004, 304:734–736.
[50] Cai, X., Schafer, A., Lu, S., Bilello, J. P., Desrosiers, R. C., Edwards, R., Raab-Traub, N., Cullen, B. R.: Epstein-Barr virus microRNAs are evolutionarily conserved and differentially expressed. *PLoS Pathog.* 2006, 2:e23.
[51] Grundhoff, A., Sullivan, C. S., Ganem, D.: A combined computational and microarray-based approach identifies novel microRNAs encoded by human gamma-herpesviruses. *RNA* 2006, 12:733–750.
[52] Hutzinger, R., Feederle, R., Mrazek, J., Schiefermeier, N., Balwierz, P. J., Zavolan, M., Polacek, N., Delecluse, H. J., Huttenhofer, A.: Expression and processing of a small nucleolar RNA from the Epstein-Barr virus genome. *PLoS Pathog.* 2009, 5: e1000547.
[53] Hammond, S. M., Boettcher, S., Caudy, A. A., Kobayashi, R., Hannon, G. J.: Argonaute2, a link between genetic and biochemical analyses of RNAi. *Science* 2001, 293:1146–1150.
[54] Samanta, M., Iwakiri, D., Kanda, T., Imaizumi, T., Takada, K.: EB virus-encoded RNAs are recognized by RIG-I and activate signaling to induce type I IFN. *EMBO J.* 2006, 25:4207–4214.
[55] Balfour, H. H. Jr, Holman, C. J., Hokanson, K. M., Lelonek, M. M., Giesbrecht, J. E., White, D. R., Schmeling, D. O., Webb, C. H., Cavert, W., Wang, D. H., Brundage, R. C. A prospective clinical study of Epstein-Barr virus and host interactions during acute infectious mononucleosis. *J. Infec. Dis.* 2005, 192:1505-1512.
[56] Grotto, I., Mimouni, D., Huerta, M., Mimouni, M., Cohen, D., Robin, G., Pitlik, S., Green, M. S.: Clinical and laboratory presentation of EBV positive infectious mononucleosis in young adults. *Epidemiol. Infect.* 2003, 131:683-689.
[57] Rea, T. D., Russo, J. E., Katon, W., Ashley, R. L., Buchwald, D. S.: Prospective Study of the Natural History of Infectious Mononucleosis Caused by Epstein-Barr Virus. *J. Am. Board Fam. Practice* 2001, 14:234-242.
[58] Gao, L. W., Xie, Z. D., Liu, Y. Y., Wang, Y., Shen, K. L.: Epidemiologic and clinical characteristics of infectious mononucleosis associated with Epstein-Barr virus infection in children in Beijing, China. *World J. Pediatr.* 2011, 7:45-49.
[59] González Saldaña, N., Torales Torales, A., Gomez Barreto, D. *Infectología Clinica Pediatrica*, Ed. Mc Graw Hill. 8ª Edition, Mexico City, Mexico 2011.
[60] Shibata, D., Tokunaga, M., Uemura, Y., Sato, E., Tanaka, S., Weiss, L. M.: Association of Epstein-Barr virus with undifferentiated gastric carcinomas with intense lymphoid infiltration. Lymphoepithelioma-like carcinoma. *Am. J. Pathol.* 1991, 139:469–474.
[61] Wong, H. L., Wang, X., Chang, R. C., Jin, D. Y., Feng, H., Wang, Q., Lo, K. W., Huang, D. P., Yuen, P. W., Takada, K.: Stable expression of EBERs in immortalized

nasopharyngeal epithelial cells confers resistance to apoptotic stress. *Mol. Carcinog.* 2005, 44:92–101.

[62] Lizasa, H., Nanbo, A., Nishikawa, J., Jinushi, M., Yoshiyama, H.: Epstein-Barr Virus (EBV)-associated gastric carcinoma. *Viruses* 2012, 4:3420–3439.

[63] Takada, K.: Epstein-Barr virus and gastric carcinoma. *Mol. Pathol.* 2000, 53:255–261.

[64] Robelo, P. H., Sirotheau, F., Brunno, S. S., Paiva, F. F., Benevenuto, B. A.: Extranodal nasal NK/T-cell lymphoma: Arare oral presentation and FASN, CD44 and GLUT-1expression. *Brazilian Dental Journal* 2013, 24:284-288.

[65] Gregory, C. D., Rowe, M., Rickinson, A. B.: Different Epstein-Barr virus-B cell interactions in phenotypically distinct clones of a Burkitt's lymphoma cell line. *J. Gen. Virol.* 1990, 71:1481–1495.

[66] Lee, J. H., Kim, S. H., Han, S. H., An, J. S., Lee, E. S., Kim, Y. S.: Clinicopathological and molecular characteristics of Epstein-Barr virus-associated gastric carcinoma: A meta-analysis. *J. Gastroenterol. Hepatol.* 2009, 24:354–365.

[67] De Paoli, P., Pratesi, C., Bortolin, M. T.: The Epstein Barr virus DNA levels as a tumor marker in EBV- associated cancers; *J. Cancer Res. Clin. Oncol.* 2007, 133:809-815.

[68] Murphy, G., Pfeiffer, R., Camargo, M. C., Rabkin, C. S.: Meta-analysis shows that prevalence of Epstein-Barr virus-positive gastric cancer differs based on sex and anatomic location. *Gastroenterology* 2009, 137:824–833.

[69] Imai, S., Koizumi, S., Sugiura, M., Tokunaga, M., Uemura, Y., Yamamoto, N., Tanaka, S., Sato, E., Osato, T.: Gastric carcinoma: Monoclonal epithelial malignant cells expressing Epstein-Barr virus latent infection protein. *Proc. Natl. Acad. Sci. US* 1994, 91:9131–9135.

[70] Chen, J. N., He, D., Tang, F., Shao, C. K.: Epstein-Barr virus-associated gastric carcinoma: A newly defined entity. *J. Clin. Gastroenterol.* 2012, 46:262–271.

[71] Gourzones, C., Busson, P., Raab-Traub, N.: *Nasopharyngeal carcinoma: keys for translational medicine and biology.* Busson, P. Ed.; Landes Bioscience and Springer Science: Villejuif, France, 2012; pp. 42–60.

[72] Epstein, M. A., Barr, Y. M., Achong, B. G.: A second virus-carrying tissue culture strain (Eb2) of lymphoblasts from burkitt's lymphoma. *Pathol. Biol.* 1964, 12:1233–1234.

[73] Luo, B., Wang, Y., Wang, X. F., Liang, H., Yan, L. P., Huang, B. H., Zhao, P.: Expression of Epstein-Barr virus genes in EBV-associated gastric carcinomas. *World J. Gastroenterol.* 2005, 11:629–633.

[74] Zhao, J., Liang, Q., Cheung, K. F., Kang, W., Lung, R. W., Tong, J. H., To, K. F., Sung, J. J., Yu, J.: Genome-wide identification of Epstein-Barr virus-driven promoter methylation profiles of human genes in gastric cancer cells. *Cancer* 2013, 119:304–312.

[75] Iezzoni, J. C., Gaffey, M. J., Weiss, L. M.: The role of Epstein-Barr virus in lymphoepithelioma-like carcinomas. *Am. J. Clin. Pathol.* 1995, 103:308–315.

[76] Zhao, J., Jin, H., Cheung, K. F., Tong, J. H., Zhang, S., Go, M. Y., Tian, L., Kang, W., Leung, P. P., Zeng, Z.: Zinc finger E-box binding factor 1 plays a central role in regulating Epstein-Barr virus (EBV) latent-lytic switch and acts as a therapeutic target in EBV-associated gastric cancer. *Cancer* 2012, 118:924–936.

[77] Xiao, P., Shi, H., Zhang, H., Meng, F., Peng, J., Ke, Z., Wang, K., Liu, Y., Han, A.: Epstein-Barr virus-associated intrahepatic cholangiocarcinoma bearing an intense lymphoplasmacytic infiltration. *J. Clin. Pathol.* 2012, 65:570–573.

[78] Hsu, J. L., Glaser, S. L.: Epstein-Barr virus-associated malignancies: Epidemiologic patterns and etiologic implications. *Crit. Rev. Oncol. Hematol.* 2000, 34:27–53.

[79] Han, A. J., Xiong, M., Zong, Y. S.: Association of Epstein-Barr virus with lymphoepithelioma-like carcinoma of the lung in southern China. *Am. J. Clin. Pathol.* 2000, 114:220–226.

[80] Begin, L. R., Eskandari, J., Joncas, J., Panasci, L.: Epstein-Barr virus related lymphoepithelioma-like carcinoma of lung. *J. Surg. Oncol.* 1987, 36:280–283.

[81] Kim do, N., Chae, H. S., Oh, S. T., Kang, J. H., Park, C. H., Park, W. S., Takada, K., Lee, J. M., Lee, W. K., Lee, S. K.: Expression of viral microRNAs in Epstein-Barr virus-associated gastric carcinoma. *J. Virol.* 2007, 81:1033–1036.

[82] Lo, A. K., Lo, K. W., Ko, C. W., Young, L. S., Dawson, C. W.: Inhibition of the LKB1-AMPK pathway by the Epstein-Barr virus-encoded LMP1 promotes proliferation and transformation of human nasopharyngeal epithelial cells. *J. Pathol.* 2013, 230:336–346.

[83] Marks, J. E., Phillips, J. L., Menck, H. R.: The national cancer data base report on the relationship of race and national origin to the histology of nasopharyngeal carcinoma. *Cancer* 1998, 83:582–588.

[84] Chen, S. J., Chen, G. H., Chen, Y. H., Liu, C. Y., Chang, K. P., Chang, Y. S., Chen, H. C.: Characterization of Epstein-Barr virus miRNAome in nasopharyngeal carcinoma by deep sequencing. *PLoS One* 2010, 5:e12745.

[85] Dawson, C. W., Port, R. J., Young, L. S.: The role of the EBV-encoded latent membrane proteins LMP1 and LMP2 in the pathogenesis of nasopharyngeal carcinoma (NPC). *Semin. Cancer Biol.* 2012, 22:144–153.

[86] Lee, S. P.: Nasopharyngeal carcinoma and the EBV-specific T cell response: Prospects for immunotherapy. *Semin. Cancer Biol.* 2002, 12:463–471.

[87] Marquitz, A. R., Mathur, A., Shair, K. H., Raab-Traub, N.: Infection of Epstein-Barr virus in a gastric carcinoma cell line induces anchorage independence and global changes in gene expression. *Proc. Natl. Acad. Sci. US* 2012, 109:9593–9598.

[88] Lerner, M. R., Andrews, N. C., Miller, G., Steitz, J. A.: Two small RNAs encoded by Epstein-Barr virus and complexed with protein are precipitated by antibodies from patients with systemic lupus erythematosus. *Proc. Natl. Acad. Sci. US* 1981, 78:805–809.

[89] Takada, K.: Role of EBER and BARF1 in nasopharyngeal carcinoma (NPC) tumorigenesis. *Semin. Cancer Biol.* 2012, 22:162–165.

[90] Iwakiri, D., Sheen, T. S., Chen, J. Y., Huang, D. P., Takada, K.: Epstein-Barr virus-encoded small RNA induces insulin-like growth factor 1 and supports growth of nasopharyngeal carcinoma-derived cell lines. *Oncogene* 2005, 24:1767–1773.

[91] Gilligan, K. J., Rajadurai, P., Lin, J. C., Busson, P., Abdel-Hamid, M., Prasad, U., Tursz, T., Raab-Traub, N.: Expression of the Epstein-Barr virus BamHI A fragment in nasopharyngeal carcinoma: Evidence for a viral protein expressed in vivo. *J. Virol.* 1991, 65:6252–6259.

[92] Robertson, E. S., Tomkinson, B., Kieff, E.: An Epstein-Barr virus with a 58-kilobase-pair deletion that includes BARF0 transforms B lymphocytes in vitro. *J. Virol.* 1994, 68: 1449–1458.

[93] Al-Mozaini, M., Bodelon, G., Karstegl, C. E., Jin, B., Al-Ahdal, M., Farrell, P. J.: Epstein-Barr virus BART gene expression. *J. Gen. Virol.* 2009, 90:307–316.

Biographical Sketch

Hugo Juarez Olguin, MSc, PhD, is currently affiliated with Instituto Nacional de Pediatria and Universidad Nacional Autonoma de Mexico (UNAM) in Mexico City. Professional Appointments: Researcher in Medical Sciences and Titular Professor of Pharmacology. Research and Professional Experience: twenty six years working as researcher in Clinical Pharmacology into Hospital of Health Ministry and Teacher of Pharmacology at Faculty of Medicine, University of Mexico. He belongs to National System of Investigators. He has published 39 publications over last 3 years.

In: Epstein-Barr Virus (EBV)
Editor: Jan Styczynski

ISBN: 978-1-63117-476-6
© 2014 Nova Science Publishers, Inc.

Chapter II

The Role of Epstein-Barr Virus in the Management of Undifferentiated Nasopharyngeal Carcinoma

Thian-Sze Wong[*], *Yu-Wai Chan and Wei Gao*
Department of Surgery, Queen Mary Hospital,
University of Hong Kong, Hong Kong

Abstract

Cancer of the nasopharynx was first documented and reported by Regaud and Schmincke separately in 1921. According to the World Heal Organization (WHO) classification, nasopharyngeal carcinoma could be classified into 3 types according to the differentiation status. Among which, type 3 undifferentiated NPC is consistently associated with Epstein-Barr virus (EBV) infection. Clinical examination relies very much on conventional imaging with the use of endoscopy and histological assessment of the endoscopic biopsy. To localize and evaluate the extent of tumor in the head and neck regions, computerized tomography (CT) scan and magnetic resonance imaging (MRI) of the skull base will be employed. These approaches however cannot be applied for routine follow-up examination and screening high-risk population for early cancer detection. In view of the close association EBV with type 3 NPC, the use of EBV-derived genes or gene products are proposed in the surveillance of undifferentiated NPC on tissues obtained with non-invasive means including nasal swabs and peripheral blood. Here, the potential application of EBV DNA and viral proteins in different clinical aspects are discussed. In light of the recent discovery of EBV-encoded microRNA in the undifferentiated NPC, the potential application of these small RNA units in the NPC patients will also be examined.

---

[*] Address for correspondence: Thian-Sze Wong; Rm 209, Housemen Quarters; Department of Surgery, Queen Mary Hospital, The University of Hong Kong; 102 Pokfulam Road, Hong Kong; Tel: (852) 2819 9604; Fax: (852) 2819 3780. E-mail: thiansze@gmail.com.

Keywords: screening, prognosis, EBV antibodies, EBV DNA, EBV-encoded small nuclear RNA, EBV microRNA, treatment strategies, deoxyribozymes

Abbreviations

BART	BamHI-A rightward transcript
BHRF1	BamHI fragment H rightward open reading frame 1
CT	Computerized tomography
DXZ	Deoxyribozymes
EA	Early Antigen
EBER	EBV-encoded small nuclear RNA
EBV	Epstein-Barr virus
IARC	International Agency for Research on Cancer
IM	Infectious mononucleosis
MRI	Magnetic resonance imaging
NPC	Nasopharyngeal carcinoma
RISC	RNA-induced silencing complex
VCA	Viral Capsid Antigen

Introduction

Epstein-Barr Virus (EBV)

EBV is a herpesvirus (HHV-4) DNA virus (172 kb linear double-stranded DNA) with the ability to infect and replicate in epithelial cells [1]. The virus was first discovered in suspended culture of African Burkitt lymphoma cells. EBV is classified as group I carcinogen under International Agency for Research on Cancer (IARC). The causal relationship of EBV with human cancer development has been demonstrated in multiple human malignancies including Hodgkin disease, non-Hodgkin's lymphoma, infectious mononucleosis (IM), lymphoepithelioma-like carcinoma, oral leukoplakia, lymphoproliferative disease, gastric cancer and nasopharyngeal carcinoma [2]. The transforming ability of EBV is also recognized in a number of cancers associated with immunocompromised patients. EBV is the first human virus found to be associated with human malignancies [3]. It is a host-specific virus and human being was found as the only target of EBV. EBV infection is ubiquitous with more than 90% adults are EBV carriers [4]. Primary infection started at childhood with no symptoms and remained persistent in the B lymphocytes [5]. EBV infection in the normal head and neck epithelia is uncommon [6]. The high degree of clonogenicity in epithelial cancer cells suggested that the tumor shares and expands from the same progenitor cell infected by EBV [7]. With the advance in molecular techniques, it is now clear that EBV have several variants, which demonstrate distinctive geographic distribution [8]. Using next generation sequencing, it was demonstrated that the NPC cells harbor unique EBV strain which is distinguishable from the EBV variants found in other human malignancies [9].

Nasopharyngeal Carcinoma (NPC)

NPC is an epithelial cancer derived from the mucosal lining of the retro-nasal area situated at skull base. The cancers are frequently found in the pharyngeal recess and the fossa of Rosenmüller (medial to the medial crus of the Eustachian tube opening) [10]. According to the International Agency for Research on Cancer 2012, NPC is a prevalent cancer in Asia (including Malaysia, Singapore, Indonesia, Vietnam, Brunei) with age-standardized rate ranged from 5.0 to 7.2 per 100,000. In America and Europe, the incidence is relatively lower with age-standardized rate ranged from 0 to 0.4 per 100,000. The World Health Organization (WHO) classified NPC into 3 histological types based on the differentiation status including Type 1 NPC (differentiated NPC), Type 2 NPC (poorly differentiated NPC) and Type 3 NPC (undifferentiated NPC). In the endemic countries including Southern China, Taiwan, and Southeast Asia, undifferentiated NPC (WHO Type 3) is the major histological subtype. To date, it is recognized that EBV are present in virtually all the WHO-2 and WHO-3 NPC cells [11]. For WHO-1 keratinizing NPC, the causal role of EBV remains unresolved as the virus could only be found in a few number of patients. EBV genome is found in all the neoplastic cells of type 3 NPC. Morphologically, the cancerous epithelial cells feature with prominent enlarged nuclei and eosinophilic nucleoli [12]. The NPC cells are scattered throughout the histological sections demonstrating loss of polarity with intraepithelial lymphoplasmacytic infiltration [13]. Early NPC is asymptomatic. For EBV associated NPC, radiotherapy is the primary treatment as the EBV-infected cells are intrinsically sensitive to radiation with good local control rate [14]. With the use of induction chemotherapy with cisplatin plus 5-fluorouracil or cisplatin plus gemcitabine followed by accelerated radiotherapy, the 5 year survival rate could reach 70%.

Latent Infection of EBV in NPC

EBV enters latency period after infecting the host cells. All the NPC cells are latently infected with EBV in latency II phase. The latently infected EBV will have a specific viral gene expression pattern. It is now known that NPC will express EBER, EBNA1, LMP2A and LMP2B during latency II phase [2]. LMP1 and LMP2 expression however is not universal in all the NPC tissues. They are expressed in about 50% of the NPC cases [15]. Reactivation and replication of EBV is found in tongue and oropharyngeal epithelial cells and are suspected to be the cellular source of EBV [16, 17]. It is suggested that the infected cells shed the virus into the saliva and spread the virus via oral secretion. In order to maintain the latent infection state in the NPC cells, EBV has to rely on the support from cellular machinery (e.g., activation of cyclin D1, regulator of G1/S transition), extracellular growth signals and tumor microenvironment [18-21].

The Role of EBV in NPC Diganosis

In clinical practice, EBV serology has long been used in NPC screening and prognosis. Further, staining the EBV gene product (e.g., EBER) is a gold standard for histological assessment of the suspicious NPC tissues as EBER is only expressed in the neoplastic cells. In view of the tight correlation of EBV with the etiology of NPC, EBV antibodies and EBV DNA has been employed as a serological indicator of tumor load of the NPC patients.

Anti-EBV Antibodies

The peripheral blood of NPC patients had a persistently high antibody titer against EBV antigens [22]. Hence, serological measurement of the circulating immunoglobulin by peptide-based anti-EBV antibody ELISA is suitable for use to evaluate the disease status at molecular level [23]. The elevation of EBV antibody titer is parallel to the increase in tumor volume [24]. The increase is not suitable to be used as an early screening tool as the EBV antibody titer will only increase after the disease onset [24]. Commonly used anti-EBV antibodies includes antibodies against both EBV early and viral capsid antigens including IgA / Early Antigen (EA), IgA / Viral Capsid Antigen (VCA), IgG / Early Antigen (EA) and IgG / Viral Capsid Antigen (VCA) [25]. Active EBV replication and expression of EBV antigen is observed in B cell lymphoma cell line but not epithelial cell line. Most EBV infected NPC cells are in latency phase and hence the lytic phase protein (such as EA & VCA) is not detected in the NPC tissues. At present, it remains unclear why the patients will develop immune response against the lytic gene product. It has been suggested that the EBV harbor in the head and neck epithelia are reactivated during caner progression and hence trigger the host's immune response [26]. In the recent years, the use of anti-EBV antibodies are gradually replaced by other EBV-derived markers in view of the fact that normal individuals could also has high circulating EBV titer. In addition, the detection sensitivity and specificity of EBV antibody titers varies greatly according to the selected antibodies. NPC is not the only human malignancy induced by EBV. Hence, the high EBV titer might not be a unique feature to NPC patients and might implied the existence of other human malignancies [27].

EBV DNA

Tumor-derived EBV DNA is regarded as a valuable diagnostic criterion as it could be detected in the plasma or serum of NPC patients with high sensitivity and specificity [28]. Meta-analysis on 1492 NPC patients and 2641 controls revealing that plasma EBV DNA has the highest diagnostic efficacy with pooled sensitivity 0.73 (range: 0.71-0.75) and pooled specificity 0.89 (range: 0.88-0.90). Plasma EBV DNA concentration is an indicator of body tumor load with high correlation to the EBER1 in the primary cancer tissues [29]. High EBV DNA concentration is observed in patients with different clinical manifestation including primary NPC (6200 copies/mL), local recurrent NPC (9200 copies/mL), and distant metastatic NPC (2050 copies/mL) [29]. Different from anti-EBV antibodies, EBV could be used as a screening marker as high level is existed in high-risk population. The circulating EBV DNA drops significantly in response to the treatment including radiotherapy and nasopharyngectomy. The circulating EBV DNA concentration will drop beyond the detection level in 1 week after radiotherapy and is suggested to be a good clinical indicator of complete remission [29-31].

EBV RNA: EBV-Encoded Small Nuclear RNA (EBER)

Undifferentiated NPC is characterized by the abundant expression of EBV non-polyadenylated RNA named EBER [32]. EBV expresses EBER in all the 3 latency period. Although EBER do not codes for any protein, it is abundantly expressed in all the neoplastic NPC cells. EBER is detected in the nucleus of NPC with high specificity [33]. Hence, high resolution in situ hybridization (ISH) of EBER is employed as detection mean in the histological evaluation of NPC tissues. EBER is a stable molecule and ISH could be applied on both frozen and paraffin-embedded tissue sections [34]. EBER expression in the NPC cells is not an absolute event. It should be noted that a small proportion of undifferentiated NPC are EBER negative in areas where NPC incidence is low [35]. In addition, differentiated NPC could also be found to be EBER positive. EBER expression level can be regarded as an indicator of tumor load and is correlated with the circulating DNA level [35]. EBER staining is used to differentiate NPC from other form of epithelial cancer in the enlarged metastatic lymph node with unknown primary [33]. At present, little is known about the function of EBER in the malignant progression of NPC. It might possibly contribute to the NPC tumorigenesis through modulating the pro-inflammatory cytokine secretion pathways [36].

Recent Development of EBV Makers and EBV-Based Therapy

Novel EBV Marker – EBV MicroRNA

MicroRNA is a group of small non-protein-coding RNA (<25 b.p. long) which functions as post-transcriptional regulators. EBV was the first human virus found to express microRNA [37]. Both NPC cells and EBV will express these group of small RNA. MicroRNA functions as epigenetic regulator by binding to specific mRNA transcripts. Partial complementary binding at the 3'UTR of the target transcript is suffice to guide the recruitment of RNA-induced silencing complex (RISC) complex and promote mRNA cleavage or hinder translation. The seed sequence (2-8 b.p. sequence located at the 5' end of the EBV microRNA) is important for the EBV microRNA to recognize the target genes in the host cells [38]. Theoretically, the oncogenic microRNA produced by the virus could hinder the function of tumor suppression genes in the host cells resulting in the malignant transformation. It is estimated that each microRNA could recognize 100 target sites and control multiple signaling pathways simultaneously [39].

In EBV genome, EBV microRNA encoding genes are located in 2 main clusters: BamHI fragment H rightward open reading frame 1 (BHRF1) and BamHI-A rightward transcript (BART). NPC patients have higher circulating EBV microRNA levels in comparison with the normal counterparts. In addition, the EBV microRNA could be detected in serological EBV DNA negative patients suggesting that circulating EBV microRNA could potentially be used as a group of sensitive surrogate makers in NPC screening. With the use of deep sequencing, it was noted that the expression levels of several EBV microRNA are equivalent to the expression levels of human microRNA [40]. In addition, EBV microRNA could share the same seed sequence with the oncogenic microRNA identified in the cancer cells suggesting that they may have similar role in the transformation process [40]. At present, the precise regulatory mechanism of EBV microRNA and the correlation with the EBV life cycle in the epithelial cells are not completely understood. It is observed that EBV will express the viral microRNA in 2 days after infecting the host cells and the virus is manage to change the microRNA expression patterns in response to the environmental changes induced by radiation and chemotherapeutic agents [41-43].

Targeting EBV Gene Product As a Treatment Strategy

In view of the proximity of NPC and EBV, several groups attempted to develop vaccine preventing NPC development by targeting the EBV gene product. Many efforts are tried to target the gp350/220 (907 amino acid polypeptide), the glycoprotein expressed on the virus envelop which mediate the entrance of the virus to the host cells [44]. The gp350/220 is a lytic phase protein. It will bind to the CD21 molecule on the B cell surface leading to the preferential infection. Other group designed their vaccine through targeting the latent proteins such as EBNA-2 and EBNA-3C [45]. At present, there is still no consensus on the most effective target genes in the development of prophylactic vaccine targeting EBV [46].

The Use of Deoxyribozymes (DXZ) As Therapeutic Oligonucleotides in NPC Treatment

Apart from targeting the viral proteins, it has been suggested that targeting the viral transcripts is also a feasible way. DXZ (also known as catalytic oligodeoxynucleotides) is a synthetic single-stranded DNA molecule which could down-regulate the target RNA based on sequence complementary. The enzyme consists of a catalytic domain of 15 nucleotides, flanked by two substrate-recognition domains of 7–10 nucleotides. It has been demonstrated that exogenous delivery of DXZ to viral-associated cancer cells is an effective way to remove the viral mRNA. For example, DXZ could be used to down-regulate HPV E6/E7 mRNA [47]. The advantage of DXZ is that it poses no toxicity to the target cells with high stability under physiological environment. DXZ targeting EBV LMP1 could also inhibit NPC cell proliferation and induce apoptosis [48].

Conclusion

EBV-infected NPC is a distinct clinical entity and the EBV-derived maker is a unique tool allowing us to monitor the disease. The diagnostic and prognostic value of EBV provides insights into the long-term monitoring schemes for secondary primary or disease recurrence. With the identification of EBV microRNA, further studies are warranted to unravel and elucidate the outcome of viral microRNA dysregulation and NPC development. An in-depth understanding on the virus will facilitate us in shaping a safe vaccination strategy against the development of NPC.

Glossary

EBV

EBV is a double-stranded DNA virus and is classified as group I carcinogen due to its causal roles in human cancers. It was first identified in Burkitt's lymphoma cells and is associated with nasopharyngeal carcinoma. It could act as a biomarker for nasopharyngeal carcinoma screening and prognosis.

Nasopharyngeal carcinoma

Nasopharyngeal carcinoma is an epithelial cancer derived from the mucosal lining of the retro-nasal area and is predominant in male. It has a high incidence in southeastern Asia. It is classified into 3 types according to the degree of differentiation and undifferentiated NPC (WHO Type 3) is closely related to EBV infection.

EBV latent infection

EBV has the ability to select two various lifestyles: latent replication and lytic replication. EBV enters latency period after infecting the nasopharyngeal carcinoma cells. During latency period, its genomic DNA displays as a closed circular plasmid. The latently infected EBV exhibits a specific viral gene expression pattern and expresses EBER, EBNA1, LMP2A and LMP2B.

EBV-encoded microRNAs

EBV genome encodes 2 main cluster of microRNA: BamHI fragment H rightward open reading frame 1 (BHRF1) and BamHI-A rightward transcript (BART). Circulating EBV microRNAs could serve as non-invasive biomarkers for nasopharyngeal carcinoma diagnosis. EBV microRNAs exert oncogenic roles in nasopharyngeal carcinoma progression.

Summary Points List

- EBV infects NPC in latency II and expresses specific viral genes including EBER, EBNA1, LMP2A and LMP2B.
- Serological EBV antibodies and EBV DNA levels have long been used in NPC screening and prognosis.
- The use of anti-EBV antibodies are gradually replaced by other EBV-derived markers in view of the fact that normal individuals could also has high circulating EBV titer.
- Tumor-derived EBV DNA is regarded as a valuable diagnostic criterion as it could be detected in the plasma or serum of NPC patients with high sensitivity and specificity.
- Staining the EBV gene product is a gold standard for histological assessment of the suspicious NPC tissues as EBER is only expressed in the neoplastic cells.
- EBV microRNA could be detected in serological EBV DNA negative patients suggesting that circulating EBV microRNA could potentially be used as a group of sensitive surrogate makers in NPC screening.

- The circulating EBV DNA drops significantly in response to the treatment including radiotherapy and nasopharyngectomy, suggesting that it is a good clinical indicator of complete remission after treatment.

Future Issue List

- To elucidate the precise regulatory mechanisms of EBV microRNA and the correlation with the EBV life cycle in the epithelial cells.
- To identify the most effective target genes in the development of prophylactic vaccine targeting EBV.

References

[1] Petrova M, Kamburov V: Epstein-Barr virus: silent companion or causative agent of chronic liver disease? *World J Gastroenterol* 2010, 16:4130-4134.
[2] Raab-Traub N: Epstein-Barr virus in the pathogenesis of NPC. *Semin Cancer Biol* 2002, 12:431-441.
[3] Moore PS, Chang Y: Why do viruses cause cancer? Highlights of the first century of human tumour virology. *Nat Rev Cancer* 2010, 10:878-889.
[4] Gullo C, Low WK, Teoh G: Association of Epstein-Barr virus with nasopharyngeal carcinoma and current status of development of cancer-derived cell lines. *Ann Acad Med Singapore* 2008, 37:769-777.
[5] Niedobitek G, Young LS: Epstein-Barr virus persistence and virus-associated tumours. *Lancet* 1994, 343:333-335.
[6] Sam CK, Brooks LA, Niedobitek G, Young LS, Prasad U, Rickinson AB: Analysis of Epstein-Barr virus infection in nasopharyngeal biopsies from a group at high risk of nasopharyngeal carcinoma. *Int J Cancer* 1993, 53:957-962.
[7] Pathmanathan R, Prasad U, Sadler R, Flynn K, Raab-Traub N: Clonal proliferations of cells infected with Epstein-Barr virus in preinvasive lesions related to nasopharyngeal carcinoma. *N Engl J Med* 1995, 333:693-698.
[8] Zeng MS, Li DJ, Liu QL, Song LB, Li MZ, Zhang RH, Yu XJ, Wang HM, Ernberg I, Zeng YX: Genomic sequence analysis of Epstein-Barr virus strain GD1 from a nasopharyngeal carcinoma patient. *J Virol* 2005, 79:15323-15330.
[9] Liu P, Fang X, Feng Z, Guo YM, Peng RJ, Liu T, Huang Z, Feng Y, Sun X, Xiong Z, Guo X, Pang SS, Wang B, Lv X, Feng FT, Li DJ, Chen LZ, Feng QS, Huang WL, Zeng MS, Bei JX, Zhang Y, Zeng YX: Direct sequencing and characterization of a clinical isolate of Epstein-Barr virus from nasopharyngeal carcinoma tissue by using next-generation sequencing technology. *J Virol* 2011, 85:11291-11299.
[10] Niedobitek G: Epstein-Barr virus infection in the pathogenesis of nasopharyngeal carcinoma. *Mol Pathol* 2000, 53:248-254.
[11] Sam CK, Brooks LA, Niedobitek G, Young LS, Prasad U, Rickinson AB: Analysis of Epstein-Barr virus infection in nasopharyngeal biopsies from a group at high risk of nasopharyngeal carcinoma. *Int J Cancer* 1993, 53:957-962.

[12] Wai Pak M, To KF, Lee JC, Liang EY, van Hasselt CA: In vivo real-time diagnosis of nasopharyngeal carcinoma in situ by contact rhinoscopy. *Head Neck* 2005, 27:1008-1013.

[13] Andersson-Anvret M, Forsby N, Klein G, Henle W: Relationship between the Epstein-Barr virus and undifferentiated nasopharyngeal carcinoma: correlated nucleic acid hybridization and histopathological examination. *Int J Cancer* 1977, 20:486-494.

[14] DeNittis AS, Liu L, Rosenthal DI, Machtay M: Nasopharyngeal carcinoma treated with external radiotherapy, brachytherapy, and concurrent/adjuvant chemotherapy. *Am J Clin Oncol* 2002, 25:93-95.

[15] Wang Y, Wang XF, Sun ZF, Luo B: Unique variations of Epstein-Barr virus-encoded BARF1 gene in nasopharyngeal carcinoma biopsies. *Virus Res* 2012, 166:23-30.

[16] Herrmann K, Frangou P, Middeldorp J, Niedobitek G: Epstein-Barr virus replication in tongue epithelial cells. *J Gen Virol* 2002, 83:2995-2998.

[17] Sixbey JW, Nedrud JG, Raab-Traub N, Hanes RA, Pagano JS: Epstein-Barr virus replication in oropharyngeal epithelial cells. *N Engl J Med* 1984, 310:1225-1230.

[18] Beck A, Päzolt D, Grabenbauer GG, Nicholls JM, Herbst H, Young LS, Niedobitek G: Expression of cytokine and chemokine genes in Epstein-Barr virus-associatednasopharyngeal carcinoma: comparison with Hodgkin's disease. *J Pathol* 2001, 194:145-151.

[19] Li J, Zhang XS, Xie D, Deng HX, Gao YF, Chen QY, Huang WL, Masucci MG, Zeng YX: Expression of immune-related molecules in primary EBV-positive Chinese nasopharyngeal carcinoma: associated with latent membrane protein 1 (LMP1) expression. *Cancer Biol Ther* 2007, 6:1997-2004.

[20] Tsang CM, Yip YL, Lo KW, Deng W, To KF, Hau PM, Lau VM, Takada K, Lui VW, Lung ML, Chen H, Zeng M, Middeldorp JM, Cheung AL, Tsao SW: Cyclin D1 overexpression supports stable EBV infection in nasopharyngeal epithelial cells. *Proc Natl Acad Sci U S A* 2012, 109:E3473-3482.

[21] Zhang G, Tsang CM, Deng W, Yip YL, Lui VW, Wong SC, Cheung AL, Hau PM, Zeng M, Lung ML, Chen H, Lo KW, Takada K, Tsao SW: Enhanced IL-6/IL-6R signaling promotes growth and malignant properties in EBV-infected premalignant and cancerous nasopharyngeal epithelial cells. *PLoS One* 2013, 8:e62284.

[22] Chien YC, Chen JY, Liu MY, Yang HI, Hsu MM, Chen CJ, Yang CS: Serologic markers of Epstein-Barr virus infection and nasopharyngeal carcinoma in Taiwanese men. *N Engl J Med* 2001, 345:1877-1882.

[23] Zeng Y: Seroepidemiological studies on nasopharyngeal carcinoma in China. *Adv Cancer Res* 1985, 44:121-138.

[24] Mazeron MC: Value of anti-Epstein-Barr antibody detection in the diagnosis and management of undifferentiated carcinoma of the nasopharynx. *Bull Cancer Radiother* 1996, 83:3-7.

[25] Tiwawech D, Srivatanakul P, Karaluk A, Ishida T: Significance of plasma IgA and IgG antibodies to Epstein-Barr virus early and viral capsid antigens in Thai nasopharyngeal carcinoma. *Asian Pac J Cancer Prev* 2003, 4:113-118.

[26] Henle G, Henle W: Epstein-Barr virus-specific IgA serum antibodies as an outstanding feature of nasopharyngeal carcinoma. *Int J Cancer* 1976, 17:1-7.

[27] Shao JY, Li YH, Gao HY, Wu QL, Cui NJ, Zhang L, Cheng G, Hu LF, Ernberg I, Zeng YX: Comparison of plasma Epstein-Barr virus (EBV) DNA levels and serum EBV

immunoglobulin A/virus capsid antigen antibody titers in patients with nasopharyngeal carcinoma. *Cancer* 2004, 100:1162-1170.

[28] Chan KC, Lo YM: Circulating EBV DNA as a tumor marker for nasopharyngeal carcinoma. *Semin Cancer Biol* 2002, 12:489-496.

[29] Shao JY, Zhang Y, Li YH, Gao HY, Feng HX, Wu QL, Cui NJ, Cheng G, Hu B, Hu LF, Ernberg I, Zeng YX: Comparison of Epstein-Barr virus DNA level in plasma, peripheral blood cell and tumor tissue in nasopharyngeal carcinoma. *Anticancer Res* 2004, 24:4059-4066.

[30] Chan AT, Lo YM, Zee B, Chan LY, Ma BB, Leung SF, Mo F, Lai M, Ho S, Huang DP, Johnson PJ: Plasma Epstein-Barr virus DNA and residual disease after radiotherapy for undifferentiated nasopharyngeal carcinoma. *J Natl Cancer Inst* 2002, 94:1614-1619.

[31] Ngan RK, Yip TT, Cheng WW, Chan JK, Cho WC, Ma VW, Wan KK, Au SK, Law CK, Lau WH: Circulating Epstein-Barr virus DNA in serum of patients with lymphoepithelioma-like carcinoma of the lung: a potential surrogate marker for monitoring disease. *Clin Cancer Res* 2002, 8:986-994.

[32] Shi W, Pataki I, MacMillan C: Molecular pathology parameters in human nasopharyngeal carcinoma. *Cancer* 2002, 94:1997-2006.

[33] Gulley ML: Molecular diagnosis of Epstein-Barr virus-related diseases. *J Mol Diagn* 2001, 3:1-10.

[34] Fan SQ, Ma J, Zhou J, Xiong W: Differential expression of Epstein-Barr virus-encoded RNA and several tumor-related genes in various typesof nasopharyngeal epithelial lesions and nasopharyngeal carcinoma using tissue microarray analysis. *Hum Pathol* 2006, 37:593-605.

[35] Kalpoe JS, Dekker PB, van Krieken JH, Baatenburg de Jong RJ, Kroes AC: Role of Epstein-Barr virus DNA measurement in plasma in the clinical management of nasopharyngeal carcinoma in a low risk area. *J Clin Pathol* 2006, 59:537-41.

[36] Takada K: Role of EBER and BARF1 in nasopharyngeal carcinoma (NPC) tumorigenesis. *Semin Cancer Biol* 2012, 22:162-165.

[37] Pfeffer S, Zavolan M, Grässer FA, Chien M, Russo JJ, Ju J, John B, Enright AJ, Marks D, Sander C, Tuschl T: Identification of virus-encoded microRNAs. *Science* 2004, 304:734-736.

[38] Stark A, Brennecke J, Russell RB, Cohen SM: Identification of Drosophila MicroRNA targets. *PLoS Biol* 2003, 1:E60.

[39] Brennecke J, Stark A, Russell RB, Cohen SM: Principles of microRNA-target recognition. *PLoS Biol* 2005, 3:e85.

[40] Chen SJ, Chen GH, Chen YH, Liu CY, Chang KP, Chang YS, Chen HC: Characterization of Epstein-Barr virus miRNAome in nasopharyngeal carcinoma by deep sequencing. *PLoS One* 2010, 5:e12745.

[41] Chan JY, Gao W, Ho WK, Wei WI, Wong TS: Overexpression of Epstein-Barr virus-encoded microRNA-BART7 in undifferentiated nasopharyngeal carcinoma. *Anticancer Res* 2012, 32:3201-3210.

[42] Choy EY, Siu KL, Kok KH, Lung RW, Tsang CM, To KF, Kwong DL, Tsao SW, Jin DY: An Epstein-Barr virus-encoded microRNA targets PUMA to promote host cell survival. *J Exp Med* 2008, 205:2551-2560.

[43] Pratt ZL, Kuzembayeva M, Sengupta S, Sugden B: The microRNAs of Epstein-Barr Virus are expressed at dramatically differing levels among cell lines. *Virology* 2009, 386:387-397.

[44] Sitompul LS, Widodo N, Djati MS, Utomo DH: Epitope mapping of gp350/220 conserved domain of epstein barr virus to develop nasopharyngeal carcinoma (npc) vaccine. *Bioinformation* 2012, 8:479-482.

[45] Lockey TD, Zhan X, Surman S, Sample CE, Hurwitz JL: Epstein-Barr virus vaccine development: a lytic and latent protein cocktail. *Front Biosci* 2008, 13:5916-5927.

[46] Cohen JI, Mocarski ES, Raab-Traub N, Corey L, Nabel GJ: The need and challenges for development of an Epstein-Barr virus vaccine. *Vaccine* 2013, 31:B194-196.

[47] Benítez-Hess ML, Reyes-Gutiérrez P, Alvarez-Salas LM: Inhibition of humanpapillomavirus expression using DNAzymes. *Methods Mol Biol* 2011, 764:317-335.

[48] You X, Yang YC, Ke X, Hong SL, Hu GH: Fluorescence Visualization Screening for EBV-LMP1-Targeted DNAzymes. *Otolaryngol Head Neck Surg* 2013.

Biographical Sketch

Stanley Thian-Sze Wong, BSc(Hon.), JD, LLM, PhD, is currently affiliated with Department of Surgery (Division: Ear, Nose and Throat / Head and Neck Surgery / Plastic and Reconstructive Surgery), Queen Mary Hospital, The University of Hong Kong and appointed as assistant professor. Professional Experience: Head and neck cancers, epigenetics, and molecular diagnostic. His research interest is related to: (1) Epigenomics of head and neck cancers including clustered hypermethylation, chromatin remodeling and anomalous microRNA expression; (2) Potential use of epigenetic markers in head and neck cancer screening, diagnosis, and prognosis; (3) Epigenetic therapies on head and neck cancers with demethylating agents, histone deacetylase and natural polyphenols. He has published 26 papers over last 3 years.

In: Epstein-Barr Virus (EBV)
Editor: Jan Styczynski

ISBN: 978-1-63117-476-6
© 2014 Nova Science Publishers, Inc.

Chapter III

Epstein-Barr Virus (EBV) – Associated B-Cell Lymphoma

Prakash Vishnu, MD, FACP[1,*]
and David M. Aboulafia, MD[1,2]
[1]Floyd and Delores Jones Cancer Institute at
Virginia Mason Medical Center, Seattle, WA, US
[2]Division of Hematology, University of Washington,
Seattle, WA, US

Abstract

Epstein-Barr virus (EBV) is an omnipresent human γ-herpesvirus that causes life-long asymptomatic infection in immunocompetent hosts, whereas, it is commonly associated with a broad spectrum of lymphomas in immune-compromised individuals including organ transplant recipients and people living with human immunodeficiency virus/acquired immunodeficiency syndrome (HIV/AIDS). Antibodies to EBV are present in all population groups; approximately 95% of adults are EBV-seropositive. The majority of primary EBV infections are subclinical, yet EBV is a double stranded DNA transforming virus that has been causally linked to a wide range of human neoplasia. The evidence for such an association is strongest for B-cell non-Hodgkin's lymphomas (NHL). EBV infects and transforms B-lymphocytes by encoding a series of products that mimic growth and anti-apoptotic transcription factors. EBV-associated lymphomas demonstrate heterogeneity at both the clinical and the molecular levels. This includes the degree by which they express EBV-encoded latent antigens. Our evolving understanding of how EBV induces molecular transformation is important for it promises new opportunities to combat lymphomagenesis. In this chapter we highlight salient molecular and clinical features of EBV-associated B-cell NHL and briefly review treatment options for these various lymphoproliferative disorders.

---

[*] Corresponding author: Prakash Vishnu, MD, FACP; Floyd and Delores Jones Cancer Institute at Virginia Mason Medical Center; 1100 9th Avenue, Seattle, WA 98101; Tel: (206) 223-6193; Fax: (206) 223-2382; E-mail: prakash.vishnu@vmmc.org.

Keywords: Epstein-Barr virus, lymphoproliferative disorder, B-cell non-Hodgkin's lymphoma, chronic antigenic stimulation, chemotherapy, monoclonal antibodies

Introduction

Epstein-Barr virus (EBV) is named after Michael Epstein and Yvonne Barr, who discovered the virus in 1964 while conducting research on suspension cultures of African Burkitt's lymphoma (BL) cells. It was the first human virus to be directly implicated in carcinogenesis [1]. In view of EBV's causal association with several different types of tumors, the World Health Organization (WHO) classified EBV as a tumor virus in 1997 [2]. EBV can cause infectious mononucleosis, also known as 'glandular fever', 'Mono' and 'Pfeiffer's disease'.

EBV is also called Human herpesvirus 4 (HHV-4). It belongs to the herpes family (which includes Herpes simplex virus and Cytomegalovirus). Its genome is composed of double stranded DNA, about 170kb in length, and the DNA is linear in the virus particle. It is characterized by its ability to immortalize human B-lymphocytes in culture.

Although herpesviruses are ubiquitous, humans are the only natural hosts for EBV. The host cells of EBV are mainly lymphocytes and epithelial cells. Though the role of epithelial cells in the life cycle of EBV is not well defined, the oropharynx represents the site of primary EBV infection, and intermittent reactivation and virus replication in the oropharyngeal epithelia allow the spreading of EBV [3]. The role of epithelial cells in the life cycle of EBV is, however, not nearly as well defined despite evidence linking EBV and cancer formation in nasopharyngeal carcinoma (NPC).

Once infected by EBV, B-lymphocytes are activated to grow and differentiate into memory B-lymphocytes via the germinal center (GC) reaction. The GC reaction is the basis of T-dependent humoral immunity against foreign pathogens and the ultimate expression of the adaptive immune response. GCs represent a unique collaboration between proliferating antigen-specific B cells, T follicular helper cells, and the specialized follicular dendritic cells that constitutively occupy the central follicular zones of secondary lymphoid organs. The primary function of GCs is to produce high-affinity antibody-secreting plasma cells and memory B cells that ensure sustained immune protection and rapid recall responses against previously encountered foreign antigens. However, the process of somatic mutation of antibody variable region genes that underpins GC function also carries significant risks in the form of unintended oncogenic mutations and generation of potentially pathogenic autoantibody specificities [4]. Although the numbers of EBV infected B-lymphocytes wane with the passage of time a small reservoir persists with the viral genome present in a latent form. Once the virus has colonized the B-lymphocyte compartment, reactivation from latency can occur at any mucosal site, such as the cervix or the oropharynx, where the B-lymphocytes reside.

The pathogenesis of EBV-associated cancers is related to the virus's latent cycle. Four types of latent gene expression have been described. In healthy individuals, EBV is latently maintained in memory B-lymphocytes, which express only the transcripts for EBV small RNAs. This state, also known as Latency 0, allows for persistence of the virus in a way that is non-pathogenic and cloaked from the immune system [5]. The other three types of latency (I,

II and III), which characterize a heterogeneous group of malignancies, are based on patterns of expression of the EBV genome [3] (Table 1). Latency I, characterized by expression of EBV nuclear antigen 1 (EBNA-1) and Epstein-Barr Early RNAs (EBERs), is associated with BL; EBV gene expression in latency II is associated with Hodgkin's lymphoma (HL). T-cell non-Hodgkin's lymphoma (NHL) and NPC are limited to EBNA-2, EBERs and latent membrane proteins (LMPs) 1 and 2. Latency III is seen mainly in the back drop of immunosuppression such as seen in post-transplant lymphoprolife-rative disorders (PTLD) and AIDS-related lymphomas. It most often involves the unrestricted expression of EBNA, EBERs and LMPs [6].

EBV latent genes induce an activated B-lymphocyte phenotype. Although these cells are not transformed, if their replication proceeds unchecked or if they acquire oncogenic mutations, they can become neoplastic. During EBV latency, B-lymphocytes are not actively dividing but various viral genes are activated and encode a series of products stimulating anti-apoptotic molecules, cytokines and signal transducers which result in dysregulated cellular pathways [7].

In immunocompetent individuals, cytotoxic T-cell responses against latent viral proteins prevent the expansion of activated B-lymphocytes. Because cytotoxic responses to EBNA-1 are rare, EBNA-1-expressing lymphocytes escape immune surveillance, ultimately becoming the viral reservoir. Intermittently, these cells may enter the lytic cycle - which is characterized by increased EBV viral replication, suppression of host protein synthesis and death of the infected cells. This lead to the release of circulating virions which are free to infect additional cells.

In the immunocompromised host, the interplay between EBV replication, latency and immune control can be disrupted, and prolonged proliferation of EBV-infected lymphocytes may result [8]. EBV-associated B-cell lymphoma (EBCL) is the result of such abnormal outgrowth of EBV infected B-lymphocytes that would normally be contained by an effective EBV-specific T-cell mediated cellular cytotoxic response. EBCL may occur most prominently in the milieu of primary and secondary immune deficiencies, as well as in individuals without overt or documented immunodeficiency.

Table 1. EBV viral gene expression and associated malignancies

Latency type	Viral gene expressed	Associated malignances
Latency 0	EBERs	None
Latency I	EBNA-1 EBERs	Burkitt's lymphoma
Latency II	EBNA-1 EBERs LMP 1 and 2	Hodgkin's lymphoma Nasopharyngeal carcinoma Peripheral T/NK-cell lymphoma
Latency III	All EBNAs EBERs LMP 1 and 2	HIV-associated lymphoma Post-transplant lymphoproliferative disorders

EBERs: EBV-encoded small RNAs; EBNA-1: EBV nuclear antigen 1; LMP: Latent membrane protein. Adapted from Thompson et al. [3].

The ability of EBV to maintain its viral genome within the B-cell, to evade the host immune response, and to activate aberrant growth and cellular differentiation are all important factors that contribute to its malignant phenotype. While EBV plays an important role in carcinogenesis, it does not work in isolation to trigger malignant transformation. Other factors such as specific defects of immune recognition, stimulation of B-cell proliferation by other mitogenic processes, and appearance of secondary genetic aberrations and mutations are also important contributors to carcinogenesis [3]. EBV is associated with 1% of the tumors worldwide. These tumors range from a variety of B- and T-cell NHLs to various carcinomas and smooth muscle tumors. Most EBV-associated NHLs are characterized clinically by rapid growth and histologically by significant necrosis. EBV-associated NHL can be divided into two broad categories - those arising in patients with immunodeficiency and those arising in individuals without overt immunodeficiency (Table 2). In an analysis of tumor tissues collected from 208 patients with B-cell lymphomas the EBV genome was identified most frequently in high-grade lymphomas, and to a much lesser degree among low-grade lymphomas [10]. Lymphomas with greater than 80% EBER-positive tumor cells were invariably either diffuse large B-cell lymphoma (DLBCL), sporadic BL or those with plasmacellular differentiation.

There are no specific dietary or lifestyle risk factors for EBCLs. However, there are areas of the world where certain EBV-related lymphomas have a much higher prevalence, including EBV-positive NK/T-cell lymphomas in parts of Asia, EBV-positive HL in Latin America, and EBV-positive BL in areas of Africa with holoendemic malaria [11]. While EBV

Table 2. Epstein-Barr virus (EBV) associated B-cell non-Hodgkin lymphoma (NHL)

Type of NHL	EBV frequency
Immunocompromised patients	
NHL associated with primary immunodeficiency	>95%
Post-transplant lymphoma	
Hematopoietic stem cell transplant	>95%
Solid organ transplant	>95%
HIV-associated lymphomas	
Primary CNS lymphoma	>95%
Primary effusion lymphoma	>95%
DLBCL	30 - 60%
Burkitt's lymphoma	30 - 60%
Immunocompetent patients	
Lymphomatoid granulomatosis	80 - 95%
Burkitt's lymphoma (endemic)	>95%
EBV-positive DLBCL	>95%
DLBCL and CD30$^+$ Ki1$^+$ anaplastic large cell lymphoma of B-cell type	10 - 35%
T-cell/histiocyte-rich B-cell lymphoma	20%
Angioimmunoblastic B-cell lymphoma	>80%

CNS: central nervous system; HIV: human immunodeficiency virus; DLBCL: Diffuse large B-cell lymphoma.
Adapted from Heslop, H. E. [9].

is detected in approximately 95% of endemic BL cases, only a minority of BL encountered outside Africa are EBV-positive [10].

EBV infection is also linked to several unique NHLs, three of which we briefly mention. The first, and perhaps best described, is pyothorax-associated lymphoma [12]. This form of DLBCL frequently develops in the pleural cavity of immunocompetent patients with at least a 20-year history of pyothorax. More than two thirds of these lymphomas carry EBV-specific DNA sequences [13].

The second unique lymphoma is 'EBV-positive DLBCL of the elderly' and is defined as an EBV-positive monoclonal large B-cell proliferation that occurs in patients greater than 50 years of age and in whom there is no known immunodeficiency or history of lymphoma. These tumors are more common in Asia but also occur in North America and Europe at a low frequency. These neoplasms exhibit a morphologic continuum, from polymorphous to monomorphous, but morphologic features do not correlate with prognosis as all patients have a clinically aggressive course [14]. Most EBV-positive DLBCL of the elderly patients have an activated B-cell immunophenotype and are characterized by prominent nuclear factor-κB activation. It was recently incorporated provisionally into the WHO 2008 classification of tumors of hematopoietic and lymphoid tissues. [14]

The third unique lymphoma occurs in the context of Richter's transformation (RT, Richter's syndrome). It was first described in 1928 by Maurice Richter as the development of an aggressive large-cell lymphoma in the setting of underlying chronic lymphocytic leukemia/small lymphocytic lymphoma (CLL/SLL). Although DLBCL is the most common histology seen in patients with RT, HL and T- cell lymphomas have also been reported less commonly. [15-17] The therapeutic strategies for RT typically include therapies developed for NHL or acute lymphoblastic leukemia. The reported response rates with these therapies are 5% to 43%, and the median survival duration ranges from 5 to 9 months. About 15-20% of cases of RT, are triggered by EBV [18].

Whereas EBV infection in these various lymphomas is firmly established, its association with other tumor entities such anaplastic large cell lymphoma and squamous cell carcinoma of the oral cavity remains controversial [19, 20].

Interaction of EBV and B-Lymphocytes: Contribution of EBV Antigens to B-Cell Transformation

Though EBV may induce proliferation of B-lymphocytes, the virus carrying state is usually asymptomatic. The harmonious coexistence between virus and host is a result of a mutual adaptation, based on variations in the viral gene expression in the infected cells and the immune response of the host [21]. While it can also infect T-lymphocytes and epithelial cells, EBV exhibits a high degree of B-lymphocyte tropism. It binds to CD21, a B lymphocyte-specific surface molecule which is a receptor for C3d fragment of the complement system. The binding of the EBV to the cell surface receptor triggers specific isoforms of protein kinase C (PKC) and protein tyrosine kinase (PTK) which mediate the activation of mitotic activity of a resting B-lymphocyte's mitotic activity [22]. These activated B-lymphocytes, also referred to as the lymphoblastoid cell lines (LCLs) *in vitro*, harbor the viral genome which is maintained in an episomal form.

The expression of EBV-derived proteins varies depending on the differentiation and activation status of the B-lymphocyte and also the status of the host's immune system. The cell transformation process is dependent on the expression of EBV nuclear and membrane proteins; six of these proteins (EBNA-1, EBNA-2, EBNA-3, EBERs, LMP1 and LMP2) are considered necessary for the activating and proliferation driving effect of the virus (Table 3).

In healthy individuals, latently infected virus-carrying cells are present in the resting memory B-lymphocyte compartment, and express only EBNA-1. The replication and stable persistence of episomes in EBV-infected proliferating B-lymphocyte is dependent on expression of EBNA-1 and it is the only EBV encoded antigen that is consistently expressed in all EBV-associated tumors [24, 25].

EBNA-1 can disrupt important cellular processes such as apoptosis, DNA repair and senescence through its interactions with cell cycle regulator proteins, leading to cell immortalization and survival. [26] EBNA-1 sequesters and destabilizes *p*53, the 'guardian of the genome', by competitively binding cellular ubiquitin-specific protease 7 (USP7) [27]. It also promotes degradation of promyelocytic leukemia (PML) nuclear bodies (NB) that control several cellular processes including apoptosis and DNA repair. EBNA-1 expression may also promote metastasis by blocking PML NB. [28] In animal models, EBNA-1 also modulates the activity of metastasis suppressor protein nucleoside diphosphate kinase/Nm23-H1 [29]. EBNA-1 has a long internal glycine-alanine repeat sequence. This repeat sequence blocks the ubiquitin and proteosome-dependent synthesis of peptides that activate MHC class I molecules; absence of these peptides secure the persistence of virus-carrying cells by circumventing the cytotoxic effects of $CD8^+$ T-lymphocytes [30].

EBNA-2 plays an important role during EBV-mediated host cell immortalization by coordinating viral and cellular gene transcription [31]. *In vitro* studies demonstrate that the expression of EBNA-2 is essential for initial growth transformation of EBV-infected B-lymphocytes [25]. It is one of the first EBV latent antigens detected after primary B-cell

Table 3. Transcription pathways used by EBV to establish and maintain infection

Type of infected B lymphocyte	Program	Genes expressed	Function of the program
Naïve cell	Growth	EBNA-1 to 6, LMP 1 and 2	Activates B lymphocyte
Germinal-center cell	Default	EBNA-1, LMP 1 and 2	Differentiates activated B-cell into memory cell
Peripheral-blood memory cell	Latency	none	Allows life-time persistence
Dividing peripheral blood memory cell	EBNA-1 only	EBNA-1	Allows viral DNA in latency program cell to divide
Plasma cell	Lytic	All lytic genes	Replicates virus in plasma cell

EBNA-1: EBV nuclear antigen 1; EBERs: EBV-encoded small RNAs; LMP: Latent membrane protein. Adapted from Thorley-lawson et al. [23].

infection, and is involved in G0 to G1 cell cycle transition. Several B-cell genes including CD21, CD23, c- myc, hes-1 and RUNX3 are each activated by EBNA-2. It also activates EBV genes including LMP1 and LMP2 which are important regulators of EBNA gene transcription.

EBNA-3 genes (3A, 3B, and 3C) are located in tandem sequence in the EBV genome [32]. Similar to EBNA-2 and LMP-1, EBNA-3 genes (3A, 3B, and 3C), are necessary for transformation of B-cells while EBNA-3B may be dispensable; all three proteins affect global transcriptional activities including viral and several cellular gene expression patterns during host cell immortalization by modulating the EBNA-2 driven transactivation process [32, 33]. In addition to their role in transcriptional regulation, EBNA-3A and 3C also play important roles in cell-cycle regulation. While EBNA-3C up regulates cellular CD21 and c-myc expression and enhances EBNA-2-driven dependent LMP1 expression, EBNA-3A and 3C together enable LCL growth through epigenetic suppression of the pro-apoptotic protein Bim and the cell cycle inhibitor p16INK4A gene expression. EBNA-3C also interacts with a wide range of cellular proteins such as cyclin A, cyclin D1, pRb, c-Myc, p53, ING4, ING5, Mdm2, p300 and histone deacetylase 1 (HDAC1), which are all involved in cell cycle, apoptosis, and epigenetic transcriptional activity; impaired activity of these proteins mediated by EBNA-3C leads to B-cell transformation [34-38].

EBER-1 and EBER-2 participate in EBV-mediated cell growth, transformation, and cancer progression by modulating the host-immune signaling activities [39]. EBERs, by their interaction with the ribosomal protein L22 and human La protein, which are stabilizers of histone mRNA, block apoptosis, suppress antiviral effects of interferon-α and induce interleukin 10 (IL-10) production, which is also mediated by binding to and blocking the function of the interferon-induced double-stranded RNA-activated protein kinase PKR [40, 41]. EBERs also may bind to RIG-I and activate its downstream signaling, which further activates type-I interferons [42]. EBERs can also induce IL-10 via NF-kB–independent IRF3 activation in BL cells [43].

LMP-1 is an integral membrane protein which has transforming potential and is necessary for B-cell immortalization by EBV [44]. LMP-1 molecules aggregate in the plasma membrane and recruit tumor necrosis factor receptor (TNFR), associated factors which are involved in the signaling cascade leading to NF-kappa B activation by LMP-1 [45]. LMP-1 has pleiotropic effects on cell cycle regulation by blocking p53-mediated apoptosis via transactivation of the anti-apoptotic factors bcl-2 and A20 and by up-regulating IL-10 expression [41, 42]. LMP-1 further modulates Janus activated kinase (JAK)/STAT, extracellular signal regulated kinase (ERK), mitogen activated protein kinase (MAPK) and Wnt signaling pathways [46]. Through these interactions, LMP-1 can affect the synthesis of both cytokines and cytokine receptors, which further alter overall angiogenesis and inflammatory responses, thereby contributing to immune escape and cancer propagation.

LMP-2, acts by blocking receptor tyrosine kinase signaling and also by inhibiting activation of the viral lytic cycle [47]. Although LMP-2 is not required for B-cell transformation, it is essential for long-term persistence for the viral episome by providing temporal growth and B-cell survival signals in the lymphoid organs [48]. LMP-2A and LMP-2B are also important in promoting persistent infection of B-lymphocytes and influencing the dynamic balance between viral latency and lytic activation [48].

EBV-Associated B-Cell Lymphomas in Immunodeficient Patients

EBCL in Primary Immunodeficiency

Several primary immunodeficiency conditions associated with abnormal T-cell function, such as severe combined immunodeficiency (SCID) and Wiskott Aldrich syndrome, are associated with an increased risk of developing EBCL [49]. Approximately 13% of individuals with Wiskott-Aldrich syndrome develop lymphoma, at an average age of 9.5 years. The risk of developing lymphoma increases with age and in the presence of autoimmune disease [50].

In addition, children with X-linked lymphoproliferative (XLP) disease are born with a defect in the gene SH2D1A. This gene encodes a small SH2 binding protein and is involved in regulation of the intense $CD8^+$ T-cell cytotoxicity stimulated by acute EBV infection [51]. Males with XLP have a selective immunodeficiency to EBV, which results in either severe infectious mononucleosis or EBCL on initial exposure to EBV. Few of these individuals survive infancy. The risk for development of EBCL in XLP is 25-30% with a mortality rate of 9 months [52].

Post-Transplant EBCL

PTLD is the most common malignancy, with the exception of skin cancer, after solid organ transplant (SOT) in adults and occurs in up to 10% of patients. The incidence varies according to the transplanted organ, and in the majority of cases, particularly those occurring less than one year after transplantation, are associated with EBV. PTLD occurs more commonly in pediatric patients than in adults.

The higher incidence in children may be related to their greater likelihood of being EBV-naïve recipients [53]. In adults, rates range from 1%–3% in kidney and liver transplants, 1%-6% in cardiac transplants, 2%-6% in combined heart-lung transplants, 4%-10% in lung transplants, and in up to 20% of small intestine transplants [53]. The variation in rates among the types of organ transplanted is likely related to the degree and duration of immunosuppression as well as the number of EBV-positive donor lymphocytes in the graft.

Duration of the post-transplant period is important because PTLD is most likely to develop in the first year following transplantation, with an incidence of 224 per 100,000, but falls to 54 per 100,000 in the second year and 31 per 100,000 in the sixth year. Late onset PTLDs following SOT are more heterogeneous and may be EBV negative [54].

After hematopoietic stem cell transplant (HSCT), the risk factors for PTLD include the degree of donor-recipient HLA mismatch, the extent to which the graft is manipulated to deplete T-lymphocytes, and the degree of immunosuppression used to prevent graft-versus-host disease (GVHD) [55]. Most of the cases of PTLD that occur after HSCT are diagnosed during the first year post-transplant, when the recipient is most severely immunocompromised.

The WHO classification schema divides PTLD into three categories: early lesions, polymorphic PTLD, and monomorphic PTLD [56] (Table 4). Early lesions are characterized by reactive plasmacytic hyperplasia. Polymorphic PTLD may be either polyclonal or monoclonal, and is characterized by the destruction of underlying lymphoid architecture, necrosis and nuclear atypia. In monomorphic PTLD, greater than 80% of cases arise from B-cells, similar to NHL in immunocompetent hosts. The most common subtype is DLBCL, but BL and plasma cell myeloma are also seen.

Rarely T-cell variants occur, which include peripheral T-cell lymphomas, gamma/delta T-cell lymphoma and T-natural killer (NK) leukemia. HL-like lymphoma is very uncommon.

EBCL in HIV Infection

HIV-associated lymphoproliferative disorders represent a diverse group of diseases, arising in the presence of HIV-induced immunodeficiency. People living with HIV-AIDS (PLWHA) are particularly vulnerable to four types of B-cell NHL each of which is associated with EBV to varying degrees (Table 2).

PLWHA have a high frequency of EBV-infected B-lymphocytes, independent of the development of lymphoma that may be related in part to their defective T-cell immune response to EBV. The risk of developing EBCL in PLWHA is greatest in those with an elevated EBV viral load and inversely proportional to the number and/or the function of EBV-specific cytotoxic T-lymphocytes (CTLs) [57]. Immunosuppression and EBV infection favor the expansion of B-cell clones, increasing the risk that these clones- which have accumulated alterations in oncogenes or tumor suppressor genes will transform to a lymphoma [58]. Other factors for lymphoma include advancing patient age, the duration of HIV infection and the cumulative period of HIV viremia [59].

Table 4. World Health Organization classification of post-transplant lymphoproliferative disorders (PTLD)

Post-transplant Lymphoproliferative Disorders
Early lesions reactive plasmacytic hyperplasia
Polymorphic PTLD
Polyclonal
Monoclonal
Monomorphic PTLD B-cell lymphomas
Diffuse large B-cell lymphoma
Burkitt's/Burkitt's-like lymphoma
Plasma cell myeloma
T-cell lymphomas
Peripheral T-cell lymphoma
Rare types (gamma/delta, T/natural killer cell)
Other types
Hodgkin's lymphoma-like
Plasmacytoma-like

Adapted from Swerdlow et al. [56].

Among PLWHA, the pathogenic role of EBV is most clearly defined in those with primary central nervous system lymphoma (PCNSL). PCNSL is associated with EBV expression in greater than 95% of cases [60]. Primary effusion lymphoma (PEL), formerly known as body cavity lymphoma, accounts for about 4% of all HIV-associated NHL [61]. By definition, cases of PEL must display evidence of infection by Kaposi's sarcoma–associated herpesvirus, otherwise known as HHV-8. In addition, most HIV-positive cases (>90%) also show evidence of EBV infection [62]. The association of EBV with other HIV-related lymphomas, including BL and DLBCL ranges from 30% to 60%. Similar to what is seen in immunocompetent individuals, there is significant variation in both the number of EBV-positive cells, and the pattern of EBV latent gene expression among these various lymphoma types [63].

HIV creates a milieu of combined immune suppression and chronic antigenic stimulation in lymph nodes [64]. This environment with dysregulated cytokine release and impaired dendritic function, along with presence of concomitant infection (e.g., EBV, HHV-8 and cytomegalovirus) may promote a permissive environment for HIV-induced polyclonal B-cell expansion and impaired T-cell immunosurveillance, culminating in lympho-proliferative disorders [65].

EBV-Associated B-Cell Lymphomas in Immunocompetent Patients

Lymphomatoid Granulomatosis

Lymphomatoid granulomatosis (LyG) is an uncommon EBV-associated systemic angio-centric-destructive lymphoproliferative disorder. It is characterized by an EBV-related B-cell proliferation associated with a reactive T-cell proliferation [66]. It is likely due to a defective host immune response to EBV. Grades I and II of LyG show rare to moderately large EBV-positive polyclonal or oligoclonal B-lymphocytes while grade III LyG demonstrates numerous large EBV-positive monoclonal B-lymphocytes, likely reflecting progressive transformation [67]. LyG is characterized by prominent pulmonary involvement but can also involve other extra nodal sites. Although the plasma EBV viral load is relatively low in most cases of LyG, alterations in immune function are present. Most notably, patients have depressed $CD8^+$ and $CD4^+$ cell counts. Patients with LyG have a clinical course marked by progressive disease and in some case series, a mortality ranging between 63-90% at 5 years; however, the clinical outcomes can be variable, with some patients experiencing spontaneous remissions [67-69].

Burkitt's Lymphoma

BL is a high-grade malignant small non-cleaved cell lymphoma. It has the fastest doubling time among human tumors with a unique clinical picture and histopathology [70]. The endemic form is found in Africa and 95% of such cases are associated with EBV. The sporadic form, which is seen elsewhere, is associated with EBV in only 20% of cases.

Nevertheless, almost all cases of both endemic and sporadic BL are characterized by constitutive activation of c-myc owing to a reciprocal chromosomal translocation between chromosome 8 and either chromosome 2, 14, or 22, which juxtaposes the proto-oncogene to one of the three immunoglobulin loci. The lack of co-stimulatory surface molecules enables the EBV-carrying BL tumor cells to evade the immune system. In addition EBNA-1, the only EBV-encoded protein they express, does not provide MHC class I-associated peptides that could be recognized by CD8$^+$ CTL [71].

EBV-Positive Diffuse Large B-Cell Lymphoma of the Elderly

EBV-positive DLBCL of the elderly, first described in 2003, is a provisional entity in the 2008 WHO classification system [72, 73]. It is defined as an EBV-positive monoclonal large B-cell proliferation that occurs in patients greater than 50 years of age, and in whom there is no known immunodeficiency or history of lymphoma. These tumors are more commonly seen in Asia, but also occur in North America and Europe at a low frequency.

These neoplasms exhibit a morphologic continuum, from polymorphous to monomorphous, but morphologic features do not correlate with prognosis as all patients have a clinically aggressive course. Most EBV-positive DLBCL of the elderly have an activated B-cell immunophenotype, which also predicts a poor prognosis, and are characterized by prominent nuclear factor-κB activation [74, 75]. Published studies of clinical series have identified a high risk of treatment failure in these patients [76].

T-Cell/Histiocyte-Rich B-Cell Lymphoma

T-cell/histiocyte-rich B-cell lymphoma (T/HRBCL) is an uncommon morphologic variant of DLBCL that disproportionately occurs in younger patients, predominantly affecting men. It is characterized by advanced stage at diagnosis and a predilection to involve spleen, liver and bone marrow at a greater frequency than does DLBCL [77].

Pathologically, it is distinguished by less than 10% malignant B-lymphocytes amongst a majority population of reactive T-lymphocytes and histiocytes [78].

Diagnosis of this entity is sometimes difficult, as it may appear similar to other lymphoid diseases, such as nodular lymphocyte-predominant HL and classic HL, but when strict morphological and immunophenotypic criteria are applied, approximately 20% of these tumors are found to be LMP-1 positive [79, 80]. Despite the unique clinical features and robust host inflammatory response, T/HRBCL follows a natural history similar to those of other DLBCLs and responds similarly to therapy.

Other EBV-Positive B-NHL

EBCL occurring in the immunocompetent host also include some cases of CD30$^+$ Ki-1$^+$ anaplastic lymphoma kinase (ALK)-positive large cell lymphoma of B-cell type. It is a rare tumor distinct in many aspects from ALK-positive anaplastic large cell lymphoma of T-cell origin.

Genetic studies demonstrate that the majority of ALK⁺ DLBCL cases are characterized by the clathrin-ALK fusion and in a few cases with rearrangement of NPM-ALK [81]. Between 10% and 35% of these tumors are EBV positive expressing a type II latency pattern, with a higher frequency seen in oral cavity lymphomas [82].

Angioimmunoblastic lymphoma is characterized by oligoclonal proliferations of T- and B-lymphocytes, and EBV is detected in many cases in either T- or B-lymphocytes. The clinical presentation usually includes systemic disease with B symptoms, while pathology reveals a polymorphous infiltrate involving lymph nodes, with a prominent proliferation of endothelial and dendritic cells. Some patients develop a secondary EBV-positive large B-cell lymphoma [83, 84].

Treatment Approach to EBV-Associated B-Cell Lymphoma

Despite the current understanding of the underlying molecular pathogenic mechanisms of EBV infection leading to the development of its related diseases, the optimal management of EBCL remains investigational. When EBCLs develop in the context of immunosuppression, remedying the immune defect can assist in the treatment of these lymphomas. In HIV-associated lymphomas, antiretroviral therapy to suppress HIV replication is appropriate, although potential drug interactions and the effects of chemotherapy on the ability to maintain combined anti-retroviral therapy must be considered with regard to the timing and type of antiretroviral therapy [85]. It is inadequate to treat AIDS-related lymphomas with just antiretroviral therapy.

The management of PTLD may also be challenging and unlike AIDS-related lymphomas, is generally without a standardized therapeutic approach that can be applied to all patients. Despite this diversity, reduction of immunosuppression (ROI) remains the cornerstone for treatment of EBV-driven B-cell PTLD, independent of histology. Starzl and colleagues were the first to suggest reduction, or withdrawal, of immunosuppression as a treatment option for PTLD in the setting of renal transplantation [86]. This strategy allows the patient's natural immunity to recover and gain control over proliferating EBV-infected cells. As many as 40% of patients will achieve a complete remission after reduction or discontinuation of immunosuppressive therapy. Patients with less aggressive or polyclonal PTLD tend to respond more favorably to this management approach, as compared to patients with clinically aggressive PTLD.

Recent studies have demonstrated promising outcomes against EBCL with combined therapeutic approaches of chemotherapy coupled with specific antiviral compounds targeting specific viral antigens, along with either targeted monoclonal antibodies or T-cell–based immunotherapy [87].

Reduction or Modification of Immunosuppression

ROI is an effective approach to the treatment of EBV-PTLD in some cases, although this strategy must be balanced against the risk of transplant rejection in patients with SOT or graft vs. host disease (GvHD) in patients with HSCT [88]. The rapidity with which an EBV-specific immune response regenerates following ROI is also unpredictable. Risk of PTLD is higher recipients of a T-cell depleted stem cell graft, or in patients treated with antibodies that specifically target T-lymphocytes, such as muromonab-CD3, antithymocyte globulin, or alemtuzumab, the later which binds to CD52, a protein present on the surface of mature lymphocytes, but not on the stem cells from which these lymphocytes are derived. After treatment with alemtuzumab, these CD52-bearing lymphocytes are targeted for destruction.

Immune reconstitution may also be delayed for several weeks even after ROI or discontinuation of immunosuppressive agents. As an alternative to ROI, modification of the immunosuppression regimen to include agents that have potential antitumor and antiviral properties is an attractive option – this allows for treatment of the EBV-PTLD while maintaining the level of immunosuppression necessary to prevent graft rejection and GvHD.

Immunosuppressive agents, such as mammalian target of rapamycin (mTOR) inhibitors have been investigated in PTLD given its potent antitumor properties. The mTOR signaling pathway is important in B-cell proliferation and early EBV-PTLD lesions are associated with activation of the mTOR pathway [89, 90]. Remissions of EBV-PTLD have been reported in SOT patients following modification of immunosuppression regimen to include an mTOR inhibitor *in lieu* of a calcineurin inhibitor [91]. *In vitro*, inhibits the proliferation of EBV-positive lymphoma cell lines, but not EBV-negative lymphoma cell lines, suggestive of possible antiviral activity as well [92].

Rituximab

Rituximab is a chimeric monoclonal antibody against the protein CD20, which is primarily found on the surface of B-lymphocytes. It destroys B-lymphocytes and is therefore used to treat diseases which are characterized by excessive number, overactive and/or dysfunctional B-lymphocytes [93]. Rituximab, either alone or coupled with the antiviral agent cidofovir, abrogates the symptoms of PTLD in greater than 60% of SOT patients [94]. Similar efficacy is also seen when rituximab is employed as a monotherapy for treatment of EBV-PTLD in HSCT patients, and is considered first-line treatment by many transplant centers [95]. A significant benefit of rituximab for EBV-PTLD is that many patients can be spared from the toxicities of combination chemotherapy and that their immunosuppression often can be continued, leading to lower risk of graft rejection and/or GvHD. Rituximab may be effective in EBV-PTLD not only because it targets the CD20$^+$ tumor but also through B-cell depletion; it shifts the ratio of EBV-infected B-lymphocytes to EBV specific CTLs in favor of an antiviral/antitumor immune response. Limitations to using rituximab for treatment of PTLD is that it may select out CD20$^-$ variants, induce profound and prolonged B-cell depletion, and impair the cellular immune response to EBV, which may be crucial for the long-term control of EBV-mediated B-cell proliferation. It can also contribute to hypogammaglobulinemia and less commonly suppression of hematopoiesis [96].

Adoptive Cellular Immunotherapy

Adoptive immunotherapy using EBV-specific CTLs in order to stimulate the host immune responses against EBCLs is particularly useful in the context of PTLDs that occur following allogeneic HSCT [97, 98]. The CTLs can be generated from a healthy donor and infused directly into the recipient patient to reinstate immunocompetence. The infusion of donor lymphocytes which have not been manipulated can result in high response rates, although there is a considerable risk of GVHD due to alloreactive CTLs. This risk can be abrogated by using EBV-specific CTLs [97].

EBCLs represent an attractive target for CTL-based immunotherapy, as the transformed B-lymphocytes express a full array of latent antigens. The relative ease to synthesize EBV-specific CTLs in large numbers using in vitro transformed EBV-positive LCLs makes it an attractive approach for treating patients who have undergone HSCT. The benefits of such an approach, however, are limited in patients with SOT who develop EBV-associated lymphoproliferative syndromes. This is perhaps due to the *in vivo* loss of adoptively transferred CTLs in SOT patients as they continue to receive high dose immunosuppression which can compromise the long-term survival of these CTLs.

Although adoptive transfer of EBV-specific CTLs may help in restoring immunocompetence, CTL function is still partially impaired by the concomitant use of immunosuppressive drugs. Current strategies to genetically modify EBV-specific CTLs for resistance against immunosuppressive drugs are being developed [99]. Generation of EBV-specific CTLs in this patient population offers various challenges compared with HSCT recipients, as the organ donor is not always HLA matched and donor organs, with the exception of renal transplantation, is typically procured after the donor has died.

Several groups have successfully administered autologous EBV-specific CTLs as prophylaxis in SOT recipients [100]. However, manufacturing autologous CTLs is not always feasible. Comparative advantages and drawbacks of adoptive T-cell transfer are listed in Table 5.

Signaling Pathway Inhibitors

LMP-2, which is present in some EBV-related lymphomas, mimics a functional B-cell receptor (BCR) and activates downstream signaling pathways, including Syk, Akt, and mTOR [102, 103]. The Lyn/Syk pathway is downstream of the BCR and, when activated, functions to promote the survival of B-lymphocytes. In murine NHL tumor models, Syk is required for tumor survival. *In vitro* and *in vivo*, tumors that do not express Syk have increased apoptosis [104]. Syk signaling leads to activation of Akt and XIAP, a caspase inhibitor, resulting in inhibition of apoptosis [105]. Anti-tumor activities of Syk inhibitors are present in patients with CLL and NHL [106]. In EBV-PTLD cell lines, inhibition of Syk leads to reduced tumor proliferation and induction of apoptosis [105]. The EBV protein LMP-1, a mimic of CD40, activates the PI3K/Akt pathway also through the non-canonical Syk signaling [107].

Several small molecule PI3K inhibitors, Akt inhibitors, and dual PI3K/mTOR inhibitors are in development. MK-2206, an Akt inhibitor, is effective in inhibiting growth of NPC cell lines. When combined with cisplatin chemotherapy a supra-additive inhibitory effect occurs

[108]. MK-2206 is being studied in Phase II clinical trials for patients with relapsed/refractory NHL, as well as recurrent NPC [109].

Table 5. Comparative advantages and disadvantages of emerging technologies for adoptive T-cell therapy

T-cell therapy technology	Benefits	Drawbacks
In vitro expanded virus-specific T-cells, stimulated with synthetic peptides/recombinant protein	Expands both $CD8^+$ and $CD4^+$ T-cells Defined antigen specificity No infectious agent in T-cell therapy	Restricted antigen specificity of T-cells Limited by the availability of appropriate peptide epitopes or protein antigens
In vitro expanded virus-specific T-cells, stimulated with viral lysate or LCLs	Expands both $CD8^+$ and $CD4^+$ T-cells Broad coverage of antigen specificity	Prolonged expansion process, especially when LCLs are used as APC. Potential risk from infectious virus in T-cell therapy
In vitro expanded virus-specific T-cells, stimulated with recombinant replication-deficient viral vectors	Expands both $CD8^+$ and $CD4^+$ T-cells Defined antigen specificity Rapid availability of T-cell therapy	Restricted antigen specificity of T-cells Limited by the antigens or epitopes included in the recombinant vector May not expand $CD4^+$ T-cells
MHC-peptide multimers selected antigen-specific T-cells	Rapid availability of T-cell therapy (1-2 days) Defined antigen specificity Enhanced *in vivo* expansion capacity	Restricted antigen specificity of T-cells Limited by the availability of MHC-peptide multimers Lack of availability of MHC class II multimers for $CD4^+$ T-cells
IFN-γ capture enriched T-cells	Rapid availability of T-cell therapy (1-2 days) Defined antigen specificity Enhanced *in vivo* expansion capacity	Restricted antigen specificity of T-cells Limited by the availability of peptides or recombinant antigens
Third party HLA matched virus-specific T-cells	Rapid availability of T-cell therapy - "off-the shelf" Defined antigen specificity Includes both $CD8^+$ and $CD4^+$ T-cells	Limited by the HLA matching of T-cells with recipient HLA alleles Decreased therapeutic efficacy with incomplete HLA matching

LCL: lymphoblastoid cell line; APC: antigen presenting cell; IFN-γ: interferon gamma.
Adapted from Khanna et al. [101].

LMP-1, by signaling through the JAK/STAT pathway, also may function to increase programmed cell death ligand 1 (PD-L1) expression in EBV-positive tumors, including EBV-PTLD. [110] EBV-transformed LCLs express high levels of JAK3-associated STAT proteins (pSTAT3 and pSTAT5) and enhanced LMP-1 leads to heightened STAT5 activity.

PD-L1 is a co-signaling molecule that inhibits the function of activated effector T-lymphocytes. PD-L1 thus acts to dampen T-cell–mediated immune responses, including antitumor immunity. PD-1 inhibition is a promising targeted therapy in hematologic malignancies and has already proven to be effective in the treatment of other solid tumor malignancies such as melanoma [111]. PD-L1 inhibition and reactivation of a dampened immune response may be especially relevant for EBV-related tumors.

As smaller molecule inhibitors are being tested in treatment of NHL, investigating these novel agents in EBV-related lymphomas may prove to be a particularly fruitful endeavor. In this context small molecule inhibitors may provide better antitumor activity compared to EBV-negative lymphomas, as intricate interactions between EBV and the various signaling pathways can be specifically abrogated by these agents.

EBV Vaccines

A vaccine to prevent EBV infection was proposed by Epstein and Achong in 1973, approximately a decade after their group discovered this human γ-herpesvirus [112, 113]. Development of an EBV vaccine, however, has been agonizingly slow because of difficulties in establishing a suitable animal model and because of disparate viewpoints about what the vaccine could or should actually achieve.

Nearly four decades after the discovery of EBV, Sokal and colleagues completed the first multicenter, randomized, placebo-controlled, double-blind trial of an EBV vaccine to prevent infectious mononucleosis [114]. During an 18-month period of observation, an adjuvant recombinant glycoprotein 350 (gp350) subunit EBV vaccine reduced the proportion of *symptomatic* primary EBV infections in teenagers and young adults from 10% (9 of 91 subjects) in the placebo group to 2% (2 of 90 subjects) in the vaccine group, according to intention-to-treat analysis.

What impact such vaccines might have in reducing the incidence of EBV-related malignancies is unknown. Symptomatic EBV infection induces a long-term deficit in T-cell responsiveness to IL-15 [115]. An important rationale for vaccine use would be to prevent EBV- induced immune dysfunction, which is considered a root-cause of subsequent immunelogic and malignant disorders.

A variety of EBV-vaccine clinical trials have recently been completed. A peptide epitope- based vaccine aimed at stimulating $CD8^+$ T-cell mediated immunity against immune-dominant latency antigens was employed to induce EBV-specific T-cell responses in healthy volunteers in an effort to prevent EBV primary infection [116]. In another trial involving pediatric patients awaiting SOT, the gp350 vaccine given pre-transplant with the hopes of improving antiviral T-cell immunity to prevent EBV-PTLD, failed to elicit a durable immune response in the majority of trial participants [117].

More recently, a phase I trial of recombinant modified vaccinia Ankara encoding EBV tumor antigens, EBNA-1/LMP-2 delivered to patients with NPC in remission following primary therapy was reported [118]. Fifteen of eighteen patients showed strong T-cell responses to one or both vaccine antigens with no dose-limiting toxicity suggesting that the vaccine was both safe and immunogenic.

Several other EBV vaccine trials (e.g., NCT00278200, NCT01094405) are underway, based on these observations and the promising results from the phase 2 gp350 vaccine trial in healthy humans [109].

Lytic Inducers Coupled with Antiherpetic Agents

To achieve a long-term harmonious co-existence with the host, EBV maintains tight control over the switch between latent and lytic gene expression. Lytic proteins, such as viral thymidine kinase, are not expressed during latency. As a result, anti-herpesvirus drugs that rely on phosphorylation by viral thymidine kinase (TK) for conversion of the prodrug to its active form are not effective during latent infection.

Pharmacologic lytic activation of EBV to render infected tumor cells susceptible to antiviral agents is a well-reviewed strategy to control B-cell lymphoproliferation. Ganciclovir, a drug that efficiently target viral TK, when administered together with arginine butyrate, which induces lytic cycle and TK production, has shown positive results in patients with PTLD [119]. Similarly, chemotherapy agents such as gemcitabine and doxorubicin may also induce lytic activation; pre-clinical studies using the combination of these agents with ganciclovir led to highly effective inhibition of EBV-driven lymphoproliferation [120]. Inhibition of EBV DNA polymerase with antiviral agents such as foscarnet and cidofovir is another opportunity to target tumor cells [119].

Lytic activation may render EBV-infected cells more susceptible to immune recognition and clearance by CTLs due to a less restricted expression of viral proteins. Lytic activation may be part of the DNA damage response or unfolded protein response to stress in the endoplasmic reticulum.

Drugs used for the treatment of various cancers can be used in a targeted way to interfere with EBV-induced cell cycling. Bortezomib, a proteasome inhibitor and antineoplastic agent currently in use for treatment of various NHLs and multiple myeloma activates EBV lytic gene expression in EBV-positive BL cell lines [121]. Histone deacetylase inhibitors (HDACi) induce lytic gene expression and sensitize EBV-positive lymphoma cell lines to ganciclovir at drug concentrations achievable in patients [122]. In a clinical trial of 15 patients with refractory EBV-positive lymphomas, 10 responded to treatment with arginine butyrate, an HDACi and lytic inducer, in combination with ganciclovir [123]. However, it remains unclear whether the response seen was due to the antitumor activity of the HDACi or truly related to lytic induction and ganciclovir sensitization of tumor cells.

Arsenic trioxide is approved by the United States Food and Drug Administration as first-line treatment of APL. When treated with arsenic trioxide EBV-positive NPC cell lines show increased lytic gene expression and decreased viability [124]. When ganciclovir is added to arsenic-treated EBV-positive cells, viability is further reduced, whereas EBV negative cells show no changes in viability after treatment with arsenic alone, ganciclovir alone, or the combination of arsenic and ganciclovir.

LMP-1-positive cells also have higher levels of PML-NB protein expression and treatment with arsenic trioxide decreases PML-NB protein levels [124]. PML-NB degradation may have an important role in the switch from latent to lytic herpesvirus gene expression and LMP-1 may increase PML-NB expression to maintain latency. EBNA-1 also mediates the switch between latency and lytic activation through alterations in PML-NB [125].

Epigenetic modifying agents, such as 5-azacytidine, also induce lytic gene expression in EBV-positive cell lines and, when combined with ganciclovir, lead to caspase-mediated apoptosis [126]. Parthenolide, a plant extract, induces lytic gene expression in EBV-positive BL cell lines and has cytotoxic activity that synergizes with ganciclovir [127].

Conclusion

EBV is a complex DNA virus whose mysteries have yet to be completely elucidated. Through a better understanding of how EBV persists *in vivo* and alters the intracellular milieu of the host cell, we are acquiring a better understanding of how EBV can cause neoplasia in general and lymphoproliferative disorders, specifically. Current knowledge of EBV-induced neoplasia provides a platform for designing better treatments, but there are few candidate antiviral drugs, and much work remains to be done to make such therapies effective and practical.

Despite the proliferation-inducing capacity of the virus in B-lymphocytes, the viral carrier state is mostly harmless in immunocompetent hosts - their immune system recognizes these cells which express the growth-promoting proteins as foreign, and eliminate them. However, the immunocompromised individuals have a higher risk for EBV-induced disease states. The most severe consequences of EBV occur when the immune system fails to control infection and/or viral oncogenesis. Further research is needed to determine means to predict who will be affected most severely and to develop therapeutic strategies to reduce symptoms.

In EBV-infected lymphoid cells the expression of virally-encoded proteins occurs in various patterns that are regulated as the cells differentiate and mature. These EBV-infected cells are not driven to proliferation by the virus, but their phenotype is modified - they acquire alterations in cellular interactions, production and response to cytokines that execute escaping of apoptosis and enhanced responsiveness to growth stimulating signals. Increasing our understanding of how specific EBV gene products and expression programs contribute to pathogenesis provides hope of more rational treatment strategies in the future.

Finally, an EBV vaccine has the potential to reduce the substantial disease burden due to primary EBV infection and possibly prevent or modify its chronic sequelae. However, development of such a vaccine has been challenging. Eventually, the combination of vaccination and immunotherapy approaches with small molecules that increase the expression of lytic cycle antigens, or target the viral proteins or the microenvironment may offer the most effective therapeutic approach to these diseases.

By devoting more research toward preventing and treating EBV infection we hope that the impact of a very common infectious disease will be minimized including the incidence of certain human malignancies, such as endemic BL and NPC.

Glossary

Herpes virus

A double-stranded DNA virus that belongs to the family of *Herpesviridae*, a large group of viruses that is distributed widely within the animal kingdom. The *Herpesviridae* family

Herpesviridae comprises of three subfamilies, namely, Alpha-, Beta- and Gamma-herpesvirinae. The gamma-herpesviruses (Epstein-Barr virus and Kaposi's sarcoma-associated herpes-virus) replicate and persist in lymphoid cells but some are capable of undergoing lytic replication in epithelial and fibroblast cells.

Lymphocytes

A type of white blood cell (WBC) that provide specific and non-specific immunity against infectious microorganisms and other foreign substances. In humans lymphocytes comprise up to one-third of the total number of WBC.

They are usually found in the circulation and also are concentrated in lymphoid organs, such as the spleen, tonsils and lymph nodes. They are divided into three main groups: B-lymphocytes, which produce antibodies in the humoral immune response, T-lymphocytes, which participate in the cell-mediated immune response and the null group, which contains natural killer cells, the cytotoxic cells that participate in the innate immune response.

Carcinogenesis

The process by which normal cells are transformed into cancer cells. It is characterized by changes at the cellular, genetic and epigenetic level that ultimately reprogram a cell to undergo uncontrolled cell division, thus forming a malignant tumor.

Lytic cycle

It is the process in which the virus overtakes a cell and uses the cellular machinery of the host to reproduce. Lytic cycle results in destruction of the infected cell and its membrane. In lytic cycle, the viral DNA exists as a separate molecule within the cell, and replicates separately from the host bacterial DNA.

Cell signaling pathways

It is part of a complex system of communication that governs basic cellular activities and orchestrates cell function. The ability of cells to perceive and correctly respond to their microenvironment is the basis of development, tissue repair, and immunity as well as normal tissue homeostasis. Errors in cellular information processing are responsible for diseases such as cancer, autoimmunity, and diabetes.

Epigenetics

It refers to the functional changes to the genome, without any change in its structure. These modifications do not change the DNA sequence, but instead, they affect how the genes are read.

The epigenetic changes may last through cell divisions for the duration of the cell's life, and may also last for multiple generations. An important role of epigenetics is the process of cellular differentiation.

Lymphoma

A cancer that originates in the cells of the immune system. There are two major categories of lymphomas - Hodgkin and non-Hodgkin. Hodgkin lymphoma is characterized by the presence of Reed-Sternberg cell, a neoplastic B-cell.

Non-Hodgkin lymphomas are a large and diverse group which can be further divided into lymphomas that have an indolent course and those that have an aggressive course. These subtypes behave and respond to treatment variably.

Both Hodgkin and non-Hodgkin lymphomas can occur in children and adults, and prognosis and treatment depend on the stage and the type of lymphoma.

Post-transplant lymphoproliferative disorders (PTLD)

PTLD are lymphoid and/or plasmacytic proliferation that occurs in the setting of solid organ or allogeneic hematopoietic stem cell transplantation as a result of immunosuppression. Majority of PTLD is of B-cell origin and associated with Epstein-Barr virus. These patients may develop infectious mononucleosis-like lesions or polyclonal polymorphic B-cell hyperplasia. Some of these B-cells may undergo mutations which eventually transform to high-grade lymphoma.

Solid-organ transplantation

A surgical procedure in which a vital organ of the body is removed from one person and placed into another person for the purpose of replacing the recipient's damaged or absent organ. Solid organs that can be transplanted include heart, lung, liver, kidney, pancreas, and intestine. The major challenges of such procedures include transplant rejection, where the host's body has an immune response to the transplanted organ, possibly leading to transplant failure.

When feasible, transplant rejection can be ameliorated through serotyping to determine the most appropriate donor-recipient match, and through the use of immunosuppressant medications.

Hematopoietic stem cell transplantation (HSCT)

A medical procedure of infusing multipotent hematopoietic stem cells derived from bone marrow, peripheral blood, or umbilical cord blood. It is often performed for patients with cancers of the blood or bone marrow, such as multiple myeloma or leukemia. Conditioning regimens using combination of chemotherapeutic agents and/or total body irradiation to eradicate patient's disease and suppress immune reactions against the graft is employed prior to infusion of hematopoietic stem cells. Allogeneic HSCT remains an arduous undertaking with many possible complications such as infection and graft-versus-host-disease and hence is reserved for patients with life-threatening diseases.

Rituximab

It is a chimeric monoclonal antibody against the protein CD20, an activated-glycosylated phosphoprotein expressed on the surface of B-cells. Rituximab destroys both normal and malignant B cells that have expression of CD20 on their surfaces, and is therefore used to treat diseases which are characterized by overactive and/or dysfunctional B-cells.

These conditions include several lymphomas, leukemias, transplant rejection and auto-immune disorders.

Adoptive cellular immunotherapy

A treatment used to help the immune system fight diseases, such as cancer and certain viral infections. The potential use adoptive of immunotherapy is to restore the immune system of patients with immune deficiencies as result of infection or chemotherapy. T cells that have a natural or genetically engineered reactivity to a patient's cancer or an infection are generated *in vitro*.

This increases the number of T cells that are able to kill cancer cells or fight infections. These T cells are given back to the patient to help the immune system fight the disease.

Vaccine

It is a biological substance used to stimulate the production of antibodies and provide immunity against a particular disease. A vaccine typically contains a preparation that resembles a disease-causing microorganism, and is often made from weakened or killed forms of the microbe, its toxins or one of its surface proteins. This stimulates the body's immune system to recognize these agents as foreign, destroy, and also keep a long term immunologic memory, so that the immune system can recognize and destroy any of these at a later encounter.

Summary Points

- Epstein-Barr virus (EBV) is an omnipresent γ-herpesvirus that infects a large proportion of human population.
- Primary infection is often asymptomatic and results in lifelong infection.
- In some people, EBV infection can result in infectious mononucleosis, and is associated with the development of B and T cell non-Hodgkin lymphomas, Hodgkin lymphoma and nasopharyngeal carcinomas, predominantly in immuno-compromised patients.
- EBV detection can be helpful for diagnostic, prognostic and therapeutic purposes.
- *In situ* hybridization of viral EBERs remains the gold standard for virus detection.
- Accumulated genetic alterations of oncogenes and tumor suppressor genes (e.g., deletions, mutations, rearrangements, and amplifications) and epigenetic changes (e.g., aberrant hypermethylation) that involve tumor suppressor genes are integral to the pathogenesis of EBV-associated lymphomas.
- Despite the current understanding of the molecular pathogenic mechanisms of EBV related diseases, the optimal management of EBV-associated lymphomas remains investigational.

Future Issues

Current knowledge of EBV-induced neoplasia provides a platform for designing better treatments, but there are very few candidate antiviral drugs, and much work remains to be done to make such therapies effective and practical.

Little is known about the virologic and immunologic events that occur during the long incubation period prior to symptoms in adults or asymptomatic individuals, especially children. Further research is needed to determine means to predict who will be affected most severely, and to develop therapeutic strategies to reduce EBV-related illnesses. Eventually, the combination of vaccination and immunotherapy approaches with small molecules that increase the expression of lytic cycle antigens, or target the viral proteins or the microenvironment may offer the most effective therapeutic approach to these diseases.

Increasing our understanding of how specific EBV gene products and expression programs contribute to pathogenesis holds promise for the development of more rational treatment strategies in the future.

References

[1] Epstein, M. A., Achong, B. G., Barr, Y. M.: Virus particles in cultured lymphoblasts from Burkitt's lymphoma. *Lancet* 1964;1:702-703.

[2] *Proceedings of the iarc working group on the evaluation of carcinogenic risks to humans*. Epstein-Barr virus and kaposi's sarcoma herpesvirus/human herpesvirus 8. Lyon, france, 17-24 june 1997. *IARC monographs on the evaluation of carcinogenic risks to humans* / World Health Organization, International Agency for Research on Cancer 1997;70:1-492.

[3] Thompson, M. P., Kurzrock, R.: Epstein-Barr virus and cancer. *Clinical cancer research: an official journal of the American Association for Cancer Research* 2004;10: 803-821.

[4] Gatto, D., Brink, R.: The germinal center reaction. *The Journal of Allergy and Clinical Immunology* 2010;126:898-907; quiz 908-899.

[5] Timms, J. M., Bell, A., Flavell, J. R., Murray, P. G., Rickinson, A. B., Traverse-Glehen, A., Berger, F., Delecluse, H. J.: Target cells of Epstein-Barr-Virus (EBV)-positive post-transplant lymphoproliferative disease: Similarities to EBV-positive hodgkin's lympho-ma. *Lancet* 2003;361:217-223.

[6] Niedobitek, G., Young, L. S., Herbst, H.: Epstein-Barr virus infection and the pathogenesis of malignant lymphomas. *Cancer Surveys* 1997;30:143-162.

[7] Pietersma, F., Piriou, E., van Baarle, D.: Immune surveillance of EBV-infected B cells and the development of non-Hodgkin lymphomas in immunocompromised patients. *Leukemia and Lymphoma* 2008;49:1028-1041.

[8] Filipovich, A. H., Mathur, A., Kamat, D., Shapiro, R. S.: Primary immunodeficiencies: Genetic risk factors for lymphoma. *Cancer Research* 1992;52:5465s-5467s.

[9] Heslop, H. E.: Biology and treatment of Epstein-Barr virus-associated non-Hodgkin lymphomas. *Hematology / the Education Program of the American Society of Hematology American Society of Hematology Education Program* 2005:260-266.

[10] Hummel, M., Anagnostopoulos, I., Korbjuhn, P., Stein, H.: Epstein-Barr virus in B-cell non-hodgkin's lymphomas: Unexpected infection patterns and different infection incidence in low- and high-grade types. *The Journal of Pathology* 1995;175:263-271.

[11] Kanakry, J. A., Ambinder, R. F.: EBV-related lymphomas: New approaches to treatment. *Current Treatment Options in Oncology* 2013;14:224-236.

[12] Loong, F., Chan, A. C., Ho, B. C., Chau, Y. P., Lee, H. Y., Cheuk, W., Yuen, W. K., Ng, W. S., Cheung, H. L., Chan, J. K.: Diffuse large B-cell lymphoma associated with chronic inflammation as an incidental finding and new clinical scenarios. *Modern Pathology,* 2010;23:493-501.

[13] Nakatsuka, S., Yao, M., Hoshida, Y., Yamamoto, S., Iuchi, K., Aozasa, K.: Pyothorax-associated lymphoma: A review of 106 cases. *Journal of Clinical Oncology* 2002; 20: 4255-4260.
[14] Ok, C. Y., Papathomas, T. G., Medeiros, L. J., Young, K. H.: EBV-positive diffuse large B-cell lymphoma of the elderly. *Blood* 2013;122:328-340.
[15] Tsimberidou, A. M., Keating, M. J.: Richter syndrome: Biology, incidence, and therapeutic strategies. *Cancer* 2005;103:216-228.
[16] Bockorny, B., Codreanu, I., Dasanu, C. A.: Hodgkin lymphoma as richter transformation in chronic lymphocytic leukaemia: A retrospective analysis of world literature. *British journal of haematology* 2012;156:50-66.
[17] Lee, A., Skelly, M. E., Kingma, D. W., Medeiros, L. J.: B-cell chronic lymphocytic leukemia followed by high grade t-cell lymphoma. An unusual variant of Richter's syndrome. *American Journal of Clinical Pathology* 1995;103:348-352.
[18] Tsimberidou, A. M., Keating, M. J.: Richter's transformation in chronic lymphocytic leukemia. *Seminars in Oncology* 2006;33:250-256.
[19] Herrmann, K., Niedobitek, G.: Epstein-Barr virus-associated carcinomas: Facts and fiction. *The Journal of Pathology* 2003;199:140-145.
[20] Herling, M., Rassidakis, G. Z., Jones, D., Schmitt-Graeff, A., Sarris, A. H., Medeiros, L. J.: Absence of Epstein-Barr virus in anaplastic large cell lymphoma: A study of 64 cases classified according to world health organization criteria. *Human Pathology* 2004; 35:455-459.
[21] Klein, G.: Epstein-Barr virus strategy in normal and neoplastic B cells. *Cell* 1994;77: 791-793.
[22] Roberts, M. L., Luxembourg, A. T., Cooper, N. R.: Epstein-Barr virus binding to CD21, the virus receptor, activates resting B cells via an intracellular pathway that is linked to B cell infection. *The Journal of General Virology* 1996;77 (Pt 12):3077-3085.
[23] Thorley-Lawson, D. A., Gross, A.: Persistence of the Epstein-Barr virus and the origins of associated lymphomas. *The New England Journal of Medicine* 2004;350:1328-1337.
[24] Babcock, G. J., Decker, L. L., Volk, M., Thorley-Lawson, D. A.: EBV persistence in memory B cells in vivo. *Immunity* 1998;9:395-404.
[25] Middeldorp, J. M., Brink, A. A., van den Brule, A. J., Meijer, C. J.: Pathogenic roles for Epstein-Barr virus (EBV) gene products in EBV-associated proliferative disorders. *Critical Reviews in Oncology/Hematology* 2003;45:1-36.
[26] Frappier, L.: Contributions of Epstein-Barr Nuclear Antigen 1 (EBNA1) to cell immortalization and survival. *Viruses* 2012;4:1537-1547.
[27] Li, M., Chen, D., Shiloh, A., Luo, J., Nikolaev, A. Y., Qin, J., Gu, W.: Deubiquitination of p53 by hausp is an important pathway for p53 stabilization. *Nature* 2002;416:648-653.
[28] Sivachandran, N., Sarkari, F., Frappier, L.: Epstein-Barr nuclear antigen 1 contributes to nasopharyngeal carcinoma through disruption of PML nuclear bodies. *PLoS Ppathogens* 2008;4:e1000170.
[29] Murakami, M., Kaul, R., Kumar, P., Robertson, E. S.: Nucleoside diphosphate kinase/ nm23 and Epstein-Barr virus. *Molecular and Cellular Biochemistry* 2009;329: 131-139.

[30] Levitskaya, J., Coram, M., Levitsky, V., Imreh, S., Steigerwald-Mullen, P. M., Klein, G., Kurilla, M. G., Masucci, M. G.: Inhibition of antigen processing by the internal repeat region of the Epstein-Barr virus nuclear antigen-1. *Nature* 1995;375:685-688.

[31] Zimber-Strobl, U., Strobl, L. J.: EBNA2 and NOTCH signalling in Epstein-Barr virus mediated immortalization of B lymphocytes. *Seminars in Cancer Biology* 2001;11:423-434.

[32] White, R. E., Groves, I. J., Turro, E., Yee, J., Kremmer, E., Allday, M. J.: Extensive co-operation between the Epstein-Barr Virus EBNA3 proteins in the manipulation of host gene expression and epigenetic chromatin modification. *PloS One* 2010;5:e13979.

[33] Anderton, E., Yee, J., Smith, P., Crook, T., White, R. E., Allday, M. J.: Two Epstein-Barr virus (EBV) oncoproteins cooperate to repress expression of the proapoptotic tumour-suppressor bim: Clues to the pathogenesis of Burkitt's lymphoma. *Oncogene* 2008;27:421-433.

[34] Bajaj, B. G., Murakami, M., Cai, Q., Verma, S. C., Lan, K., Robertson, E. S.: Epstein-Barr virus nuclear antigen 3c interacts with and enhances the stability of the c-myc oncoprotein. *Journal of Virology* 2008;82:4082-4090.

[35] Yi, F., Saha, A., Murakami, M., Kumar, P., Knight, J. S., Cai, Q., Choudhuri, T., Robertson, E. S.: Epstein-Barr virus nuclear antigen 3c targets p53 and modulates its transcriptional and apoptotic activities. *Virology* 2009;388:236-247.

[36] West, M. J.: Structure and function of the Epstein-Barr virus transcription factor, EBNA 3c. *Current Protein and Peptide Science* 2006;7:123-136.

[37] Saha, A., Halder, S., Upadhyay, S. K., Lu, J., Kumar, P., Murakami, M., Cai, Q., Robertson, E. S.: Epstein-Barr virus nuclear antigen 3c facilitates g1-s transition by stabilizing and enhancing the function of cyclin d1. *PLoS Pathogens* 2011;7:e1001275.

[38] Kaul, R., Murakami, M., Lan, K., Choudhuri, T., Robertson, E. S.: EBNA3c can modulate the activities of the transcription factor necdin in association with metastasis suppressor protein nm23-h1. *Journal of Virology* 2009;83:4871-4883.

[39] Lung, R. W., Tong, J. H., To, K. F.: Emerging roles of small Epstein-Barr virus derived non-coding rnas in epithelial malignancy. *International Journal of Molecular Sciences* 2013;14:17378-17409.

[40] Elia, A., Vyas, J., Laing, K. G., Clemens, M. J.: Ribosomal protein l22 inhibits regulation of cellular activities by the Epstein-Barr virus small RNA EBER-1. *European Journal of Biochemistry / FEBS* 2004;271:1895-1905.

[41] Tu, Y. C., Yu, C. Y., Liang, J. J., Lin, E., Liao, C. L., Lin, Y. L.: Blocking double-stranded RNA-activated protein kinase PKR by Japanese encephalitis virus nonstructural protein 2a. *Journal of Virology* 2012;86:10347-10358.

[42] Samanta, M., Iwakiri, D., Kanda, T., Imaizumi, T., Takada, K.: EB virus-encoded rnas are recognized by rig-i and activate signaling to induce type I IFN. *The EMBO Journal* 2006;25:4207-4214.

[43] Iwakiri, D., Takada, K.: Role of EBERs in the pathogenesis of EBV infection. *Advances in Cancer Research* 2010;107:119-136.

[44] Gires, O., Zimber-Strobl, U., Gonnella, R., Ueffing, M., Marschall, G., Zeidler, R., Pich, D., Hammerschmidt, W.: Latent membrane protein 1 of Epstein-Barr virus mimics a constitutively active receptor molecule. *The EMBO Journal* 1997;16:6131-6140.

[45] Soni, V., Cahir-McFarland, E., Kieff, E.: Lmp1 trafficking activates growth and survival pathways. *Advances in Experimental Medicine and Biology* 2007;597:173-187.
[46] Graham, J. P., Arcipowski, K. M., Bishop, G. A.: Differential B-lymphocyte regulation by CD40 and its viral mimic, latent membrane protein 1. *Immunological Reviews* 2010; 237:226-248.
[47] Lynch, D. T., Zimmerman, J. S., Rowe, D. T.: Epstein-Barr virus latent membrane protein 2b (lmp2b) co-localizes with lmp2a in perinuclear regions in transiently transfected cells. *The Journal of General Virology* 2002;83:1025-1035.
[48] Babcock, G. J., Thorley-Lawson, D. A.: Tonsillar memory B cells, latently infected with Epstein-Barr virus, express the restricted pattern of latent genes previously found only in Epstein-Barr virus-associated tumors. *Proceedings of the National Academy of Sciences of the US* 2000;97:12250-12255.
[49] Shapiro, R. S.: Malignancies in the setting of primary immunodeficiency: Implications for hematologists/oncologists. *American Journal of Hematology* 2011;86:48-55.
[50] Schurman, S. H., Candotti, F.: Autoimmunity in Wiskott-Aldrich syndrome. *Current Oopinion in Rheumatology* 2003;15:446-453.
[51] Parvaneh, N., Filipovich, A. H., Borkhardt, A.: Primary immunodeficiencies predisposed to Epstein-Barr virus-driven haematological diseases. *British Journal of Haematology* 2013;162:573-586.
[52] Booth, C., Gilmour, K. C., Veys, P., Gennery, A. R., Slatter, M. A., Chapel, H., Heath, P. T., Steward, C. G., Smith, O., O'Meara, A., Kerrigan, H., Mahlaoui, N., Cavazzana-Calvo, M., Fischer, A., Moshous, D., Blanche, S., Pachlopnik Schmid, J., Latour, S., de Saint-Basile, G., Albert, M., Notheis, G., Rieber, N., Strahm, B., Ritterbusch, H., Lankester, A., Hartwig, N. G., Meyts, I., Plebani, A., Soresina, A., Finocchi, A., Pignata, C., Cirillo, E., Bonanomi, S., Peters, C., Kalwak, K., Pasic, S., Sedlacek, P., Jazbec, J., Kanegane, H., Nichols, K. E., Hanson, I. C., Kapoor, N., Haddad, E., Cowan, M., Choo, S., Smart, J., Arkwright, P. D., Gaspar, H. B.: X-linked lymphoproliferative disease due to sap/sh2d1a deficiency: A multicenter study on the manifestations, management and outcome of the disease. *Blood* 2011;117:53-62.
[53] LaCasce, A. S.: Post-transplant lymphoproliferative disorders. *The Oncologist* 2006;11: 674-680.
[54] Van Leeuwen, M. T., Grulich, A. E., Webster, A. C., McCredie, M. R., Stewart, J. H., McDonald, S. P., Amin, J., Kaldor, J. M., Chapman, J. R., Vajdic, C. M.: Immunosuppression and other risk factors for early and late non-Hodgkin lymphoma after kidney transplantation. *Blood* 2009;114:630-637.
[55] Chen, D. B., Song, Q. J., Chen, Y. X., Chen, Y. H., Shen, D. H.: Clinicopathologic spectrum and EBV status of post-transplant lymphoproliferative disorders after allogeneic hematopoietic stem cell transplantation. *International Journal of Hematology* 2013;97:117-124.
[56] Swerdlow, S. H., Campo, E., Harris, N. L., Jaffe, E. S., Pileri, S. A., Stein, H., Thiele, J., Vardiman, J. W.: *World Health Organization classification of tumours of haematopoietic and lymphoid tissues.* Lyon, IARC Press, 2008.
[57] Van Baarle, D., Hovenkamp, E., Callan, M. F., Wolthers, K. C., Kostense, S., Tan, L. C., Niesters, H. G., Osterhaus, A. D., McMichael, A. J., van Oers, M. H., Miedema, F.: Dysfunctional Epstein-Barr virus (EBV)-specific CD8(+) T lymphocytes and increased

EBV load in HIV-1 infected individuals progressing to AIDS-related non-Hodgkin lymphoma. *Blood* 2001;98:146-155.

[58] Johannessen, I., Perera, S. M., Gallagher, A., Hopwood, P. A., Thomas, J. A., Crawford, D. H.: Expansion in SCID mice of Epstein-Barr virus-associated post-transplantation lymphoproliferative disease biopsy material. *The Journal of General Virology* 2002;83:173-178.

[59] Vishnu, P., Aboulafia, D. M.: AIDS-related non-Hodgkin's lymphoma in the era of highly active antiretroviral therapy. *Advances in Hematology* 2012;2012:485943.

[60] Cingolani, A., De Luca, A., Larocca, L. M., Ammassari, A., Scerrati, M., Antinori, A., Ortona, L.: Minimally invasive diagnosis of acquired immunodeficiency syndrome-related primary central nervous system lymphoma. *Journal of the National Cancer Institute* 1998;90:364-369.

[61] Chen, Y. B., Rahemtullah, A., Hochberg, E.: Primary effusion lymphoma. *The Oncologist* 2007;12:569-576.

[62] Ascoli, V., Lo-Coco, F.: Body cavity lymphoma. *Current Opinion in Pulmonary Medicine* 2002;8:317-322.

[63] Gloghini, A., Dolcetti, R., Carbone, A.: Lymphomas occurring specifically in HIV-infected patients: From pathogenesis to pathology. *Seminars in Cancer Biology* 2013; 23:457-467.

[64] Knowles, D. M.: Etiology and pathogenesis of AIDS-related non-Hodgkin's lymphoma. *Hematology/Oncology Clinics of North America* 2003;17:785-820.

[65] Epeldegui, M., Vendrame, E., Martinez-Maza, O.: HIV-associated immune dysfunction and viral infection: Role in the pathogenesis of AIDS-related lymphoma. *Immunologic Research* 2010;48:72-83.

[66] Wilson, W. H., Kingma, D. W., Raffeld, M., Wittes, R. E., Jaffe, E. S.: Association of lymphomatoid granulomatosis with Epstein-Barr viral infection of B lymphocytes and response to interferon-alpha 2b. *Blood* 1996;87:4531-4537.

[67] Katzenstein, A. L., Doxtader, E., Narendra, S.: Lymphomatoid granulomatosis: Insights gained over 4 decades. *The American Journal of Surgical Pathology* 2010;34:e35-48.

[68] Katzenstein, A. L., Carrington, C. B., Liebow, A. A.: Lymphomatoid granulomatosis: A clinicopathologic study of 152 cases. *Cancer* 1979;43:360-373.

[69] Castrale, C., El Haggan, W., Chapon, F., Reman, O., Lobbedez, T., Ryckelynck, J. P., Hurault de Ligny, B.: Lymphomatoid granulomatosis treated successfully with rituximab in a renal transplant patient. *Journal of Transplantation* 2011;2011:865957.

[70] De Leval, L., Hasserjian, R. P.: Diffuse large B-cell lymphomas and Burkitt lymphoma. *Hematology/Oncology Cclinics of North America* 2009;23:791-827.

[71] Masucci, M. G., Zhang, Q. J., Gavioli, R., De Campos-Lima, P. O., Murray, R. J., Brooks, J., Griffin, H., Ploegh, H., Rickinson, A. B.: Immune escape by Epstein-Barr virus (EBV) carrying Burkitt's lymphoma: In vitro reconstitution of sensitivity to ebv-specific cytotoxic t cells. *International Immunology* 1992;4:1283-1292.

[72] Oyama, T., Nakamura, S.: [Senile EBV-associated b-cell lymphoproliferative disorder]. *Uirusu* 2003;53:211-216.

[73] Campo, E., Swerdlow, S. H., Harris, N. L., Pileri, S., Stein, H., Jaffe, E. S.: The 2008 WHO classification of lymphoid neoplasms and beyond: Evolving concepts and practical applications. *Blood* 2011;117:5019-5032.

[74] Anderson, J. J., Fordham, S., Overman, L., Dignum, H., Wood, K., Proctor, S. J., Crosier, S., Angus, B., Culpin, R. E., Mainou-Fowler, T.: Immunophenotyping of diffuse large B-cell lymphoma (DLBCL) defines multiple sub-groups of germinal centre-like tumours displaying different survival characteristics. *International Journal of Oncology* 2009;35:961-971.

[75] Bavi, P., Uddin, S., Bu, R., Ahmed, M., Abubaker, J., Balde, V., Qadri, Z., Ajarim, D., Al-Dayel, F., Hussain, A. R., Al-Kuraya, K. S.: The biological and clinical impact of inhibition of NF-kappaB-initiated apoptosis in diffuse large B cell lymphoma (DLBCL). *The Journal of Pathology* 2011;224:355-366.

[76] Park, S., Lee, J., Ko, Y. H., Han, A., Jun, H. J., Lee, S. C., Hwang, I. G., Park, Y. H., Ahn, J. S., Jung, C. W., Kim, K., Ahn, Y. C., Kang, W. K., Park, K., Kim, W. S.: The impact of Epstein-Barr virus status on clinical outcome in diffuse large B-cell lymphoma. *Blood* 2007;110:972-978.

[77] Tousseyn, T., De Wolf-Peeters, C.: T cell/histiocyte-rich large B-cell lymphoma: An update on its biology and classification. *Virchows Archiv* 2011;459:557-563.

[78] Abramson, J. S.: T-cell/histiocyte-rich B-cell lymphoma: Biology, diagnosis, and management. *The Oncologist* 2006;11:384-392.

[79] Axdorph, U., Porwit-Macdonald, A., Sjoberg, J., Grimfors, G., Bjorkholm, M.: T-cell-rich b-cell lymphoma - diagnostic and therapeutic aspects. *APMIS: Acta Pathologica, Microbiologica, et Immunologica Scandinavica* 2002;110:379-390.

[80] Loke, S. L., Ho, F., Srivastava, G., Fu, K. H., Leung, B., Liang, R.: Clonal Epstein-Barr virus genome in T-cell-rich lymphomas of B or probable B lineage. *The American Journal of Pathology* 1992;140:981-989.

[81] Rudzki, Z., Rucinska, M., Jurczak, W., Skotnicki, A. B., Maramorosz-Kurianowicz, M., Mruk, A., Pirog, K., Utych, G., Bodzioch, P., Srebro-Stariczyk, M., Wlodarska, I., Stachura, J.: ALK-positive diffuse large B-cell lymphoma: Two more cases and a brief literature review. *Polish Journal of Pathology* 2005;56:37-45.

[82] Kuze, T., Nakamura, N., Hashimoto, Y., Abe, M., Wakasa, H.: Clinicopathological, immunological and genetic studies of CD30+ anaplastic large cell lymphoma of B-cell type; association with Epstein-Barr virus in a Japanese population. *The Journal of Pathology* 1996;180:236-242.

[83] Skugor, N. D., Peric, Z., Vrhovac, R., Radic-Kristo, D., Kardum-Skelin, I., Jaksic, B.: Diffuse large B-cell lymphoma in patient after treatment of angioimmunoblastic T-cell lymphoma. *Collegium Antropologicum* 2010;34:241-245.

[84] Yang, Q. X., Pei, X. J., Tian, X. Y., Li, Y., Li, Z.: Secondary cutaneous Epstein-Barr virus-associated diffuse large B-cell lymphoma in a patient with angioimmunoblastic T-cell lymphoma: A case report and review of literature. *Diagnostic Pathology* 2012;7:7.

[82] Rubinstein, P. G., Aboulafia, D. M., Zloza, A.: *Malignancies in HIV/AIDS: From epidemiology to therapeutic challenges.* AIDS 2014.

[86] Starzl, T. E., Nalesnik, M. A., Porter, K. A., Ho, M., Iwatsuki, S., Griffith, B. P., Rosenthal, J. T., Hakala, T. R., Shaw, B. W., Jr., Hardesty, R. L., et al.: Reversibility of lymphomas and lymphoproliferative lesions developing under cyclosporin-steroid therapy. *Lancet* 1984;1:583-587.

[87] Heslop, H. E., Ng, C. Y., Li, C., Smith, C. A., Loftin, S. K., Krance, R. A., Brenner, M. K., Rooney, C. M.: Long-term restoration of immunity against Epstein-Barr virus

infection by adoptive transfer of gene-modified virus-specific T lymphocytes. *Nature Medicine* 1996;2:551-555.

[88] Lee, T. C., Savoldo, B., Rooney, C. M., Heslop, H. E., Gee, A. P., Caldwell, Y., Barshes, N. R., Scott, J. D., Bristow, L. J., O'Mahony, C. A., Goss, J. A.: Quantitative ebv viral loads and immunosuppression alterations can decrease ptld incidence in pediatric liver transplant recipients. *American Journal of Transplantation* 2005;5:2222-2228.

[89] Nelson, B. P., Wolniak, K. L., Evens, A., Chenn, A., Maddalozzo, J., Proytcheva, M.: Early posttransplant lymphoproliferative disease: Clinicopathologic features and correlation with mtor signaling pathway activation. *American Journal of Clinical Pathology* 2012;138:568-578.

[90] El-Salem, M., Raghunath, P. N., Marzec, M., Wlodarski, P., Tsai, D., His, E., Wasik, M. A.: Constitutive activation of mtor signaling pathway in post-transplant lymphoproliferative disorders. *Laboratory Investigation*; 2007;87:29-39.

[91] Garcia, V. D., Bonamigo Filho, J. L., Neumann, J., Fogliatto, L., Geiger, A. M., Garcia, C. D., Barros, V., Keitel, E., Bittar, A. E., Ferrera des Santos, A., Roithmann, S.: Rituximab in association with rapamycin for post-transplant lymphoproliferative disease treatment. *Transplant International* 2003;16:202-206.

[92] Vaysberg, M., Balatoni, C. E., Nepomuceno, R. R., Krams, S. M., Martinez, O. M.: Rapamycin inhibits proliferation of Epstein-Barr virus-positive b-cell lymphomas through modulation of cell-cycle protein expression. *Transplantation* 2007;83:1114-1121.

[93] Keating, G. M.: Rituximab: A review of its use in chronic lymphocytic leukaemia, low-grade or follicular lymphoma and diffuse large B-cell lymphoma. *Drugs* 2010;70:1445-1476.

[94] Hanel, M., Fiedler, F., Thorns, C.: Anti-CD20 monoclonal antibody (rituximab) and cidofovir as successful treatment of an EBV-associated lymphoma with CNS involvement. *Onkologie* 2001;24:491-494.

[95] Styczynski, J., Einsele, H., Gil, L., Ljungman, P.: Outcome of treatment of epstein-barr virus-related post-transplant lymphoproliferative disorder in hematopoietic stem cell recipients: A comprehensive review of reported cases. *Transplant Infectious Disease* 2009;11:383-392.

[96] Fanale, M. A., Younes, A.: Monoclonal antibodies in the treatment of non-Hodgkin's lymphoma. *Drugs* 2007;67:333-350.

[97] Doubrovina, E., Oflaz-Sozmen, B., Prockop, S. E., Kernan, N. A., Abramson, S., Teruya-Feldstein, J., Hedvat, C., Chou, J. F., Heller, G., Barker, J. N., Boulad, F., Castro-Malaspina, H., George, D., Jakubowski, A., Koehne, G., Papadopoulos, E. B., Scaradavou, A., Small, T. N., Khalaf, R., Young, J. W., O'Reilly, R. J.: Adoptive immunotherapy with unselected or EBV-specific T cells for biopsy-proven EBV+ lymphomas after allogeneic hematopoietic cell transplantation. *Blood* 2012;119:2644-2656.

[98] Heslop, H. E., Slobod, K. S., Pule, M. A., Hale, G. A., Rousseau, A., Smith, C. A., Bollard, C. M., Liu, H., Wu, M. F., Rochester, R. J., Amrolia, P. J., Hurwitz, J. L., Brenner, M. K., Rooney, C. M.: Long-term outcome of EBV-specific T-cell infusions to prevent or treat EBV-related lymphoproliferative disease in transplant recipients. *Blood* 2010;115:925-935.

[99] Vera, J. F., Brenner, M. K., Dotti, G.: Immunotherapy of human cancers using gene modified T lymphocytes. *Current gene therapy* 2009;9:396-408.

[100] Comoli, P., Labirio, M., Basso, S., Baldanti, F., Grossi, P., Furione, M., Vigano, M., Fiocchi, R., Rossi, G., Ginevri, F., Gridelli, B., Moretta, A., Montagna, D., Locatelli, F., Gerna, G., Maccario, R.: Infusion of autologous Epstein-Barr virus (EBV)-specific cytotoxic T cells for prevention of EBV-related lymphoproliferative disorder in solid organ transplant recipients with evidence of active virus replication. *Blood* 2002;99: 2592-2598.

[101] Khanna, R., Smith, C.: Cellular immune therapy for viral infections in transplant patients. *Indian J. Med. Res.* 2013;138:12.

[102] Chen, J.: Roles of the pi3k/akt pathway in Epstein-Barr virus-induced cancers and therapeutic implications. *World Journal of Virology* 2012;1:154-161.

[103] Incrocci, R., McCormack, M., Swanson-Mungerson, M.: Epstein-Barr virus LMP2a increases IL-10 production in mitogen-stimulated primary B-cells and B-cell lymphomas. *The Journal of General Virology* 2013;94:1127-1133.

[104] Young, R. M., Hardy, I. R., Clarke, R. L., Lundy, N., Pine, P., Turner, B. C., Potter, T. A., Refaeli, Y.: Mouse models of non-Hodgkin lymphoma reveal syk as an important therapeutic target. *Blood* 2009;113:2508-2516.

[105] Hatton, O., Phillips, L. K., Vaysberg, M., Hurwich, J., Krams, S. M., Martinez, O. M.: Syk activation of phosphatidylinositol 3-kinase/akt prevents htra2-dependent loss of x-linked inhibitor of apoptosis protein (XIAP) to promote survival of Epstein-Barr virus+ (EBV+) B cell lymphomas. *The Journal of Biological Chemistry* 2011;286:37368-37378.

[106] Friedberg, J. W., Sharman, J., Sweetenham, J., Johnston, P. B., Vose, J. M., Lacasce, A., Schaefer-Cutillo, J., De Vos, S., Sinha, R., Leonard, J. P., Cripe, L. D., Gregory, S. A., Sterba, M. P., Lowe, A. M., Levy, R., Shipp, M. A.: Inhibition of syk with fostamatinib disodium has significant clinical activity in non-Hodgkin lymphoma and chronic lymphocytic leukemia. *Blood* 2010;115:2578-2585.

[107] Hatton, O., Lambert, S. L., Krams, S. M., Martinez, O. M.: Src kinase and syk activation initiate pi3k signaling by a chimeric latent membrane protein 1 in epstein-barr virus (EBV)+ B cell lymphomas. *PloS One* 2012;7:e42610.

[108] Ma, B. B., Lui, V. W., Hui, C. W., Lau, C. P., Wong, C. H., Hui, E. P., Ng, M. H., Tsao, S. W., Li, Y., Chan, A. T.: Preclinical evaluation of the akt inhibitor mk-2206 in nasopharyngeal carcinoma cell lines. *Investigational New Drugs* 2013;31:567-575.

[109] Clinicaltrials.Gov, 2013.

[110] Green, M. R., Rodig, S., Juszczynski, P., Ouyang, J., Sinha, P., O'Donnell, E., Neuberg, D., Shipp, M. A.: Constitutive AP-1 activity and EBV infection induce PD-l1 in Hodgkin lymphomas and posttransplant lymphoproliferative disorders: Implications for targeted therapy. *Clinical Cancer Research* 2012;18:1611-1618.

[111] Ramsay, A. G.: Immune checkpoint blockade immunotherapy to activate anti-tumour T-cell immunity. *British Journal of Haematology* 2013;162:313-325.

[112] Epstein, M. A., Barr, Y. M.: Cultivation in vitro of human lymphoblasts from Burkitt's malignant lymphoma. *Lancet* 1964;1:252-253.

[113] Epstein, M. A., Achong, B. G.: The EB virus. *Annual Review of Microbiology* 1973;27: 413-436.

[114] Sokal, E. M., Hoppenbrouwers, K., Vandermeulen, C., Moutschen, M., Leonard, P., Moreels, A., Haumont, M., Bollen, A., Smets, F., Denis, M.: Recombinant gp350 vaccine for infectious mononucleosis: A phase 2, randomized, double-blind, placebo-controlled trial to evaluate the safety, immunogenicity, and efficacy of an Epstein-Barr virus vaccine in healthy young adults. *The Journal of Infectious Diseases* 2007;196: 1749-1753.

[115] Sauce, D., Larsen, M., Curnow, S. J., Leese, A. M., Moss, P. A., Hislop, A. D., Salmon, M., Rickinson, A. B.: EBV-associated mononucleosis leads to long-term global deficit in T-cell responsiveness to IL-15. *Blood* 2006;108:11-18.

[116] Elliott, S. L., Suhrbier, A., Miles, J. J., Lawrence, G., Pye, S. J., Le, T. T., Rosenstengel, A., Nguyen, T., Allworth, A., Burrows, S. R., Cox, J., Pye, D., Moss, D. J., Bharadwaj, M.: Phase I trial of a CD8+ T-cell peptide epitope-based vaccine for infectious mononucleosis. *Journal of Virology* 2008;82:1448-1457.

[117] Rees, L., Tizard, E. J., Morgan, A. J., Cubitt, W. D., Finerty, S., Oyewole-Eletu, T. A., Owen, K., Royed, C., Stevens, S. J., Shroff, R. C., Tanday, M. K., Wilson, A. D., Middeldorp, J. M., Amlot, P. L., Steven, N. M.: A phase i trial of Epstein-Barr virus gp 350 vaccine for children with chronic kidney disease awaiting transplantation. *Transplantation* 2009;88:1025-1029.

[118] Hui, E. P., Taylor, G. S., Jia, H., Ma, B. B., Chan, S. L., Ho, R., Wong, W. L., Wilson, S., Johnson, B. F., Edwards, C., Stocken, D. D., Rickinson, A. B., Steven, N. M., Chan, A. T.: Phase I trial of recombinant modified vaccinia ankara encoding Epstein-Barr viral tumor antigens in nasopharyngeal carcinoma patients. *Cancer Research* 2013;73: 1676-1688.

[119] Israel, B. F., Kenney, S. C.: Virally targeted therapies for EBV-associated malignancies. *Oncogene* 2003;22:5122-5130.

[120] Feng, W. H., Hong, G., Delecluse, H. J., Kenney, S. C.: Lytic induction therapy for Epstein-Barr virus-positive B-cell lymphomas. *Journal of Virology* 2004;78:1893-1902.

[121] Shirley, C. M., Chen, J., Shamay, M., Li, H., Zahnow, C. A., Hayward, S. D., Ambinder, R. F.: Bortezomib induction of c/ebpbeta mediates Epstein-Barr virus lytic activation in burkitt lymphoma. *Blood* 2011;117:6297-6303.

[122] Ghosh, S. K., Perrine, S. P., Williams, R. M., Faller, D. V.: Histone deacetylase inhibitors are potent inducers of gene expression in latent EBV and sensitize lymphoma cells to nucleoside antiviral agents. *Blood* 2012;119:1008-1017.

[123] Perrine, S. P., Hermine, O., Small, T., Suarez, F., O'Reilly, R., Boulad, F., Fingeroth, J., Askin, M., Levy, A., Mentzer, S. J., Di Nicola, M., Gianni, A. M., Klein, C., Horwitz, S., Faller, D. V.: A phase 1/2 trial of arginine butyrate and ganciclovir in patients with Epstein-Barr virus-associated lymphoid malignancies. *Blood* 2007;109:2571-2578.

[124] Sides, M. D., Block, G. J., Shan, B., Esteves, K. C., Lin, Z., Flemington, E. K., Lasky, J. A.: Arsenic mediated disruption of promyelocytic leukemia protein nuclear bodies induces ganciclovir susceptibility in Epstein-Barr positive epithelial cells. *Virology* 2011; 416:86-97.

[125] Sivachandran, N., Wang, X., Frappier, L.: Functions of the Epstein-Barr virus EBNA1 protein in viral reactivation and lytic infection. *Journal of Virology* 2012;86:6146-6158.

[126] Jung, E. J., Lee, Y. M., Lee, B. L., Chang, M. S., Kim, W. H.: Lytic induction and apoptosis of Epstein-Barr virus-associated gastric cancer cell line with epigenetic modifiers and ganciclovir. *Cancer Letters* 2007;247:77-83.

[127] Li, Y., Zhang, Y., Fu, M., Yao, Q., Zhuo, H., Lu, Q., Niu, X., Zhang, P., Pei, Y., Zhang, K: Parthenolide induces apoptosis and lytic cytotoxicity in Epstein-Barr virus-positive Burkitt lymphoma. *Molecular Medicine Reports* 2012;6:477-482.

Biographical Sketch

Prakash Vishnu, MD, FACP, is currently affiliated with Floyd and Delores Jones Cancer Institute, Virginia Mason Medical Center, Seattle, WA, USA, and appointed as Consultant and Attending Physician. He obtained MB.BS., degree in Medicine and Surgery in Bangalore Medical College, Bangalore University, India, and a PG Diploma in Molecular Medicine at Molecular Medicine and Cancer Therapeutics in University of Auckland, Auckland, New Zealand. He completed residency program in internal medicine in Detroit Medical Center, Wayne State University, Michigan and a fellowship program in medical oncology and hematology in Mayo Graduate School of Medicine, Mayo Clinic. He is a member of American College of Physicians, American Society of Hematology, American Society of Clinical Oncology, American Association of Cancer Research and Washington State Medical Oncology Society. He is honored with a number of Awards from American Society of Hematology, American Association of Cancer Research, American College of Physicians, South East Michigan Center for Medical Education, Detroit Medical Center/Wayne State University, 12th World Conference on Lung Cancer, and ASCO Breast Cancer Symposium. He has published 27 papers over last 3 years.

In: Epstein-Barr Virus (EBV)
Editor: Jan Styczynski

ISBN: 978-1-63117-476-6
© 2014 Nova Science Publishers, Inc.

Chapter IV

The Role of the Epstein-Barr Virus in the Pathogenesis of Post-Transplant Lymphoproliferative Disorders

Julie Morscio[1*] *and Thomas Tousseyn*[1,2]
[1]KU Leuven, Department of Imaging and Pathology, Translational
Cell and Tissue Research, Leuven, Belgium;
[2]University Hospitals KU Leuven,
Department of Pathology, Leuven, Belgium

Abstract

The Epstein-Barr virus (EBV) is regarded as an oncogenic human Herpesvirus and is associated with infectious mononucleosis and a number of biologically different cancers, mainly lymphoproliferations of B-cell origin. EBV-positive lymphoproliferations occur primarily in patients that are immunocompromised and originate from several B-cell developmental stages. These give rise to a variety of lesions ranging from reactive infiltrations to overt malignant lymphoma subtypes like diffuse large B-cell lymphoma, Burkitt lymphoma or plasmablastic lymphoma, presumably in a multistage evolutionary process. Although many different mechanisms by which EBV proteins contribute to lymphomagenesis have been defined, it is currently unclear what role EBV plays in the pathogenesis of these biologically diverse disorders. Clues for the different impact of EBV are given by the distinct patterns of expression of viral latency proteins in different lymphoma subtypes. Molecular studies have demonstrated interactions between EBV proteins and the apoptosis-related BCL-2 family. EBV-encoded microRNAs have been shown to promote cell survival and to suppress the induction of the viral lytic cycle. Via induction of host microRNAs, EBV indirectly alters host innate immune responses. In addition, EBV is capable of manipulating the host immune response via expression of viral IL-10. The tumor microenvironment seems to play an important role in the course of

---

[*] Address for correspondence: Julie Morscio, KU Leuven, Department of Imaging and Pathology. Minderbroedersstraat 12, blok Q, B-3000 Leuven, Belgium. Tel: +32/16 336622. Fax: +32/16 336548. E-mail: julie.morscio@med.kuleuven.be.

disease representing a local niche that can allow antitumor immune responses even in an immunocompromised host.

The aim of this chapter is to give an overview of the known mechanisms that contribute to lymphoma development in the context of the immune status of the host, in particular the role of EBV. Five types of lymphoproliferative disorders (LPDs) associated with immunodeficiency are recognized by the World Health Organization: (1) post-transplant lymphoproliferative disorders (PTLDs), (2) lymphomas associated with HIV infection, (3) methotrexate-associated LPDs seen most frequently in patients with autoimmune disease, (4) LPDs associated with primary immune disorders and (5) the provisional category of LPDs associated with age-related immunosenescence.

In this chapter we focus in particular on PTLDs as this is the focus of our research. Regarding PTLDs, many studies do not discriminate between EBV-positive and -negative cases which considerably impedes the analysis and interpretation of the role of EBV in pathogenesis and prognosis. Based on the available data and our microarray study we propose that EBV-positive and -negative PTLDs are molecular-genetically distinct. In our model, oncogenic signaling by EBV-encoded proteins and (tolerant) immune responses are the main drivers of malignant EBV-positive PTLDs. Malignant EBV-negative PTLDs on the other hand could be mainly induced by chronic immune triggering by the graft and accumulating genetic alterations. Interestingly, EBV-negative PTLDs seem to be biologically similar to EBV-negative lymphomas arising in the general population suggesting these PTLDs are coincidental lymphomas that arise following transplantation.

Indications for a prognostic role of EBV are scare although some may point to a positive impact on outcome. The differences between EBV-positive and -negative PTLDs may have important implications for the development future targeted therapies which may considerably improve the prognosis of EBV-positive lymphomas.

Keywords: Immunodeficiency, organ transplantation, lymphomagenesis, lymphoid neoplasia, PTLD, HIV-associated lymphomagenesis, lymphoma in primary immunodeficiency

Abbreviations

A20	Tumor necrosis factor, alpha-induced protein (TNFAIP3)
ABC	Activated B-cell
AICDA	Activation-induced cytidine deaminase
AIDS	Acquired immunodeficiency syndrome
Ala	Alanine
ALCL	Anaplastic large cell lymphoma
ALK	Anaplastic lymphoma kinase
ATR	Ataxia telangiectasia and Rad3 related
AURK	Aurora kinase
B2M	Beta2 microglobulin
BACH	BTB and CNC homology 1, basic leucine zipper transcription factor
BART	BamA rightward transcripts
BCL	B-cell lymphoma
BCR	B-cell receptor
BHRF	Bam HI fragment H rightward open reading frame

BIM	Bcl-2 Interacting Mediator Of Cell Death
BIRC	Baculoviral IAP repeat containing
BL	Burkitt lymphoma
BLIMP1	B-lymphocyte-induced maturation protein 1
BLNK	B-cell linker
BTG	BTG family, member
BUB1	BUB1 mitotic checkpoint serine/threonine kinase
CARD	Caspase recruitment domain family
CCL	Chemokine (C-C motif) ligand
CCR	Chemokine (C-C motif) receptor
CD	Cluster of differentiation
CDCA	Cell division cycle associated
CDKN	Cyclin-dependent kinase inhibitor
CENP	Centromere protein
C-FLIP	Cellular FLICE-like inhibitory protein 2
CGH	Comparative genomic hybridization
CHOP	Cyclophosphamide-Adriamycin-Vincristin-Prednisone
CIITA	Class II, major histocompatibility complex, transactivator
CKS	CDC28 protein kinase regulatory subunit
CMV	Cytomegalovirus
C-MYC	Cellular myelocytomatosis viral oncogene
CNS	Central nervous system
CNV	Copy number variation
CREBBP	CREB binding protein
CSR	Class switch recombination
CT	Computed tomography
CTL	Cytotoxic T-lymphocyte
CTLA	Cytotoxic T-lymphocyte antigen
CVID	Common variable immunodeficiency
CXCL	Chemokine (C-X-C motif) ligand
CXCR	Chemokine (C-X-C motif) receptor
DAP-K	Death-associated protein kinase
DLBCL	Diffuse large B-cell lymphoma
DNA	Deoxyribonucleic acid
ds	Double-stranded
EBER	Epstein-Barr virus-encoded RNA
EBF	Early B-cell factor
EBI	Epstein-Barr virus-induced
EBNA	Epstein-Barr virus nuclear antigen
EBV	Epstein-Barr virus
ECOG	Eastern Cooperative Oncology Group
ENKTCL	Extranodal nasal-type NK/T-cell lymphoma
EP300	E1A binding protein p300
E-PTLD	Early post-transplant lymphoproliferative disorder
ERK	Extracellular signal-regulated kinase
EZH2	Enhancer of zeste homolog 2

FANCL	Fanconi anemia, complementation group L
FDG	Fluoro-deoxy-glucose
FFH	Florid follicular hyperplasia
FLT	Fluorothymidine
FOXP	Forkhead box protein P
FRA	Fragile site
GC	Germinal center
GCB	Germinal center B-cell
GEP	Gene expression profiling
Gly	Glycine
GM-CSF	Granulocyte-monocyte colony stimulating factor
gp	Glycoprotein
GVHD	Graft-versus-host-disease
HAART	Highly active antiretroviral therapy
HAT	Histone acetyltransferase
HERC	ECT and RLD domain containing E3 ubiquitin protein ligase
HHV	Human Herpesvirus
HIV	Human immunodeficiency virus
HL	Hodgkin lymphoma
HLA	Human leukocyte antigen
HMT	Histone methyltransferase
HSC	Hematopoietic stem cell
HSCT	Hematopoietic stem cell transplantation
HSTCL	Hepatosplenic T-cell lymphoma
IA	Immunomodulatory agent
IAR-LPD	Immunomodulatory agent-related lymphoproliferative disorder
IDO	Indoleamine-2,3-dioxygenase
IFI	Interferon, alpha-inducible protein
IFIT	Interferon-induced protein with tetratricopeptide repeats 3
IFN	Interferon
Ig	Immunglobulin
IgH	Immunoglobulin heavy chain
IgV	Immunoglobulin variable chain
IL	Interleukin
IM	Infectious mononucleosis
IPI	International prognostic index
IRF	Interferon regulatory factor
ISH	*In situ* hybridization
ITK	IL2-inducible T-cell kinase
KLRD	Killer cell lectin-like receptor subfamily D, member
LCK	Lymphocyte-specific protein tyrosine kinase
LCL	Lymphoblastoid cell line
LCP	Lymphocyte cytosolic protein
LDH	Lactate dehydrogenase
LMP	Latency membrane protein
LOH	Loss of heterozygosity

LP	Leader protein
LPD	Lymphoproliferative disorder
LPS	Lipopolysaccharide
LYN	V-yes-1 Yamaguchi sarcoma viral related oncogene homolog
MALT	Mucosa-associated lymphoid tissue
MAPK	Mitogen-activated protein kinase
MHC	Major histocompatibility complex
miRNA	microRNA
MGMT	O6-methylguanine-DNA methyltransferase
MLL	Mixed lineage leukemia
M-PTLD	Monomorphic post-transplant lymphoproliferative disorder
MRI	Magnetic resonance imaging
MSI	Microsatellite instability
MUM	Melanoma-associated antigen (mutated)
MX	Myxovirus (influenza virus) resistance
NF	Nuclear factor
NHL	Non-Hodgkin lymphoma
NK-cell	Natural killer cell
NKG	Natural killer cell group
NOS	Not otherwise specified
NUP37	Nucleoporin 37kDa
OAS	2'-5'-oligoadenylate synthetase
ORI	Origin of replication
p	Short arm of a chromosome
PAX	Paired box
PBL	Plasmablastic lymphoma
PBMC	Peripheral blood mononuclear cell
PCNSL	Primary central nervous system lymphoma
PCR	Polymerase chain reaction
PDL	Programmed death ligand
PET	Positron emission tomography
PH	Plasmacytic hyperplasia
PID	Primary immunodeficiency
PIM	Pim-1 oncogene
PLK	Polo-like kinase
PMBCL	Primary mediastinal large B-cell lymphoma
P-PTLD	Polymorphic post-transplant lymphoproliferative disorder
PRDM	PR domain containing 1, with ZNF domain
PTCL	Peripheral T-cell lymphoma
PTLD	Post-transplant lymphoproliferative disorder
q	Long arm of a chromosome
RHOH	Ras homolog family member H
RIS	Reduction of immunosuppression
RNA	Ribonucleic acid
RS	Reed-Sternberg
SCID	Severe combined immunodeficiency syndrome

SH3BP	SH3-binding domain protein
SHM	Somatic hypermutation
SNP	Single nucleotide polymorphism
SOT	Solid organ transplantation
SYK	Spleen tyrosine kinase
TCL	T-cell leukemia
TCR	T-cell receptor
TERT	Telomerase reverse transcriptase
TGF	Transforming growth factor
TIA	T-cell-restricted intracellular antigen
TNF	Tumor necrosis factor
TP53	Tumor protein p53
Treg	Regulatory T-cell
UCB	Umbillical cord blood
UD	Uniparental disomy
UTR	Untranslated region
VCA	Viral capsid antigen
VEGF	Vascular endothelial growth factor
VRK	Vaccinia-related kinase
VSIG	V-set and immunoglobulin domain containing
WHIM	Warts, hypogammaglobulinemia, infections, myelokathexis
WHO	World Healt Organization
X	X chromosome
XLP	X-linked lymphoproliferative disease
ZAP70	Zeta-chain (TCR) associated protein kinase 70kDa
ZEBRA	Z Epstein-Barr virus replication activator

1. Introduction

Until the 1960s, the association between infection and cancer remained a rather unexplored field of research while recent estimates suggest that over 15% of cancers could be attributed to viral infections. One of the most widely spread oncogenic viruses is the Epstein-Barr virus (EBV), a gamma human Herpesvirus with a seroprevalence of 90-95% of adults worldwide. EBV has been associated with lymphoproliferative disease, both benign (such as infectious mononucleosis also known as 'Kissing Disease') and malignant (such as Burkitt lymphoma). The acquired immunodeficiency syndrome (AIDS) epidemic and the increasing number of organ transplantations have shown that mainly immunocompromised individuals are susceptible to the deleterious effects of EBV [1]. Post-transplant lymphoproliferative disorders (PTLDs) are among the most severe complications of solid organ and hematopoietic stem cell transplantation (SOT and HSCT). The first cases were described in renal transplant recipients shortly after the introduction of chronic immunosuppressive drugs in the 1960s [2]. PTLDs cover a continuous spectrum ranging from benign lymphoproliferations resembling inflammation to overt lymphoma associated with a poor outcome. Currently, little is known about the pathogenesis of PTLD, mainly because of its rarity. However, the rising number of transplantations together with prolonged survival of transplant recipients result in a steadily increasing incidence of PTLD.

The majority of PTLDs is of B-cell origin rather than T-cell origin and most commonly presents as extranodal diffuse large B-cell lymphoma (DLBCL). Post-transplant lymphoma is morphologically nearly indistinguishable from lymphoma occurring in immunocompetent individuals but an intriguing difference between these two is their EBV status, the former being strongly associated with EBV. Despite this strong association, the role of EBV in lymphomagenesis is currently obscure and so far it is not completely clear how EBV-positive and EBV-negative lymphomas differ biologically as well as clinically.

This chapter aims at giving a thorough insight in the pathogenetic mechanisms that drive B-cell PTLD, and in particular in the role of EBV.

2. PTLD Histology

Since PTLDs reflect a wide spectrum of histologically diverse lymphoproliferative disorders different classification systems have been developed [3] of which the one proposed by the World Health Organization (WHO) is the most commonly used (Table 1). Three types of morphological lesions are recognized: polyclonal early lesions (E-PTLD), polymorphic PTLD (P-PTLD) and malignant monoclonal monomorphic PTLD (M-PTLD) [4]. These three kinds of lesions are assumed to represent consecutive stages in the pathogenesis of PTLD but this process of evolution remains poorly understood. The interval between transplantation and the onset of E-, P- or M-PTLD is not clearly delimited and may overlap. Generally, E-PTLD and P-PTLD arise earlier following transplantation then M-PTLD supporting the hypothesis that M-PTLD arises gradually from these lesions. It is feasible that also lymphoma in the immunocompetent population originates from a similar multi-step process but so far no evidence exists to support this hypothesis.

E-PTLDs comprise reactive proliferations that cannot be distinguished from reactive proliferations in an immunocompetent host (compare Figure 1A-C and Figure 1D). These lesions most commonly occur in the first year following transplantation in tonsils or lymph nodes. Preservation of the normal tissue architecture is crucial. Three E-PTLD subtypes are discriminated: plasmacytic hyperplasia (PH)-like PTLD, infectious mononucleosis (IM)-like paracortical hyperplasia and florid follicular hyperplasia (FFH). PH-like PTLD is characterized by an extensive polytypic plasma cell proliferation and the presence of a few immunoblasts. In IM-like paracortical hyperplasia immunoblasts are more prominent and the paracortical regions are markedly expanded. In contrast, in FFH the lymph node follicles are significantly enlarged. Except for EBV infection, these early lesions have no known etiology.

P-PTLDs represent morphological lesions that are almost exclusively observed in the context of immunosuppression [5]. These lesions comprise a mixture of B-cells of all differentiation stages and an extensive proliferation of stromal immune cells resulting in effacement of the lymphoid architecture. Few oligoclonal or monoclonal B-cells and Reed-Sternberg (RS)-like cells (reminiscent of RS cells in classic Hodgkin lymphoma) may be present (Figure 1E-F).

Like E-PTLDs most P-PTLDs are EBV-positive and arise within one year following transplantation. When clonal B-cell populations are detected P-PTLD may be more similar to lymphoma than to a benign reactive lesion.

M-PTLDs consist of B-cell or T/NK-cell malignancies and are classified according to the WHO classification of lymphomas in the general population (Table 1). In the Western world the vast majority of M-PTLDs are of B-cell origin, while T/NK-cell PTLDs are more prevalent in Asia [6]. Within the group of B-cell malignancies non-Hodgkin lymphomas (NHL) represent over 80% of the cases. Like for lymphomas in the immunocompetent population the histological subtypes of M-PTLD can be traced back to a particular stage in the normal T-cell (in)dependent B-cell activation process (*infra*, 8.1.1 B-cell biology). Post-transplant diffuse large B-cell lymphoma (DLBCL) is the most frequently occurring lymphoma subtype and is characterized by diffuse sheets of large clonal B-cells that destroy the typical follicular structure of the lymphoid tissue (compare Figure 1G and Figure 1J). The most common morphological variants are centroblastic (medium-sized to large tumor cells with two to four nucleoli), immunoblastic (large tumor cells with a single central nucleolus) and anaplastic (large to very large round, oval to polygonal tumor cells with pleiomorphic nuclei) DLBCL. The centroblastic and immunoblastic variants largely correspond to the molecular subtypes (germinal center B-cell, GCB versus activated B-cell, ABC subtypes) identified in DLBCL (*infra*, 8.1.1 B-cell biology and 8.2.1 Lymphoma in immunocompetent individuals) and have been reported in PTLD patients [7]. Burkitt lymphoma (BL) is the second most common post-transplant lymphoma and consists of sheets of small/medium-sized tumoral B-cells and dispersed tingible body-containing macrophages resulting in a typical starry-sky background. A very high mitotic rate demonstrated by numerous mitotic figures is characteristic for BL (compare Figure 1H and Figure 1K). Plasmablastic lymphoma (PBL) is a more uncommon M-PTLD and consists of large tumor cells with immunoblastic to plasmacytic morphology. PBL was originally described in the oral cavity of human immunodeficiency virus (HIV)-positive individuals but has increasingly been reported in transplant recipients [8] (compare Figure 1I and Figure 1L). It is important to note that M-PTLDs are almost exclusively aggressive lymphomas like DLBCL, BL and PBL. Indolent lymphomas like follicular lymphoma and small cell lymphomas are very rarely encountered following transplantation and are still not considered as real PTLDs according to the WHO [4].

Monomorphic T/NK-cell lymphomas make up less than 15% of M-PTLDs in Western countries and include many types that share the morphological and immunophenotypical features of similar lymphomas in the immunocompetent population (Table 1). T-cell PTLDs are less well studied and the current classification does not cover a spectrum from benign to malignant lymphoproliferations as is the case for B-cell PTLD, excluding post-transplant polyclonal T-cell proliferations from the diagnosis PTLD. As a consequence (bi)clonal T-cell expansions that are frequently present in E- and P-PTLD are not considered as T-cell PTLDs [9]. In total only about 160 cases of T-cell PTLD have been described (since the first reported case in 1987) and recently these published cases have been reviewed by our and another independent research group [6, 10]. The most common T-cell PTLD subtypes are peripheral T-cell lymphoma not otherwise specified (PTCL, NOS, 19% of the cases), hepatosplenic T-cell lymphoma (HSTCL, 12%) and anaplastic large cell lymphoma (ALCL, 12%), either ALK-positive, ALK-negative, systemic or primary cutaneous.

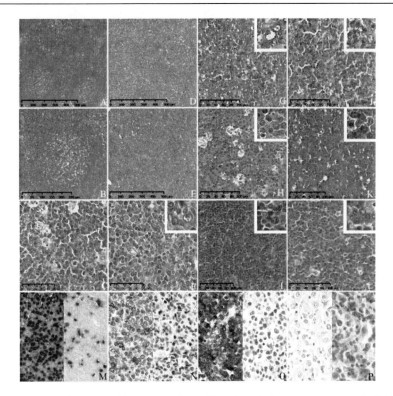

Figure 1. Histology of reactive and malignant lymphoproliferations in immunocompetent individuals and transplant recipients

A-C. Reactive lymph node from an immunocompetent individual. In A. two secondary follicles characterized by a germinal center and the surrounding mantle zone are shown. In B. the structure of one of the secondary follicles is more clearly shown. In C. the tingible body macrophages in the germinal center are clearly visible together with large centroblasts and small, darker centrocytes.

D. An early PTLD lesion: the lymph node architecture is preserved illustrated by the reactive secondary follicle.

E-F. A polymorphic PTLD lesion: the lymph node architecture is effaced by an extensive proliferation of immune cells. In F. the florid mixture of different cell types and large Reed-Sternberg-like cells is shown. Inset: a Reed-Sternberg-like cell with a bilobed nucleus and an prominent eosinophilic nucleolus in each lobe.

G-I. Histology of post-transplant diffuse large B-cell lymphoma (DLBCL, G), Burkitt lymphoma (BL, H) and plasmablastic lymphoma (PBL, I). In the insets the different morphological features of the tumor cells of each subtype are clearly visible.

J-L. Histology of diffuse large B-cell lymphoma (DLBCL, J), Burkitt lymphoma (BL, K) and plasmablastic lymphoma (PBL, L) of immunocompetent individuals. In the insets, the different morphological features of the tumor cells of each subtype are clearly visible.

Comparison of G-I and J-L shows that lymphomas in transplant recipients and immunocompetent individuals are morphologically very similar. DLBCL is characterized by large tumor cells and prominent lymphocytic infiltration. BL is characterized by a starry-sky appearance caused by the presence of dispersed tingible body macrophages (see also C) and relatively small to medium-sized tumor cells. In PBL, the tumor cells have a typical eccentric nucleus, a paranuclear hof and basophilic cytoplasm.

M-P. Epstein-Barr virus-encoded RNA *in situ* hybridization (EBER ISH) and the staining patterns of the three EBV latency types. Figure M. shows the variability of EBER-positive staining which can range from 100% (left) to 10% of the tumor cells (right). N-P show stainings of the Epstein-Barr viral proteins LMP1 (left) and EBNA2 (right) that are used to define the EBV latency profile: latency III (LMP1+/EBNA2+, N), latency II (LMP1+/EBNA2-, O), latency I (LMP1-/EBNA2-, P).

True NK-cell PTLDs are very rare and include NK-cell lymphoma and/or leukemia (6 cases reported) and extranodal NK/T-cell lymphoma, nasal-type (8 cases reported) [6]. Whereas up to 80% of monomorphic B-cell PTLDs are positive for EBV, this is the case for only about a third of monomorphic T-cell PTLDs. Because of the rarity of T-cell PTLD and because only a minority of T-cell PTLDs are EBV-driven, B-cell PTLD will be the main focus of this chapter. Unless clearly stated otherwise, the paragraphs refer to B-cell PTLD.

Table 1. Classification of mature non-Hodgkin B-cell, T-cell and NK-cell lymphoproliferations (WHO 2008)

Mature B-cell lymphoproliferations	Mature T-cell and NK-cell lymphoproliferations
Chronic lymphocytic leukemia/ small lymphocytic lymphoma	T-cell prolymphocytic leukemia
B-cell prolymphocytic leukemia	T-cell large granular lymphocytic leukemia
Splenic marginal zone lymphoma	**Aggressive NK-cell lymphoma/leukemia**
Hairy cell leukemia	Hydroa vacciniforme-like lymphoma
Splenic lymphoma/leukemia, unclassifiable	Adult T-cell leukemia/lymphoma
Lymphoplasmacytic lymphoma	**Extranodal NK/T-cell lymphoma, nasal type**
Waldenström macroglobulinemia	Enteropathy-associated T-cell lymphoma
Heavy chain diseases	**Hepatosplenic T-cell lymphoma**
Plasma cell myeloma	Subcutaneous panniculitis-like T-cell lymphoma
Solitary plasmacytoma of bone	Mycosis fungoides
Extraosseous plasmacytoma	Sézary syndrome
Extranodal marginal zone lymphoma of mucosa-associated lymphoid tissue (MALT lymphoma)	Primary cutaneous CD30+ T-cell lymphoproliferative disorders
Nodal marginal zone lymphoma	**Peripheral T-cell lymphoma, NOS**
Follicular lymphoma	Angioimmunoblastic T-cell lymphoma
Primary cutaneous follicular center lymphoma	**Anaplastic large cell lymphoma**
Mantle cell lymphoma	
Diffuse large B-cell lymphoma, NOS	**Post-transplant lymphoproliferative disorders**
Primary mediastinal (thymic) large B-cell lymphoma	**Florid follicular hyperplasia**
Intravascular large B-cell lymphoma	**Plasmacytic hyperplasia**
ALK+ large B-cell lymphoma	**Infectious mononucleosis-like paracortical hyperplasia**
Plasmablastic lymphoma	**Polymorphic PTLD**
Primary effusion lymphoma	**Monomorphic PTLD (B and T/NK-cell types)**
Burkitt lymphoma	**Hodgkin lymphoma-like PTLD**
	Classic Hodgkin lymphoma-type PTLD

Abbreviations: ALK: anaplastic lymphoma kinase; DLBCL: diffuse large B-cell lymphoma; NK-cell: natural killer cell; NOS: not otherwise specified. Rare subtypes and provisional categories from the WHO classification (2008) are left out of the table. Lymphoproliferations that occur as PTLD are indicated in **bold**.

A fourth PTLD category contains miscellaneous lesions that mostly resemble Hodgkin lymphoma (HL) and which are nearly always EBV-positive. Conventionally, HL-like PTLD lesions are grouped with classic HL-type PTLD in this category. However clinical, immunophenotypic, and molecular-genetic differences have been described raising the question whether HL-like PTLD is truly a form of HL or actually more closely resembles non-Hodgkin B-cell PTLD [11, 12]. One study suggested that the EBV+/CD15+

/CD30+/CD45- phenotype supports the diagnosis of classic HL-type PTLD whereas EBV+/CD15-/CD30+/CD45+ would be suggestive for HL-like PTLD [13]. If these disorders really represent different entities, distinction may be important for clinical management as classic HL requires a particular treatment approach [11].

It is important to note that different morphological subtypes can be encountered within one single biopsy specimen or within several syn- or metachronously taken biopsies, further complicating classification and treatment planning of PTLD patients.

3. Risk Factors for PTLD

Due to the diversity of the risk factors that are associated with PTLD development the prevalence of PTLD is highly variable (ranging from 1%-15% in solid organ and 0.5%-24% in hematopoietic stem cell recipients) [14]. As a result it is impossible to accurately predict which transplant recipients will ultimately develop PTLD and after what time interval following transplantation. Iatrogenic suppression of the immune system in combination with primary infection or reactivation of EBV after transplantation are regarded as the main predisposing factors for development of PTLD. Different studies have shown that individuals who are EBV-naive at the moment of transplantation and who therefore lack cellular immunity against EBV are highly susceptible to graft-mediated EBV primo-infection which may result in early-onset PTLD (within 12 months following transplantation) [15]. This process probably mainly affects pediatric transplant recipients as only 50% of the children in developed countries are carriers of EBV by the age of five [16, 17]. Nevertheless, the increased risk for PTLD development does not outweigh a life-saving transplantation. Ideally, the EBV status of both graft donor and recipient should be known for PTLD risk assessment. The EBV status of the recipient is always determined pre-transplantation by measurement of anti-EBV IgM and IgG antibodies and quantification of EBV DNAemia (*infra*). However, the EBV status of the organ donor is frequently not known compromising the estimation of the PTLD risk.

Similarly to EBV-naivety, hematopoietic stem cell transplantation (HSCT) preceded by ablation of the patient's bone marrow and resulting in elimination of any existing cellular immunity against EBV is associated with early-onset PTLD. Indeed, the occurrence of PTLD within one year following transplantation is remarkably higher for HSCT than for solid organ transplantation (SOT) [18, 19]. This has been attributed to the more profound depletion of (EBV-specific) cytotoxic T-lymphocytes (CTLs) post-HSCT compared to post-SOT [20].

Individuals who are latently infected with EBV at the moment of transplantation are prone to reactivation of EBV followed by active production of viral particles as a result of iatrogenic immunosuppression. Subsequent B-cell infection by newly synthesized virions may result in uncontrolled B-cell proliferation because of suppressed EBV-specific CTLs. This process may eventually advance to malignancy. However, the fact that not all transplant recipients develop a PTLD despite the prevalence of EBV indicates that the etiology is much more complex. Except for the immunosuppressive regimen and EBV, also the type of solid organ graft has been shown to influence the risk for PTLD development. Grafts containing a substantial amount of lymphoid tissue (e.g., small intestine) resulting in transfer of (potentially EBV-infected) donor lymphocytes may contribute to PTLD development. Also grafts that require an intensive immunosuppressive regimen (e.g., heart) are considered as risk factors [21, 22]. This is illustrated by the different rates of PTLD development for different grafts: the highest B-cell PTLD incidence is associated with intestinal and multivisceral transplants (5%-20%), followed by heart and lung transplants (2%-10%) and kidney and liver transplants (1%-5%) [23, 24].

In contrast to B-cell PTLD, T-cell PTLD arises most frequently after kidney transplantation (63%), followed by heart or heart-lung (19%), liver (9%), hematopoietic or peripheral blood stem cell (7%), lung (1%) and multivisceral transplantation (<1%) [6]. Intriguingly, these data show that multivisceral transplantation, which is the graft associated with the highest risk of B-cell PTLD development (*supra*), very rarely gives rise to T-cell PTLD. Conversely, kidney transplantation is more strongly associated with T-cell PTLD compared to B-cell PTLD. A possible explanation could be the intensity of immunosuppression that differs for different grafts: profound immunosuppression (for visceral transplants) results in severe suppression of T-cells minimizing the risk for T-cell PTLD development. In contrast, more mild immunosuppression (for kidney transplants) may allow a certain level of chronic T-cell stimulation (by the graft) which could eventually evolve to malignancy.

Regarding HSCT, the highly variable incidence of PTLD is mainly dependent on manipulation of the graft and the intensity of immunosuppression which is related to the origin of the HSC. Autologous HSCT (meaning the donor of the graft is also the recipient) is associated with a very low PTLD incidence, mainly because no intense immunosuppressive therapy is used like following allogeneic HSCT (meaning the donor and the recipient are two different individuals). T-cell depletion of the graft may increase the risk for PTLD development even following autologous HSCT suggesting that T-cell deficiency plays an important role. The importance of an active T-cell response is also supported by the better prognosis of PTLD following autologous compared to allogeneic HSCT which likely reflects the more rapid recovery of cellular immunity in the former [25].

Because of rapid availability, limited alloreactivity and a low risk of graft-versus-host-disease (GVHD) and transmission of the Cytomegalovirus (all risk factors for PTLD development, *infra*) umbillical cord blood (UCB) is now frequently used as an alternative source of stem cells for allogeneic transplantation. Because UCB yields a limited dose of stem cells compared to bone marrow it is mainly used in pediatric patients and it takes a relatively longer time for engraftment and hematopoietic reestablishment [26].

Overall the PTLD incidence after UCB transplantation and allogeneic HSCT is similar. An interesting finding is that PTLD following UCB transplantation is more frequently of host origin while the majority of PTLDs following HSCT is of donor origin (*infra*). This observation has been correlated with the engraftment status as in all reported cases of host-derived PTLD following UCB engraftment was incomplete at the moment of PTLD diagnosis [27]. Interestingly, similar results have been reported for PTLD following HSCT: the few cases of PTLD post-HSCT that originate from the host have been associated with chimerism or failed engraftment [28, 29].

Not surprisingly, human leukocyte antigen (HLA) mismatching is associated with a higher risk for PTLD both after SOT and HSCT [30-32]. HLA genes encode major histocompatibility complexes (MHC) which are important for cell-surface antigen presentation. Two clusters of MHC proteins are distinguished, namely MHC I (expressed on all nucleated cells and encoded by HLA A, B, and C) and MHC II (expressed only on specialized antigen-presenting cells and encoded by HLA DP, DM, DOA, DOB, DQ, and DR). HLA mismatching is the main cause of graft rejection. As not everyone has the same set of HLA loci (i.e., haplotype), incompatible MHC proteins expressed in a graft induce an immune response of the graft recipient resulting in rejection. Although HLA mismatching may promote PTLD development, the type of donor (matched family donor, mismatched family donor, matched unrelated donor, mismatched unrelated donor) is not associated with PTLD-related mortality [33].

For both pediatric and adult organ recipients, the cumulative incidence of PTLD rises over time regardless of the transplant organ type. Importantly, the incidence in children is systematically higher compared to the adult population (53% versus 15% respectively) [23].

Over 90% of post-SOT PTLDs arise from host lymphocytes suggesting that chronic B-cell stimulation by the solid organ graft (*infra*, 11.2 Chronic antigen stimulation) together with endogenous EBV reactivation or EBV infection via donor lymphocytes plays a role in PTLD development rather than transformation of an EBV-infected donor B-cell [34].

As previously mentioned, post-HSCT PTLDs most frequently arise from donor lymphocytes potentially resulting from chronic graft-versus-host disease (GVHD) which is caused by reactive donor T-cells. To prevent GVHD T-cells are usually depleted in the graft (using antibodies targeting T-cells e.g., the anti-CD3 OKT3 antibody), however this can result in rejection of the graft by the host's residual immune cells and increases the risk for PTLD development because of uncontrolled proliferation of EBV-infected donor B-cells. If these donor B-cells are also removed from the graft or if the organ recipient is depleted from both T- and B-cells (e.g., using alemtuzumab, a monoclonal anti-CD52 antibody) and receives a graft from an EBV-negative donor, than the risk for PTLD development is reduced [31, 35].

The implications of the origin of PTLD (host or donor) have been examined in a series of liver [36] and kidney transplants [37]. In both studies, donor-derived PTLD was associated with earlier onset following transplantation and a higher rate of EBV infection compared to host-derived PTLD. The former also more frequently involved the allograft, had polymorphic morphology and showed a trend for better prognosis [37]. This is in line with the tendency for more persistent and recurrent disease in case of host-derived PTLD compared to donor-derived disease [38]. It is possible that host-derived PTLD remains subclinical for a longer time and is more persistent in contrast to donor-derived PTLD, which may more rapidly become symptomatic but will also be more easily recognized and removed by the residual immune system.

More controversial PTLD risk factors are (1) a chronically high EBV viral load following transplantation which may be caused by primary infection or reactivation of latent EBV infection [39, 40], (2) Cytomegalovirus, Herpesvirus 6 and Herpesvirus 8 infection, and (3) the individual type of drug administered following transplantation.

The EBV viral load is quantified based on the amount of viral DNA in peripheral blood and it has been reported that the EBV viral load rises during PTLD development [41]. EBV titers are frequently quantified in transplant patients and used as a means to estimate the risk for PTLD. The rise of the viral load has been attributed to an increased number of peripheral EBV-infected cells rather than to an increase in the copy number of viral genomes per infected cell (which is similar to the copy number in blood cells of healthy EBV carriers). Notably, virus-infected cells in the blood of PTLD patients are phenotypically similar to latently infected resting memory B-cells in healthy EBV carriers suggesting that there is no expansion of immunoblasts-like cells in the peripheral blood of PTLD patients [42].

Except for its role in the assessment of PTLD risk the EBV viral load is taken into account during treatment planning and management of PTLD [16, 43]. Nevertheless, many controversies still exist such as whether to use peripheral blood monocytes (PBMCs), plasma or whole blood to quantify the viral load, how frequently the viral load should be monitored and which threshold value is clinically relevant [44, 45].

Viral load quantification based on peripheral blood cells requires distinction of normal and malignant EBV-infected cells resulting in lower specificity compared to when plasma is used [46]. The few studies that examined the specificity and sensitivity of quantification of the EBV viral load as a diagnostic test for PTLD indicated good sensitivity for detecting EBV-positive PTLD but poor specificity resulting in a high number of false positives [47-50]. In most transplant centers (including ours) real-time PCR (polymerase chain reaction) of the EBV DNA in whole blood is the most commonly used practice [51]. In our view, the best approach would be to standardize this method worldwide to facilitate the comparison and interpretation of data from different transplant centers. Subsequently, prospective trials should be set up to determine the most reliable EBV DNA threshold value that can be used as an indicator for initiation of (pre-emptive) therapy. However, even if such an endeavor would be successful unexpected events such as a spontaneous decrease of EBV DNAemia cannot be excluded [52].

To recognize transplant patients at risk for PTLD development a number of different EBV viral load thresholds have been proposed; the ones most commonly used are ≥ 10.000 or ≥ 40.000 viral genome copies/ml blood [51, 53]. Strikingly however, a recent study showed that allogeneic stem cell transplant recipients with symptomatic PTLD frequently had a viral load far below these thresholds (45% and 23% had a viral load ≤ 40.000 and ≤ 10.000 viral genome copies/ml respectively) [54].

Regarding the role of the EBV viral load in the assessment of response to therapy also no consensus exists. In HSC transplants a decrease in EBV viral load (in most cases measured in whole blood or plasma) in patients treated with rituximab was shown to be predictive of a good prognosis [33]. However, another study showed that a decrease of the *cellular* viral load (i.e., the amount of EBV-infected PBMCs) is not predictive of clinical response in patients treated with rituximab. A possible explanation is that EBV-positive PBMCs are more sensitive to rituximab than lymphoma cells explaining why in that study PTLD patients progressed despite a steep decrease in viral load [42].

Together, these findings stress that relying solely on the EBV viral load in peripheral blood is insufficient and unreliable to evaluate (1) suspicion of PTLD and (2) response of PTLD to therapy. Therefore both final diagnosis of PTLD and assessment of therapy response should be supported by additional clinical, pathological and radiological data.

A more reliable marker than the viral load may be the EBV-specific CTL response which has been shown to be very low in patients prone to/with PTLD [55, 56]. Alternatively, CD30, IL-6, CXCL13 and NK-cells have been proposed as potential new markers but their clinical relevance is still under investigation [57].

Apart from EBV infection also the Cytomegalovirus (CMV), a beta human Herpesvirus residing in T-cells and macrophages, has been implicated in PTLD development. The severity of disease caused by CMV has been put forward as a possible risk factor for PTLD development in liver recipients who underwent primary EBV infection following transplantation [58]. Independently of the proposed association between CMV and PTLD, CMV reactivation *per se* results in a higher mortality rate of transplant patients [59]. For these reasons and because it cannot be excluded that CMV contributes to PTLD development (e.g., via chronic antigen stimulation), it may be useful to take CMV into account in the overall assessment of PTLD risk. A third human Herpesvirus, namely HHV6 has been associated with reactivation of CMV in liver transplant patients and may act as an indirect co-factor in PTLD [60]. Also HHV8, which is found in all primary effusion lymphomas and Castleman-associated lymphomas has been proposed as a potential cause of PTLD. It has been suggested that these (and other) viruses could play a role in the pathogenesis of (part of) the EBV-negative PTLDs although this is highly debated (*infra*, 11. Pathogenesis of monomorphic PTLD).

In a retrospective study Birkeland *et al.* concluded that there is no evidence to assume that a specific class of immunosuppressive drugs would be preferentially associated with PTLD development [61]. In contrast several studies have associated different immunosuppressive drugs with an increased (cyclosporin, tacrolimus [62]) or decreased risk (antimetabolites azathioprine and mycophenolate mofetil, anti-CD52 antibody alemtuzumab) for PTLD development although some of these results have again been argued [63].

It is generally accepted that in most cases not a particular drug but rather the dose and the associated overall level of immunosuppression are the true risk factors for PTLD development. This should probably be nuanced for drugs specifically depleting T-cells as these are strongly associated with the development of PTLD, most likely because of their direct effect on immunological EBV control. For instance betalacept, a fusion protein composed of a human IgG1 Fc fragment linked to the extracellular domain of CTLA-4 that blocks T-cell activation, has been associated with an exceptionally high risk for EBV-driven PTLD in EBV-negative patients [64-66]. Nevertheless, since the primary goal following transplantation is to preserve the graft, suppression of T-cell responses will always be indispensable in order to prevent rejection. Therefore, it may be beneficial to simultaneously suppress B-cells in transplant patients to diminish the risk for PTLD development.

4. Diagnosis of PTLD

Because PTLDs are very heterogeneous disorders, a high index-of-suspicion and a standardized diagnostic approach are crucial. Due to the close follow-up of transplant patients, some PTLDs can be diagnosed at an early stage and the incidence of disseminated disease seems to decrease. Clinical parameters such as blood concentration of lactate dehydrogenase (LDH, which is raised in many cancer patients) and EBV titers are determined routinely [67] and may give an indication of which transplant patients are at higher risk for PTLD development (together with the other aforementioned risk factors).

Radiographic imaging using magnetic resonance imaging (MRI), computed tomography (CT) and/or positron emission tomography (PET) are commonly performed as part of the initial assessment of PTLD [68]. In particular imaging of the head is recommended considering the predilection of central nervous system (CNS) localization in PTLD patients (*infra* 6. Prognostic factors in PTLD) [16]. In the past years, 18-fluoro-deoxy-glucose-positron emission tomography (FDG-PET) in combination with CT scanning has proven to be the most sensitive imaging modality for both diagnosis and staging of (non-)Hodgkin lymphoma. Recently, our group demonstrated that FDG-PET is also valuable for detection of

PTLD [68]. Since changes in tumor metabolism occur much earlier after therapy than the anatomic size reduction of the tumor, one of the major advantages of this technique is the earlier detection of therapy response compared to anatomical imaging by CT alone. However, false negative findings still may occur in small (remnant) tumor while false positive findings may occur in inflammatory lesions since inflammatory cells also show a high FDG-metabolism. The latter may represent a significant limitation for early response assessment because early after therapy a temporary influx of inflammatory cells can be seen as a result of effective therapy and FDG-PET may underestimate treatment response. PET imaging with the thymidine analogue 18F-fluorothymidine (FLT) has been shown to be superior to FDG-PET for very early response prediction in lymphoma treated with targeted therapy [68, 69]. Whether this is also true regarding PTLD still needs to be confirmed.

For definite diagnosis of PTLD, histopathological examination is considered as the gold standard. Guided by imaging techniques biopsies are taken for morphological, immunohistochemical and molecular-genetic analyses. Because of the importance of the tissue architecture for evaluation and diagnosis, excisional biopsies of the tumor lesion are preferred over needle biopsies. An important caveat is that the histology may differ significantly depending on the anatomical location of the affected lymph node(s). In addition, a bone marrow biopsy or a lumbar puncture may be performed to examine potential bone (marrow) and CNS involvement.

Because histological examination alone is insufficient for accurate diagnosis of PTLD, the use of ancillary tests such as (1) immunophenotyping to determine the cell lineage using a set of antibodies, (2) clonality assessment by PCR of the B-cell or T-cell receptor and (3) detection of EBV are required.

The main techniques for detection of EBV infection in tissues are immunohistochemistry for staining of viral proteins (latency membrane proteins, LMPs and Epstein-Barr virus nuclear antigens, EBNAs, *infra*) and *in situ* hybridization of Epstein-Barr virus-encoded RNAs (EBER ISH). The latter is considered as the gold standard as it is the most sensitive and reliable method. EBERs are always expressed in EBV-infected cells independently of the viral life cycle stage, in contrast to viral proteins. Moreover, EBERs are more highly expressed than the viral DNA [16]. The RNA preservation and quality in the biopsy should always be assessed when evaluating EBER ISH to prevent that PTLDs are mistakenly diagnosed as EBV-negative due to RNA degradation.

In EBV-positive cases EBER expression may be highly variable and can range from 10% to nearly 100% of the tumor cells (Figure 1M). Currently, there is no fixed threshold to discriminate between EBER-positive and –negative lesions but if the EBER ISH staining is reliable, EBV-positive lymphoproliferative disorders can usually be discriminated easily from EBV-negative cases. An important caveat is however that also non-neoplastic bystander cells (e.g., memory cells) may be positive for EBV but should be distinguished from the transformed cells. This may be challenging especially in P-PTLD lesions.

Although EBV is strongly associated with PTLD, according to the current WHO criteria EBER-positivity is not required to diagnose PTLD as 20% to 30% of PTLD cases are EBV-negative (mainly late-onset monomorphic PTLDs or NK/T-cell lymphomas). Currently PTLDs are not (always) differentiated according to their EBV status however based on the molecular divergence (*infra*) it may be suggested that EBV-positive and -negative PTLDs should be regarded as separate entities.

In the absence of a staging system that is tailored for PTLD, the Ann Arbor classification system (with the Cotswold's modifications), the international prognostic index (IPI) and the Murphy system (for children) [70], which have originally been developed for immunocompetent lymphoma patients, have been applied to PTLD patients. Although the validity of IPI in PTLD has been confirmed [71, 72] the current staging system may (sometimes) be suboptimal for PTLD patients. IPI was developed based on data derived from 3273 immunocompetent patients with newly diagnosed aggressive lymphoma. It provides an estimation for a lymphoma patient's response to treatment, progression and overall survival based on five adverse prognostic factors (age >60 years; ECOG performance status >1; elevated serum LDH; clinical Ann Arbor stage III or IV; and extranodal sites >1) [73]. However, in a study involving 60 PTLD patients IPI could not discriminate between low- and intermediate-risk PTLD patients. A PTLD-adjusted IPI index taking into account only the patient's age (≥60 years versus <60 years), performance status (ECOG performance status <2 versus ≥2), and serum LDH concentration (within normal range versus elevated) clearly distinguished low-, intermediate- and high-risk patients [74]. Similar results were reported in another study that used an adjusted index including only the ECOG performance status and the number of extranodal site [75]. These analyses illustrate that caution is warranted when staging systems based on immunocompetent lymphoma patients are extrapolated to PTLD patients. Moreover, based on the data presented in this chapter one may consider to include the EBV status in a PTLD-tailored staging system.

5. Treatment Options for PTLD

5.1. Reduction of Immunosuppression, Chemotherapy and Rituximab

Many different treatment approaches for PTLD have been developed largely due to the clinical heterogeneity of these disorders. Reduction of immunosuppression (RIS, usually down to 25%-50% of baseline immunosuppression) for (partial) restoration of immunity is generally considered for all patients presenting with PTLD [23]. The underlying reasoning is that RIS allows recovery of EBV-specific CTLs resulting in anti-tumor immune responses. Complete cessation of immunosuppressive therapy is not frequently applied as it dramatically increases the risk for graft rejection. In addition, the type of graft and the availability of replacement therapy (e.g., dialysis for renal transplant patients) are taken into account to determine the safety and applicability of RIS [76]. The success rate of RIS in patients with polyclonal or monoclonal EBV-driven PTLD is variable (23%-86%) [77]. Importantly, monoclonal lymphoma and EBV-negative lesions are less likely to respond to RIS than early polyclonal and EBV-positive lesions. This observation suggests that the presence of EBV can significantly influence response to therapy and prognosis. RIS has been associated with reduced PTLD-related mortality in a retrospective study involving 144 allogeneic HSCT-related PTLDs [33] but the usefulness of RIS is poorly supported by prospective data. A phase 2 clinical trial involving 16 patients associated RIS with partial response in only 6% and documented progressive disease during RIS in 50% of the patients (the EBV status of the lesions was not taken into account) [78]. A more recent prospective trial reported that although RIS may prevent unnecessary treatment of PTLD patients, subsequent treatment should be started as soon as disease progression is detected [79].

For E-PTLD, treatment is generally limited to RIS whereas for P-PTLD, RIS can be combined with chemotherapy and rituximab (a monoclonal anti-CD20 antibody). For malignant M-PTLD, the main treatment strategy is based on rituximab and a cocktail of chemotherapeutics (cyclophosphamide, hydroxyldaunorubicin, oncovin and prednisone, or CHOP therapy) [23]. This is also the standard therapy for PTLD refractory to RIS. However caution is required as chemotherapy is associated with more treatment toxicity in PTLD patients compared to immunocompetent lymphoma patients because of its immunosuppressive effects (and the subsequent infectious complications) resulting in treatment-related mortality of 25% or more [80-82]. Low-dose chemotherapy may prevent such complications and has shown promising results, mainly in pediatric PTLD patients. A potential explanation is that –in contrast to most adult PTLD patients– pediatric PTLD patients may benefit from a primary immune response against EBV [83].

The introduction of rituximab has significantly changed the way PTLD is treated and significantly improved the prognosis of B-cell PTLD patients. Because of the limited toxicity associated with rituximab, it seemed an attractive alternative for cytotoxic therapy: three clinical trials reported complete response in 21%-60% of patients treated with rituximab as monotherapy [84-86]. However, a meta-analysis of two of these clinical trials demonstrated disease progression in 57% of the patients 12 months after completing the first-line treatment [74, 84, 86]. Several other studies have reported high relapse rates to rituximab ranging from 20%-26% [86, 87]. As a single agent first-line treatment rituximab may be suboptimal for intermediate- and high-risk patients [74]. Attempts have been made to find markers to predict response to rituximab such as the change of the EBV viral load (*supra*, 3. Risk factors in PTLD) or polymorphisms in the Fc receptor that binds the antibody gamma heavy chain [88]. No markers are generally recognized and so far there are also no known biological markers that predict relapse to rituximab [74]. Therefore, it is currently not possible to predict which PTLD patients will respond well to rituximab and which patients will be non-responders. To overcome this problem it has been suggested (based on clinical trial data from a recent phase 2 trial) that in case of disease progression during RIS, rituximab treatment should be initiated and followed by CHOP within a few weeks. This approach has been associated with a lower rate of treatment-related mortality. A possible explanation is that a lower tumor burden in rituximab-responders results in decreased chemotherapy-induced toxicity [79].

So far, it is not clear whether the EBV status of PTLD influences the response to rituximab or chemotherapy, mainly because in most studies PTLDs are not discriminated based on their EBV status [86]. Although not confirmed by all studies [85] both a retrospective study and a recent prospective trial reported a trend for better response to rituximab of EBV-positive compared to EBV-negative PTLD [84, 89].

Because of the high rate of treatment-related mortality following chemotherapy compared to rituximab it is more difficult to determine whether the EBV status also affects the response to CHOP. In a recent clinical trial, patients with EBV-positive PTLD received fewer treatment cycles and lower doses of chemotherapy than patients with EBV-negative PTLD and both groups performed equally well [79]. Based on these findings EBV might be considered as a predictor of good response to therapy.

5.2. Alternative Treatment Approaches

Because the current PTLD treatment regimens do not give the desired result alternative treatment strategies have been developed mainly focusing on EBV-positive PTLD.

As many PTLDs are EBV-related, it has been hypothesized that antivirals might be effective therapeutic agents. Acyclovir and ganciclovir both inhibit EBV lytic DNA replication *in vitro* by acting as chain terminators in viral DNA synthesis but their efficiency in PTLD patients is limited. This lack of therapeutic results has mainly been attributed to restricted lytic activity of EBV in PTLD tissues although the latter is still debated (*infra*, 9.1 EBV lytic infection in PTLD). More promising results have been reported for the use of arginine butyrate (which induces the switch from the EBV latent to lytic cycle and promotes tyrosine kinase expression in tumor cells) in combination with ganciclovir (which is phosphorylated by tyrosine kinase and subsequently acts as a chain terminator). In a phase 1/2 clinical trial involving 15 patients, administration of arginine butyrate and ganciclovir resulted in a complete or partial response in 27% and 40% of the patients respectively [90]. Also bortezomib, a proteasome inhibitor that is currently used for the treatment of multiple myeloma, has been shown to induce the EBV lytic cycle *in vitro* [91] and could in theory be used in combination with antivirals.

The importance of CTLs in controlling EBV infection and the suppression of these cells post-transplantation provided reason to believe that infusion of CTLs would be beneficial in PTLD patients. Cellular therapy with donor CTLs has been successfully applied to treat PTLD following HSCT as in these patients PTLDs mostly arise from donor lymphocytes [92]. Application of this strategy in post-SOT PTLD presents more difficulties as autologous CTLs (i.e., originating from the PTLD patient) are required (because most post-SOT PTLDs arise from host lymphocytes, *supra*). Furthermore many PTLD patients are EBV-naive before transplantation and have a defective T-cell response after transplantation. Despite these hurdles, *ex vivo* activation of recipient CTLs against EBV followed by reinfusion was shown to be feasible and effective in prevention of PTLD development in high risk patients [93]. Alternatively, infusion of HLA-matched donor CTLs has also shown promising results leading to a 52% response rate in a study involving 33 patients [94]. Although the results of these studies are encouraging, the laborious nature of the protocols currently impede large-scale application of cellular therapy for PTLD patients. Moreover, for infusion of CTLs to be effective expression of the target viral antigens is crucial but this differs for different tumor types further limiting the applicability of such immunotherapy.

Attempts have been made to treat PTLD with various other types of immunotherapy among which cytokine therapy. IFN-alpha had potential because of its antiviral and antitumoral effects, but due to poor tolerance and frequent graft rejection this strategy has been largely abandoned [95]. IL-6 is a B-cell growth factor and is known to also stimulate proliferation of EBV-positive malignant B-cells [96]. Rising IL-6 plasma levels have been associated with uncontrolled PTLD in patients that do not respond to therapy suggesting an effect of IL-6 on disease progression [97]. A role for IL-6 in PTLD was confirmed by a phase 1/2 clinical trial involving 12 PTLD patients: treatment with an antibody targeting IL-6 was associated with an overall response rate of 67%. The results of this study mainly apply to patients with polymorphic PTLD as only a minority had monomorphic disease (3/12 compared to 9/12 with P-PTLD). Of note, all cases were EBV-positive (based on LMP1 or EBER detection) and anti-IL6 therapy was associated with a decrease of the EBV viral load

[98]. Before the introduction of rituximab, other potentially therapeutic antibodies have been explored, mainly anti-CD21 and anti-CD24, however these are no longer available [99, 100].

All therapeutic strategies discussed so far apply to B-cell PTLD. In contrast, T-cell PTLD is much more uncommon and very limited data are available concerning the optimal first line treatment. No clinical trials have been set up to optimize the treatment of T-cell PTLD and the therapeutic regimens are largely limited to the conventional approaches (chemotherapy, radiotherapy and surgery). Although RIS may be successfully applied, most cases of T-cell PTLD are resistant. Also response to chemotherapy is usually poor necessitating the development of new therapies. One case report described successful treatment of refractory T-cell PTLD with bexarotene [101], a retinoid analog that is used for the treatment of cutaneous T-cell lymphoma [102] but its mechanisms of action have not yet been defined in detail. Except for this compound no other new treatment approaches have been reported.

Despite intensive treatment regimens, B-cell PTLD is still associated with poor survival. Mortality rates range from 25%-60% [75] and survival estimates vary considerably with 56%-73% of the patients surviving one year and 40%-61% surviving five years [103-106]. These wide ranges can be partly attributed to the diverse presentation of the disease and the high rate of non-PTLD-related deaths (due to infection, other malignancies) [107]. Additional interventions such as administration of growth factors like GM-CSF (granulocyte-monocyte colony stimulating factor) may help to minimize mortality. Nevertheless, development of new PTLD treatment strategies based on increasing insight in the molecular pathogenesis is required for better management of PTLD.

6. Prognostic Factors in PTLD

In both retrospective and prospective studies a number of prognostic factors associated with PTLD have been identified including: LDH concentration in peripheral blood, the ECOG performance status, the age at diagnosis, the interval between transplantation and PTLD onset, the number of disease sites, CNS involvement and the cell of origin (B-cell or T-cell).

Overall, young PTLD patients have a better prognosis than older individuals [103] possibly because they better support intense chemotherapy.

Early-onset PTLD (<1 year following transplantation) usually has a better outcome than late-onset disease (>1 year following transplantation) [78]. This is probably due to the fact that lesions that arise early are mainly of E-PTLD and P-PTLD morphology whereas most late-onset lesions are M-PTLDs. Early lesions primarily involve lymph nodes or tonsils while M-PTLDs arise predominantly extranodally, either localized or systemic. Involvement of liver, lung and gastro-intestinal tract is common resulting in more severe disease. Involvement of the graft itself is also frequent and may complicate diagnosis since graft rejection should be excluded [75]. Notably, the central nervous system (CNS) is commonly affected in PTLD patients with a reported prevalence ranging from 15% [108] to 50% [109]. In many CNS PTLD cases the CNS is the only site of disease. Reasons for the predilection of CNS involvement in PTLD are unclear. Because the CNS is an immunoprivileged organ it is possible that unrestrained proliferation of EBV in that location more easily results in malignancy [110]. CNS PTLD seems to be associated with the type of graft: the highest incidence is reported in kidney transplants (72%) followed by lung (18%), heart (5%), and pancreas (5%) transplants [111]. It is unclear whether this observation is confounded by the transplantation rates of the different grafts (kidney transplantations are generally most frequently performed). CNS involvement has been associated with a poor outcome [75, 112], but some studies reported survival beyond two years following diagnosis [113, 114]. Prolonged survival may be due to RIS-induced tumor regression, which can be achieved in CNS PTLD patients although not as readily as in patients with PTLD involving other organs [110]. This is probably why prolonged survival of patients with CNS PTLD is the exception rather than the rule.

T-cell PTLDs are associated with a median overall survival of 6 months (ranging from 2 to 18 months depending on the histological subtype) and are usually more aggressive than B-cell PTLDs [6, 9]. The reason for this is unclear.

The possible impact of EBV on the prognosis of PTLD patients is still obscure potentially because EBV-positive and –negative lymphomas are treated with essentially the same protocols (with the exception of infusion of CTLs in some cases of EBV-positive PTLD). The few available studies document no [112] or a positive [75, 79] prognostic significance of EBV in PTLD. Several findings also suggest that EBV-positive monomorphic PTLD is clinically different from EBV-negative monomorphic PTLD. EBV-positive PTLD has been associated with (1) more extranodal localizations and involvement of graft and kidney, (2) a significantly earlier onset after transplantation, (3) younger age at onset and (4) a poorer performance compared to EBV-negative PTLD [79].

7. Prevention of PTLD

Preemptive treatment strategies (i.e., treatment of a person with EBV DNAemia without proven EBV-disease) that aim at preventing PTLD development have mainly focused on prevention or control of EBV infection and comprise (1) active (vaccination) and passive (infusion of CTLs) immunoprophylaxis, and (2) chemoprophylaxis (the use of antivirals).

A potential approach to reduce the high risk of PTLD development in EBV-naive (pediatric) organ recipients is to induce seroconversion prior to transplantation using an EBV vaccine. A commercial EBV vaccine is currently not available but a few potential candidates have been tested in clinical trials. A vaccine based on soluble EBV gp350 membrane protein was shown to reduce the incidence of infectious mononucleosis but did not affect the rate of EBV infection [115]. This suggests that a vaccine consisting of several viral antigens is required to effectively prevent infection (and EBV-associated malignancy). EBV vaccination can also be useful in patients with established EBV-associated disease: a vaccine based on an EBNA1/LMP2 fusion protein showed promising results as an adjuvant treatment for EBV-associated nasopharyngeal carcinoma [116]. EBNA3 and LMP2 represent other potentially interesting candidates for vaccine development [17, 117].

Despite the obvious advantages of EBV vaccination, the development of a vaccine and the setup of clinical trials are impeded by a number of problems, namely (1) little interest from the industry partly because the socio-economic benefits are not clear [118], (2) the lack of a good biomarker for EBV-associated malignancy (*supra,* 3. Risk factors for PTLD) and (3) the long interval between EBV infection and the onset of malignancy in the general population. A potential solution could be to assess the validity of a vaccine in EBV-negative individuals prior to organ transplantation. However, chronic organ disease could render this population less susceptible to seroconversion.

A number of approaches that are used for the treatment of PTLD can also be applied in an attempt to prevent PTLD. Promising results have been reported for prophylactic infusion of CTLs: in a long-term study none of 101 HSC transplant patients developed PTLD and persistent CTLs were detected up to nine years following infusion [119]. Antivirals (acyclovir and ganciclovir) that block EBV lytic replication may also help to prevent PTLD however evidence for their efficacy is largely based on retrospective studies [120, 121]. The only published trial that prospectively evaluated the impact of antivirals on prevention of PTLD reported no benefit. Nevertheless, these therapeutics are still routinely used in most transplant centers because of their hypothetical activity against EBV [57].

8. Pathogenesis of Lymphoma

8.1. The Role of the Epstein-Barr Virus in the Development of Lymphoma

In order to understand how B-cell lymphoma can arise and how the Epstein-Barr virus can play a part in this process it is important to have insight in the biology of B-cells and the infectious life cycle of EBV.

8.1.1. B-Cell Biology

The highly variable presentation of PTLD can be partly explained by the complex development of B-cells, the cell type that gives rise to the majority of PTLDs. Upon encounter of antigen a naive B-cell either (1) stays in the extrafollicular regions of the lymph node and matures into a short-lived plasma or memory cell or (2) becomes an activated blast that migrates into a nodal primary follicle where it forms a germinal center (GC). How these faith decisions are regulated is poorly understood although the nature, dose and form of the antigen are known to play a role [122]. Antigens that act as mitogens (e.g., lipopolysaccharide, LPS, from Gram-negative bacteria) can cause a naive B-cell to directly differentiate into a plasma cell without passing through the germinal center. These plasma cells only secrete IgM antibodies [122]. Overall, the majority of activated B-cells forms a GC. Upregulation of BCL-6 is required for the B-cell to enter the centroblast stage and licenses GC formation [123].

In the GC, the activated blast becomes a centroblast that transiently downregulates its B-cell receptor (BCR) and undergoes a GC reaction involving somatic hypermutation (SHM) and class switching, both regulated by the AICDA (activation-induced cytidine deaminase) enzyme. During SHM, the antigen-binding variable region of the BCR is randomly mutated followed by selection of the BCR with highly enhanced antigen specificity. Centroblasts are characterized by an extremely high proliferation rate despite the occurrence of mutations and deletions induced by AICDA. Normally, DNA damage results in cell cycle arrest or apoptosis but it has been shown that BCL-6 indirectly diminishes DNA damage sensing [123]. The goal of class switching, also referred to as class switch recombination (CSR), is to alter the pool of molecules the antibody can interact with. During this process, the antibody isotype is changed by replacement of the IgM constant region with the IgG, IgE or IgA constant region. Importantly, the variable region is conserved so the antibody specificity remains unchanged during CSR [124].

After several rounds of cell division, centroblasts migrate to a lighter and more heterogeneous zone in the GC composed of T-cells, follicular dendritic cells and macrophages. Here, they differentiate into centrocytes and acquire a mature BCR. During normal B-cell differentiation, centrocytes are selected based on the interaction of their BCR with T-helper cells and antigens bound by complement receptors on follicular dendritic cells. Only the BCRs with the highest affinity are able to interact with their corresponding antigen which provides the required signals for the centrocytes to survive and proliferate. These survival signals mainly involve upregulation of BCL-2, a central anti-apoptotic protein that is downregulated during the initial stages of the germinal center reaction to allow apoptosis of inadequate B-cells that fail to interact with their target antigen [123, 125].

During the GC reaction, the genome of the differentiating B-cells is very fragile and susceptible to translocations. Furthermore, B-cell lymphomas that arise from a GC B-cell can be continuously exposed to aberrant SHM leading to additional mutations in genes that are usually not targeted by SHM (*infra*, 8.2 Pathogenetic mechanisms of lymphomagenesis in the context of the immune status of the host) [126]. In a normal immune response, germinal center B (GCB) cells that have undergone successful affinity maturation of their immunoglobuline differentiate further into plasma cells or memory B-cells, referred to as post-GC or activated B-cells (ABCs).

Molecular studies provide more insight in the strictly regulated processes that enable B-cell activation. A recent study demonstrated an opposite expression pattern of BCL-6 (germinal center cells) and FOXP1 (non-germinal center cells) which was correlated with antagonistic gene expression regulation. FOXP1 is highly expressed in a subset of ABC lymphomas but its exact role is still obscure. It has been suggested that impairment of B-cell activation processes by aberrant FOXP1 expression contributes to lymphomagenesis [127]. During B-cell infection EBV exploits many features of the B-cell differentiation process unnoticed. Only in case of loss of homeostasis can EBV infection predispose to deregulation of physiological B-cell behavior and lymphomagenesis.

8.1.2. Epidemiology and Transmission of EBV

The Epstein-Barr virus, named after its discoverers, was first detected in 1964 in a Burkitt lymphoma cell line [128]. EBV infects over 90% of the world's population, primarily during childhood and can be considered as the most successful known human pathogen [129]. It is a member of the gamma Herpesvirus subfamily that typically persists in lymphoid cells [17, 35]. Transmission occurs very efficiently via saliva and it is estimated that every carrier hosts up to 5.10^5 EBV-infected cells (or $1/10^6$ of all B-cells) [17, 129]. This indicates that once infected, the immune system can never completely eliminate EBV [115, 130].

Despite the ubiquity and lifelong persistence of EBV, only a selected group of infected individuals eventually develops disease following infection, pointing to a crucial role for environmental and genetic factors [131]. Infectious mononucleosis (IM) occurs in 35% to 69% of individuals who become infected during adolescence or young adulthood [4, 115]. Although in most cases IM resolves within one month, about 10% of the affected individuals experience fatigue for 6 months or longer. Severe complications of EBV infection (including encephalitis, hepatitis, severe hemolytic anemia or thrombocytopenia) are seen in about 1% of infected individuals [118].

8.1.3. Infectious Life Cycle of EBV

Like all human Herpesviruses, EBV is an enveloped dsDNA (173 kb) virus that consists of an icosahedral nucleocapsid and tegument. EBV shows tropism for B-cells, but can also infect other cell types [132, 133]. Evidence on whether or not EBV infects epithelial cells *in vivo* has long been conflicting [134-137]. A morphologic study of reactive human tonsils has demonstrated that EBV infection of normal epithelial cells in tonsillar crypts from immunocompetent hosts may occur (rarely) [138]. However, contradictory reports have been published about whether or not (nasopharyngeal) epithelial cells, located in Waldeyer's ring (the lymphoid tissue in the back of the oral cavity), are the primary site of EBV infection, followed by lytic replication [17, 125, 139]. Experiments by Tugizov *et al.* identified a receptor for EBV in normal nasopharyngeal epithelial cells and it has been shown that they are infected *in vivo* [140, 141]. However, because this receptor is expressed at the basolateral surface, epithelial cells are most probably infected from the underlying lymphoid tissue and not from the saliva. It is more likely that epithelial cells are a site of replication during shedding of EBV, as has been shown for oral hairy leukoplakia [129].

The lymphoid tissue present underneath the tonsillar epithelium consists of numerous naive lymphocytes. Entry of B-cells occurs mainly through interaction of EBV's major envelope glycoproteins gp350 and gp42 with the membrane receptor CD21 and the human leukocyte antigen (HLA) class I molecules serving as a co-receptor, respectively. The exact process of infection is not yet entirely clear but the main hypothesis states that EBV first infects a naive B-cell and then takes advantage of the normal process of B-cell differentiation to become persistent in memory B-cells [125]. Upon B-cell infection, the linear viral genome circularizes and is maintained as a nuclear episome that very rarely integrates into the host genome [125, 142, 143]. It encodes a series of proteins that are homologous to or interact with cellular anti-apoptotic proteins, signal transducers and cytokines (e.g., viral IL-10 and anti-apoptotic BCL-2) and that mediate the pathogenic and oncogenic effects of EBV [67, 144]. Viral episomes are usually tethered to the host chromatin by viral proteins [143].

Primary EBV infection is associated with an extensive cellular immune response that mainly targets viral lytic proteins [145]. In a subset of individuals, this response together with the release of (viral) antigens from destructed cells may result in the clinical symptoms of IM (fever, sore throat, myalgia, fatigue, lymphadenopathy, hepatosplenomegaly) accompanied by high titers of IgM and IgG antibodies directed against the viral capsid and envelope (gp350) proteins. After recovery from primary infection, EBV establishes latency in the infected B-cells and is kept under control by a steady antibody response (anti-capsid and anti-gp350) together with 10^3 to 10^4 memory HLA class I-restricted CD8-positive CTLs. B-cells containing lytic EBV are eliminated by these humoral and cellular immune responses so only latently infected B-cells can persist. Notably, cytotoxic responses from HLA class II-restricted CD4-positive T-cells have also been detected [35].

In contrast to most viruses (e.g., HIV, Influenza), EBV has a relatively stable genome and does not vary its epitopes [146]. As a consequence, antibodies can nearly always prevent infection after viral shedding and newly infected B-cells are rapidly killed by CTLs. Therefore re-infection probably does not play a significant role in the maintenance of the pool of infected B-cells and stable latent infection of memory B-cells likely depends primarily on homeostatic cell division [129]. Nevertheless, IgG antibodies that target the viral capsid and gp350 are continuously detected in healthy carriers, indicating that lytic replication still takes place in order to sustain viral shedding and transmission [35]. Epitope conservation guarantees that cells that aberrantly express the broad latency program and fail to differentiate are always targeted by the immune system. This way the host is protected from uncontrollably proliferating lymphoid cells [147].

The life cycle of EBV is characterized by an alteration between the lytic phase and a longer period of latency [148]. Three different latency expression profiles are recognized, each characterized by a specific combination of expressed viral proteins [142]. Within 16 hours after infection the most elaborate latency program (termed latency III, broad latency or the growth program) is activated (Figure 1N and Figure 2), triggering the expression of 9 viral proteins: 6 EBV nuclear antigens (EBNA 1, 2, 3A-C and EBNA-Leader Protein) and 3 latency membrane proteins (LMP 1, 2A-B) together with BamA rightward transcripts (BARTs). BARTs encode two large clusters of microRNAs (miRNAs), which are small non-coding RNAs that (mainly) negatively regulate gene expression post-transcriptionally [149]. Two EBV-encoded RNAs (EBERs) are expressed continuously and used as markers of EBV infection (*supra*, 4. Diagnosis of PTLD). As a result, the B-cell is activated as if it was responding to antigen [129].

The primary role of EBNA1 is to maintain the EBV episome when the infected B-cells divide. It binds the origin of replication (ORI) of the episome and joins it with mitotic chromosomes. EBNA1 is the only viral protein that is detected in virtually all EBV-associated malignancies. Remarkably, EBNA1 contains Gly-Ala repeats that prevent proteasomal degradation and subsequent HLA class I presentation to CTLs [150].

EBNA2 serves as a master transcriptional factor and regulates the expression of the 9 viral genes as well as several cellular genes (*C-MYC, CD21, CD23*). It prevents B-cell differentiation by mimicking Notch signaling and it is essential for transformation [151]. EBNA2 and EBNA-Leader Protein (EBNA-LP) both enhance transcription by decreasing histone deacetylation. The role of EBNA2 as a transactivator of LMP1 and LMP2 expression renders it indispensable for cellular transformation [152]. EBNA3A-C cooperate with EBNA2 and 3A and 3C are required for immortalization of B-cells. Also, EBNA3C can interact with cyclin proteins resulting in disruption of cell cycle checkpoints.

LMP1 is a functional homologue of CD40, a transmembrane costimulatory protein required for activation of antigen-presenting cells (i.e., dendritic cells, macrophages and B-cells). It is the major EBV oncogene and it can activate both the canonical (involved in immune responses) and alternative (important in development and survival of lymphoid cells) NF-κB pathway [153]. As a result of NF-κB induction A20, an inhibitor of the NF-κB pathway, and anti-apoptotic BCL-2 are expressed [154]. *In vitro* studies have shown that LMP1-induced A20 may block TP53-directed apoptosis. Notably, also TERT (telomerase reverse transcriptase) is activated by LMP1 via NF-κB (and MAPK, ERK1/2 pathways). Telomerase is involved in the maintenance of the chromosomal telomere length, which normally decreases with each cell division. Aberrant expression of TERT enables cells to replicate limitlessly [155] but also induces resistance to apoptosis and blocks induction of the lytic cycle [156].

LMP1 signaling plays an important role in survival of infected B-cells going through the GC reaction. It induces c-FLIP (an apoptosis inhibitor) together with IL-10 that functions as an autocrine B-cell lymphoma growth factor. Via induction of HIF-1 and subsequently VEGF (vascular endothelial growth factor) LMP1 can promote angiogenesis [157]. Based on blockage of the GC reaction observed in a transgenic lymphoma mouse model in which LMP1 was constitutively expressed in B-cells it was stated that EBV-driven B-cell differentiation does not occur in the GC but rather takes place extrafollicularly [158]. Yet in reality, expression of LMP1 is tightly controlled by the expression of LMP2, known to stimulate GC development of gut mucosal B-cells [159]. Consequently, in this experiment overexpression of LMP1 by itself was probably the cause of GC blockade [147].

LMP2A is localized in the B-cell membrane and is similar to a constitutively active BCR. It binds tyrosine kinases eventually impairing BCR-mediated activation and entry of the lytic phase. To ensure survival of the infected cells, LMP2A can induce the vital signals normally provided by BCR signaling. In addition, LMP2A prevents reactivation of EBV in latently infected B-cells. LMP2B is thought to be a modulator of LMP2A [35].

The two EBERs are expressed in all latency programs but their function remains largely unknown. In EBV-positive Burkitt Lymphoma (BL) they are thought to inhibit apoptosis (induced by *C-MYC* translocation) and to induce IL-10 expression [160, 161]. Importantly, EBERs have been shown to induce IFN-gamma expression [162] and could account for the IFN-gamma-induced inflammatory responses observed in EBV-positive but not in EBV-negative post-transplant DLBCL (*infra,* 9.2 Pathogenesis of EBV-negative PTLD and the difference with EBV-positive cases).

Fourty-four viral miRNAs encoded by the EBV BHRF (in the 3' UTR of BHRF) and BART clusters have been documented and can regulate cellular genes, possibly conferring resistance to apoptosis. Interestingly, the BHRF protein is the viral homolog of BCL-2. Furthermore, EBV miRNAs can downregulate viral proteins such as LMP1 and LMP2A representing a possible mechanism for immune escape (reviewed in [163]). BHRF-encoded miRNAs are associated with the growth program, whereas BART miRNAs are more variably expressed [164]. Studies have shown that EBV-encoded miRNAs are shed via exosomes, possibly interfering with the immune response against EBV-infected cells [165]. BART11-5p transcriptionally downregulates EBF1 (early B-cell factor 1), an important B-cell transcription factor that regulates PAX5, BCR, CD40 and the germinal center reaction [166]. In an epithelial cancer cell line, BART miRNAs were associated with downregulation of pro-apoptotic BIM and inhibition of etoposide-induced apoptosis [167] suggesting they play a role in cell survival.

It has been postulated that EBNA1, 2, 3A and 3C are critical mediators of the effects of EBV on cell proliferation and survival while EBNA3B, EBERs, and BARTs may be less important (studies cited in [167]) but this has again been argued [161]. Most likely, the coordinated expression of all viral molecules is required to mimic activation of the B-cell resulting in proliferation [125]. Studies have shown that EBV-infected lymphoid B-cells are indeed phenotypically and morphologically similar to antigen-activated B-cells.

EBNA3A, 3B and 3C are highly immunogenic and in healthy individuals the induced proliferation of infected B-cells is countered by a potent CTL and antibody response. Escaping lymphoid B-cells migrate to lymphoid B-cell follicles where the second latency program (also called intermediate latency or the default program, Figure 2) is established. This pattern is characterized by the coordinated expression of LMP1 and 2A, which stimulate the infected B-cells to form a GC, EBNA1 and EBER [147]. Together, these viral gene products enable survival and differentiation of the lymphoid B-cells without the need for interaction with antigen, follicular dendritic cells or T-helper cells [129].

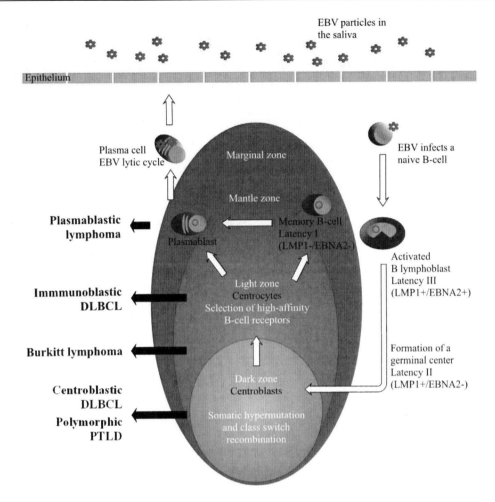

Figure 2. The infectious life cycle of the Epstein-Barr virus and the associated post-transplant lymphoproliferative disorders

After droplet infection, the Epstein-Barr viral particles cross the epithelial barrier of the tonsils. When a naive B-cell is infected, the viral broad latency program is established. Because EBV infection mimics antigen-induced B-cell activation, the infected naive B-cell becomes an activated blast and enters a primary follicle in the lymph node. Upon B-cell proliferation, a germinal center (GC) is formed in the follicle, which is now called a secondary follicle composed of three distinct regions. The marginal zone consists mainly of activated B-cells and plasma cells. The mantle zone or corona comprises lymphocytes that surround the GC. In the GC the intermediate latency profile is expressed and infected B-cell blasts undergo somatic hypermutation and class switch recombination. After leaving the GC, the centrocytes differentiate into plasmablasts and plasma cells or (mainly) memory cells. When an EBV-infected plasma cell is activated by antigen EBV enters the lytic cycle resulting in the production of new virons and viral shedding.

In all stages, the viral episome (red circle) is maintained. During each stage of B-cell development, a B-cell can give rise to malignancy resulting in different lymphoma subtypes that have features of their normal counterpart. Here the stages at which lymphoma may arise are shown for the most common post-transplant lymphoproliferations.

Abbreviations: DLBCL: diffuse large B-cell lymphoma; EBNA: Epstein-Barr virus nuclear antigen; EBV: Epstein-Barr virus; LMP: latency membrane protein; PTLD: post-transplant lymphoproliferative disorder.

First, LMP2 incites B-cells in concert with LMP1 to migrate to a lymphoid follicle and to form a germinal center where it induces somatic hypermutation (SHM) and class switch recombination (CSR) (*supra*, 8.1.1 B-cell biology). BCL-6 is the main transcription factor in the regulation of the germinal center phenotype and in centroblasts (and lymphoma cells) BCL-6 can repress ATR, a crucial protein in the detection of single-stranded DNA damage. By this mechanism, DNA damage is temporarily not detected, allowing SHM of the antibody variable regions during affinity maturation. Uncontrolled activation of BCL-6 however could result in accumulation of genetic alterations promoting lymphomagenesis. Notably, *BCL-6* translocations are among the most frequently reported genetic aberrations in P-PTLD and M-PTLD (*infra*, 10. Pathogenesis of early and polymorphic PTLD, 11. Pathogenesis of monomorphic PTLD). In normal conditions, downregulation of BCL-6 eventually causes centrocytes to leave the germinal center and to differentiate to plasma cells or (mainly) memory B-cells [123].

Table 2. EBV-encoded gene products are expressed in different latency patterns associated with different lymphoproliferative diseases

Latency	Expressed EBV gene products	Normal B-cell stage	Associated disease
Broad latency III	EBER 1-2, EBNA1-3C, EBNA-LP, LMP1-2B	Activated B lymphoblast	PTLD AIDS-related lymphoma EBV-positive DLBCL of the elderly Acute Infectious Mononucleosis
Intermediate latency II	EBER 1-2, EBNA1, LMP1-2A	B-cell undergoing the GC reaction	PTLD Classic Hodgkin lymphoma, Nasopharyngeal carcinoma, EBV-positive DLBCL of the elderly NK/T-cell lymphoma
Restricted latency I	EBER 1-2, EBNA1	Memory B-cell	EBV-positive (post-transplant) Burkitt Lymphoma

Abbreviations: EBV: Epstein-Barr virus; EBER: EBV-encoded RNA; EBNA: EBV nuclear antigen; LP: leader protein; LMP: latency membrane protein; GC: germinal center; PTLD: post-transplant lymphoproliferative disorder; AIDS: acquired immunodeficiency syndrome; DLBCL: diffuse large B-cell lymphoma.

In these memory cells that circulate primarily between the blood and Waldeyer's ring [130] the final latency program (latency I or restricted latency) is expressed, characterized by the expression of only EBERs and EBNA1 for the maintenance of the viral episome (Figure 2). The virtual absence of viral protein expression in the restricted latency profile renders the infected cells hardly immunogenic, allowing the virus to escape host immune responses. For this purpose, EBNA1 has evolved to be a very weak antigen.

It is generally assumed that each EBV-positive B-cell tumor is derived from a B-cell that has been blocked at a specific stage. Therefore, the tumor is thought to express the latency program characteristic of the differentiation stage of its cell of origin (Table 2). One may wonder why EBV needs LMP1 and 2A to drive B-cell differentiation if it can persist in normal antigen-selected B cells that undergo that process anyway. A possible explanation is that these viral proteins give a selective advantage to infected GCB cells in order to increase their chances of entering the pool of memory cells [129].

Latent EBV enters the lytic cycle when infected B-cells are stimulated to differentiate into plasma cells. BCR signaling results in the expression of the viral genes ZEBRA and EBV viral capsid antigen (VCA). In the tonsils, these plasma cells migrate to the epithelium where the viral particles are released and eventually shed into the saliva (Figure 2) [142]. Of note, two different EBV strains are distinguished (Type A and Type B EBV) based on polymorphisms in EBNA proteins and EBER. Intriguingly, type B has a greater potential to initiate EBV lytic replication (*infra*).

8.1.4. NK/T-Cell Biology

Because of the natural cellular tropism of EBV for B-cells and epithelia, the association of EBV with NK/T-cell lymphoma is not straightforward. However, T-cell expression of CD21, the receptor for EBV infection, has been reported [168] and NK-cells may acquire CD21 via interaction with EBV-infected B-cells (at least *in vitro*) [169] providing a potential mechanism for infection of these cells. Nevertheless, in a normal host EBV infection of NK or T-cells is very rare [170] and has only been observed in tonsillar T-cells or NK-cells especially during infectious mononucleosis [138]. The scarcity of natural *in vivo* infection probability explains the rarity of NK/T-cell lymphomas.

8.2. Pathogenetic Mechanisms of Lymphomagenesis in the Context of the Immune Status of the Host

Because of the rarity of post-transplant lymphoma, little is known about the underlying molecular characteristics. Therefore, insight in lymphomagenesis in the immunocompetent population may improve our understanding of PTLD. Because part of PTLDs are EBV-negative an intriguing question is if EBV-negative DLBCLs biologically differ depending on the immune status of the host.

8.2.1. Lymphoma in Immunocompetent Individuals

DLBCL is the most common adult lymphoma, accounting for 40% of non-Hodgkin lymphoma (NHL) cases. DLBCL comprises tumors that are morphologically, genetically and clinically heterogeneous of which still 20%-30% is defined solely based on the nuclear size/morphological characteristics of the tumor cells [4, 171]. Gene expression profiling studies revealed that this heterogeneity is also apparent at the molecular level. In 2000, groundbreaking microarray experiments by Alizadeh *et al.* revealed that there are at least two molecularly distinct genetic profiles of DLBCL with clinical significance. These profiles could be correlated with the signatures of germinal center (GCB) and non-germinal center B-cells respectively [172]. A third profile corresponded to that of primary mediastinal large B-cell lymphoma (PMBCL), a rare but aggressive lymphoma that presumably arises from a thymic B-cell and presents as a mediastinal mass [173]. Germinal-center B cell (GCB) DLBCL is characterized by the expression profile of normal GCB cells. Non-GCB DLBCL is genetically similar to B-cells that are activated upon BCR stimulation and is therefore also referred to as post-GCB DLBCL or activated B-cell (ABC) DLBCL (100). The cell origin of DLBCL significantly correlates with survival: in the study of Alizadeh *et al.* 76% of GCB

DLBCL patients were still alive after 5 years compared to only 16% of ABC DLBCL patients [172]. It should be noted that within the ABC and GCB groups, responsiveness to chemotherapy significantly varies [174]. The group of Kreisel stated that a classification based on predicted chemoresponsiveness might therefore be more clinically relevant [175]. Additionally ABC DLBCL is associated with a higher likelihood of relapse compared to GCB DLBCL [176]. A possible explanation lies in the distinct genetic aberrations found in GCB and ABC DLBCL respectively. Genetic lesions primarily associated with GCB DLBCL are translocations of *C-MYC* (a transcription factor involved in proliferation, differentiation and apoptosis) and mutations in *EZH2* [177, 178]. ABC DLBCL on the other hand is more frequently associated with inactivation of *PRDM1* (which encodes BLIMP-1, a transcription factor that regulates plasma cell differentiation) [179], or translocation of *BCL-6* [180]. Interestingly, loss of BLIMP-1 was shown to be mutually exclusive with *BCL-6* translocations [175]. A hallmark of ABC DLBCL is constitutive activation of the NF-κB transcription factor, a master regulator in normal B-cell development. Both the canonical and the alternative NF-κB pathway may be affected in DLBCL [181]. The proliferative effect of NF-κB is presumably mediated by IRF4/MUM1, a protein also used as a marker of activated B-cells, and CyclinD2, which drives cell cycle progression and is typically expressed in ABC DLBCL [182]. Aberrant NF-κB signaling is frequently caused by mutations in *CARD11, CD79A* (2 members of the BCR complex that influence PI3K and MAPK signaling), *MYD88, BCL-2, A20* [181] and disruption of terminal B-cell differentiation [183].

Via epigenetic modifications of DNA, histone and non-histone targets, gene transcription is fine-tuned and tightly controlled. Apart from genetic mutations, aberrant epigenetic modifications can contribute to the development of malignancy. Recent genome-wide studies revealed a key role for alterations of histone/chromatin-modifying enzymes, in particular methyltransferases (mainly MLL2, mutated in 30% of DLBCLs) and acetyltransferases (mainly CREBBP and EP300, mutated in 35% of DLBCLs) [184, 185] in the pathogenesis of DLBCL. Mutations in CREBBP, which acetylates both histone and non-histone substrates, have been associated with decreased acetylation of BCL-6 resulting in its constitutive activation [186]. MLL2 regulates transcription via trimethylation of lysine-4 on histone 3 (H3K4), a hallmark of actively transcribed chromatin [187], and could function as a haploinsufficient tumor suppressor [188]. Also EZH2, a histone methyltransferase and member of the polycomb group of transcriptional repressors is a frequent target of mutation associated with aberrant gain of function in DLBCL. The identification of mutations in chromatin-modifying enzymes may have implications for future DLBCL treatment: preclinical studies have already demonstrated the therapeutic potential of histone acetyltransferases inhibitors [189] and blocking of EZH2 [190].

Another interesting disease mechanism in DLBCL is the appearance of point mutations in the 5' regulatory regions of genes by aberrant somatic hypermutation (SHM, *supra* 8.1.1 B-cell biology). Pasqualucci *et al.* reported that in DLBCL loci of *C-MYC, PAX5, PIM1* and *RHOH*, four proto-oncogenes, are targeted by aberrant SHM and contain mutations not found in normal B-cells transiting the GC [126]. Recently, a genome-wide approach revealed mutation hotspots in genes previously not known to be mutated (*BACH2, BTG2, CXCR4, CIITA, EBF1, PIM2, TCL1A*) with potentially deleterious effects on transcriptional activity [191]. The preference for transitions (i.e., exchange of a purine for a purine or a pyrimidine for a pyrimidine) over transversions (i.e., exchange of a purine for a pyrimidine or *vice versa*) (the expected transition/transversion ratio is 0.5) and mutations in *CpG* islands and *CG/GC* dinucleotides suggest a role for enzyme-induced deamination of 5-methylcytosine residues e.g., by AICDA that normally mediates SHM during GC transition (*supra*, 8.1.1 B-cell biology) [183]. The regions affected by aberrant SHM are also frequently involved in translocations supporting the hypothesis that aberrant SHM can generate translocations through double-strand DNA breaks [192].

The importance of microRNAs (miRNAs) in oncogenesis has been highlighted by He *et al.* who demonstrated that overexpression of the miR-17-92 miRNA cluster is associated with *C-MYC* deregulation and GCB lymphomagenesis in mice [193]. Several other miRNAs have been implicated in lymphoid malignancy (miR-15a, miR-16-1, miR-155 [194, 195]) and different DLBCL subtypes are correlated with distinct miRNA signatures [196]. The clinical impact of miRNA expression patterns in lymphoma is poorly understood but a recent study suggests that expression of Drosha, involved in miRNA processing, may be related to response to chemotherapy [197].

Two other important processes in the onset of DLBCL are disrupted immune recognition and antigen presentation. Beta2 microglobulin (B2M), a polypeptide component of the MHC class I proteins normally found on all nucleated cells, is frequently lost in DLBCL. This event may be implicated in loss of MHC I class expression. (Tumor) cells lacking MHC I cannot be killed by CTLs enabling them to evade the immune system more easily. Other proteins that recurrently harbor mutations are CD58, a ligand of CD2 involved in the activation of T-cells and NK-cells [198]; TNFSF9 involved in T-cell activation and antigen presentation; CIITA, the master regulator of MHC class II expression [199] and PDL-1 and 2 that decrease CTL proliferation and can induce T-cell apoptosis via BCL-2 signaling [200].

The tumor microenvironment signature has been associated with the outcome of DLBCL patients [201]. This signature represents the global gene expression pattern of the surrounding stroma and infiltrating immune cells and can in many ways influence lymphomagenesis. A limited host immune response and production of immunosuppressive cytokines such as IDO-1, IL-10 or TGF-beta can promote tumor cell survival [202, 203]. The frequent alterations in (the expression of) genes involved in immune recognition and immune responses suggest a central role for immune evasion of tumoral cells in DLBCL pathogenesis.

EBV seems of limited importance in lymphomagenesis in the general population. In the immunocompetent Japanese and Korean population, 10% of DLBCLs is thought to be EBV-positive [204, 205] whereas in the Western world less than 5% of DLBCLs in immunocompetent individuals is EBV-driven (Table 3). As the majority of these cases occur in elderly patients, the degree in which these patients are immunosuppressed due to immunosenescence remains under investigation. Currently, the possible impact of EBV on the prognosis of DLBCL patients is not clear. In a Japanese study, EBV-positive DLBCL was associated with a median overall survival of 2 years and a 5-year survival of approximately 25% [206]. In a Korean study involving 380 immunocompetent DLBCL patients, EBV-positive lymphoma was associated with older age (>60 years), more extranodal involvement, a higher IPI index and poorer response to initial treatment compared to EBV-negative lymphoma [205]. Similar results have been published for other DLBCL series [207, 208]. In one Japanese case series, EBV was not predictive of prognosis [204]. Overall, these studies suggest a negative impact of EBV on the prognosis of DLBCL patients. However these studies mainly comprise Asian and Hispanic populations and elderly patients which may confound the results. In our meta-analysis of 102 cases of immunocompetent plasmablastic lymphoma (PBL, a terminally differentiated variant of DLBCL) (Morscio *et al.*, accepted by

AJSP 2013) EBV-positivity was a good prognostic factor, also within the group of immunocompetent PBL patients ≥50 years of age. The discrepancy between the reported studies and our meta-analysis may be explained by (1) the influence of the biology of different DLBCL subtypes on the prognostic impact of EBV and (2) the overrepresentation of elderly patients in the EBV-positive lymphoma series of the aforementioned studies but not in our PBL meta-analysis (the median age of the immunocompetent patients with EBV-positive and –negative PBL was almost similar: 66 years and 63 years respectively).

Table 3. Association of EBV with lymphoma in the context of the host's immune status

LPDs in the general population	
-Diffuse large B-cell lymphoma	<5%-10%
-Primary CNS lymphoma	9%-14%
-EBV-positive DLBCL of the elderly	100%
Organ transplantation-related LPDs	
-Early and polymorphic lesions	80%-100%
-Monomorphic lesions	60%-80%
HIV/AIDS-related LPDs	
-Primary CNS lymphoma	100%
-Diffuse large B-cell lymphoma	80%
-Burkitt lymphoma	30%-50%
-Plasmablastic lymphoma	60%
Immunomodulatory agents-related LPDs	
-Reactive lesions	10%-?
-Diffuse large B-cell lymphoma	50%-?
Primary immunodeficiency-related LPDs	
-Diffuse large B-cell lymphoma	30%-60%

LPDs in immunocompromised patients are more strongly associated with EBV than LPDs in the general population, however the association is still variable and may differ for reactive versus malignant lesions and also for different subtypes of malignant lymphoma.
Abbreviations: AIDS: acquired immunodeficiency syndrome; CNS: central nervous system; EBV: Epstein-Barr Virus; HIV: Human immunodeficiency virus; LPDs: lymphoproliferative disorders.

8.2.2. Lymphoma in Immunocompromised Individuals

Except for PTLDs the WHO currently discriminates four other types of lymphoproliferative disorders (LPDs) associated with immunodeficiency: (1) lymphomas associated with HIV infection, (2) methotrexate-associated LPDs seen most frequently in patients with autoimmune disease, (3) LPDs associated with primary immune disorders and (4) the provisional category of LPDs associated with age-related immunosenescence. Common features of these LPDs are a predominant B-cell origin, extranodal involvement, a morphological spectrum ranging from benign LPDs to different types of lymphoma and the involvement of oncogenic viruses, mainly EBV (Table 3) [4]. Insight in the mechanisms involved in the expansion of EBV-infected B-cells in each of these immunodeficiency-associated LPDs is helpful in understanding EBV-driven PTLD.

8.2.2.1. Lymphoma in Human Immunodeficiency Virus (HIV)-Infected Patients

After the first case of human immunodeficiency virus (HIV)-related lymphoma was documented in 1985, it became clear that the impaired immunosurveilllance against EBV due to destruction of T-cells made HIV patients susceptible to EBV-related LPDs ranging from benign disorders to Hodgkin and non-Hodgkin lymphoma (NHL). Overall, the incidence of NHL is 60-200 fold higher in HIV-infected individuals compared to the general population [209, 210]. Currently NHL is still one of the main causes of death of AIDS patients [211]. The most common AIDS-associated NHLs are DLBCL, plasmablastic lymphoma (PBL), Burkitt lymphoma (BL), and primary CNS lymphoma (PCNSL). CNS involvement typically affects the most severely immunocompromised patients [212] and is markedly more common in HIV (and PTLD) patients than in immunocompetent lymphoma patients (*supra*).

Lymphomagenesis following HIV infection is associated with the amount of HIV RNA copies and CD4-positive T-cells (the risk increases dramatically at >100,000 HIV-1 RNA copies/ml and/or <50 CD4-positive T-cells/µl, [213]). Interestingly, CD4-positive (cytotoxic) T-cells may play an important role in controlling EBV infection. Products released by activated cells (among which IL-21) may limit EBV-positive B-cell proliferation by downregulating EBNA2 [214].

With the introduction of highly active antiretroviral therapy (HAART) the adjusted incidence of NHL decreased from 6.2% pre-HAART (1992–1999) to 3.2% in the HAART era (1997–1999) [209]. However, the view that immunodeficiency *per se* is not the only cause of malignancy is illustrated by the striking rise in incidence of Hodgkin lymphoma in AIDS patients in the HAART era compared to the pre-HAART era [215, 216].

The association of EBV with AIDS-related non-Hodgkin lymphomas depends on the histologic variant: the association is strongest for PCNSL (100% EBV-positive), followed by immunoblastic DLBCL (80% EBV-positive) and Burkitt lymphoma (30%-50% EBV-positive) [217, 218]. Notably, type A and type B EBV (*supra*, 8.1.1 B-cell biology) are equally prevalent in HIV-related NHL, although the latter is associated with later-onset disease. A possible explanation could be that type B is less oncogenic due to its increased ability to lyse the host cell [219].

Chronic immune system activation is a hallmark of HIV pathogenesis and potentially contributes to lymphomagenesis by inducing expansion of EBV-infected B-cells (reviewed in [212]) similarly to chronic immune stimulation by the graft in transplant patients or by *Helicobacter pylori* in gastric MALT lymphoma [220]. Studies have demonstrated that HIV can directly induce polyclonal B-cell expansion [221] and can modulate expression of cytokines by the lymphoma cells that interact with HIV proteins [222].

A study of the microenvironment of AIDS-related DLBCL demonstrated increased tumor vascularization and a higher number of infiltrating CTLs in EBV-positive lymphomas compared to EBV-negative cases. This suggests that despite their compromised immune system, HIV patients can still mount immune responses against virus-infected tumor cells [223]. Regarding gene expression EBV-negative AIDS-related NHLs were indistinguishable from lymphomas in the immunocompetent population [224] (we found similar results for EBV-negative lymphoma in transplant and immunocompetent patients; *infra*, 9.2 Pathogenesis of EBV-negative PTLD and the difference with EBV-positive cases). Importantly, since the introduction of HAART the incidence of mainly EBV-positive AIDS-related DLBCL decreased [223] suggesting that partial restoration of the immune system by anti-retroviral therapy may prevent the development of EBV-associated lymphomas.

8.2.2.2. Lymphoma in Patients Treated with Immunomodulatory Agents

Autoimmune diseases such as reumathoid arthritis, inflammatory bowel disease, and psoriasis are locally or systemically treated with immunosuppressive corticosteroids (prednisone, dexamethasone, *etc*) or non-steroid drugs (azathioprine, cyclophosphamide, sirolimus, methotrexate, *etc*). For aggressive disease refractory to these regimens, targeted therapies have been developed including monoclonal antibodies (targeting TNF-alpha, CD25) and receptor antagonists (targeting IL-1 receptor). These drugs are generally referred to as immunomodulatory agents (IA). They may suppress the autoimmune inflammatory reaction and prevent further tissue damage by blocking the activation of auto-reactive cells and the production of inflammatory cytokines.

Despite their different mechanisms of action, a number of IAs (mainly methotrexate and azathioprine) have been associated with an increased risk for lymphoproliferative disorders (immunomodulatory agent-related lymphoproliferative disorders, IAR-LPD) however these data are not supported by definite epidemiological evidence. *In vitro* studies have shown that methotrexate can reactivate EBV from latently infected lymphoblastoid cell lines (LCLs). Additionally, higher viral loads of EBV have been demonstrated in patients treated with methotrexate [225] and (especially EBV-positive) methotrexate-associated LPDs often (partially) regress after methotrexate withdrawal. Reactivation of EBV together with the immunosuppressive effects of methotrexate could explain the (rare) occurrence of lymphomas. Also targeted agents may pose a risk even without directly causing immunosuppression. For example blocking of TNF-α may impair GC formation which interferes with normal B-cell development and potentially contributes to lymphomagenesis [226, 227].

One study reported that patients treated with IAs can present with a variety of lymphoproliferations, including (non-)Hodgkin and T-cell lymphoma. Interestingly, EBV was strongly associated with B-cell lymphoma (6/11 cases expressed EBER) in contrast to more benign lymphoid proliferations (1/6 cases expressed EBER) [227].

Together with the observation that withdrawal of the IA may result in regression of the lymphoproliferation [228] these findings support the hypothesis that modulation of immune reponses can lead to LPDs. Importantly, monoclonal IA-related lymphoma is less likely to respond to cessation of therapy [226] similarly to monoclonal PTLD.

8.2.2.3. Lymphoma in Patients with Primary Immunodeficiency

Primary immunodeficiencies (PIDs) are inherited or *de novo* genetic conditions, i.e., not caused by another disease, drug treatment or environmental exposure to toxins. Compared to the general population PID patients have a higher risk of lymphoma, which accounts for 60% of PID-associated malignancies [229].

PIDs are rare (1/10.000 live births) and heterogeneous. The subtypes most commonly associated with LPDs are B- and T-cell deficiencies (e.g., severe combined immunodeficiency, SCID), antibody deficiencies (e.g., common variable immunodeficiency, CVID), immune dysregulation (e.g., X-linked lymphoproliferative disease, XLP), defects in innate immunity (e.g., WHIM, an acronym for warts, hypogammaglobulinemia, infections, and myelokathexis), autoinflammatory disorders (e.g., familial mediterranean fever) and complement deficiencies. Due to the rarity of PID-associated lymphoma and the variety of PIDs (there are over 175 subtypes [230]), not much is known about the underlying disease mechanisms. Similarly to PTLDs, lymphoma in PID patients is commonly of B-cell origin (most frequently DLBCL), arises extranodally (frequently the CNS and gastro-intestinal tract are affected) and associated with EBV in 30%-60% of the cases [231].

Interestingly, XLP is associated with fulminant infectious mononucleosis, a potentially fatal exacerbated immune response to primary EBV infection due to defective EBV-specific immunity. In XLP, fulminant infectious mononucleosis is associated with mutations in SAP (SLAM-associated protein) that abrogate T-B-cell interactions impairing T-cell activation by EBV-infected B-cells. Due to limited data and PID case series therapy of PID patients is tailored taking into account the specific clinical and histological characteristics of each case. So far, allogeneic SCT has been successfully applied for the treatment of PID-related lymphomas suggesting that the underlying immune disorder is the main risk factor [5].

8.2.2.4. EBV-Positive DLBCL in Elderly Patients

In 2003, Oyama *et al.* reported 22 immunocompetent elderly patients over 60 years of age diagnosed with EBV-associated LPDs and suggested that age-related immunosenescence was at the basis of disease [232]. Although not all immune functions are affected with age (e.g., innate immunity is re-enforced [217]) several studies have supported this hypothesis. Fagnoni *et al.* studied the association between the number of circulating naive CD8-positive T-cells and age and discovered that in elderly people these cells are significantly reduced [233]. Another study demonstrated that the frequency of CD8-positive T-cells bearing a receptor specific for an immunodominant EBV lytic epitope was surprisingly higher in older compared to younger subjects. However, the fraction of these cells that could produce IFN-gamma was significantly lower in older individuals suggesting that with age defective T-cells accumulate [234]. Combined, these events could contribute to immunosuppression associated with aging and more specifically to a decrease in T-cell function. This may eventually facilitate uncontrolled proliferation of EBV-positive B-cells [235].

Because DLBCLs in patients with "acknowledged immunodeficiency" (mainly AIDS patients, transplant recipients) and in elderly patients have common features (morphological heterogeneity, association with EBV, extranodal involvement, *supra*) EBV-positive DLBCL of the elderly has been recognized as a provisional entity of immunodeficiency-associated lymphoma in the WHO classification of Tumors of Hematopoietic and Lymphoid Tissues (2008). It is defined as 'a blastic proliferation of a B-cell clone in association with EBV occurring in patients over 50 years of age' [4]. Cases of EBV-positive DLBCL in younger patients without evidence of immunodeficiency have also been reported [206, 207] underlining that the proposed age limit is not absolute. The incidence of EBV-positive DLBCL of the elderly seems to depend on the geographical location and/or ethnicity. The incidence is highest in Asian countries (5-11%) compared to Europe and the United States (<5%) [4].

Similarly to PTLDs different histological subtypes of EBV-positive DLBCL of the elderly have been described. Reactive polyclonal proliferations with an intact nodal architecture are associated with a limited number of EBV-positive cells and are frequently self-limiting. Histologic transformation to classic Hodgkin lymphoma (cHL) has been described. cHL may arise from Reed-Sternberg-like cells that are commonly detected in reactive lesions of elderly individuals [236]. EBV-positive cells are more frequent in nodal or extranodal (mainly EBV-associated mucocutaneous ulcer) polymorphous lesions that consist of neoplastic B-cells of all stages of B-cell maturation and infiltrations of small lymphocytes and Reed-Sternberg-like cells, reminiscent of P-PTLD (*supra*, 2. PTLD histology) [237]. The third subtype comprises monomorphic lesions characterized by more uniform neoplastic cells with a minimal or no residual reactive infiltrate. In both polymorphous and monomorphic lesions, the underlying lymph node structure is effaced by the tumor cells and frequently shows areas of extensive necrosis, which is usually associated with EBV infection.

Most commonly, cases of senile EBV-positive lymphoproliferations show mixed histology with numerous mitoses and tingible body macrophages containing apoptotic bodies [238].

Regarding overall survival, localized reactive and extranodal polymorphic lesions have a good outcome (respectively 100% and 93% of the patients survive for 5 years). Nodal polymorphic and monomorphic lesions behave aggressively (respectively 57% and 25% of the patients survive for 5 years) [232, 236]. The difference in prognosis may be partly related to the presence of clonal B-cell populations, which may be a sign of disease progression. Such B-cell populations are markedly more frequent in nodal polymorphic and monomorphic lesions than in reactive and extranodal lesions. Another potential explanation is the accumulation of clonal B-cells due to reduced development of new naïve B-cells in aging individuals [236]. Similarly, restricted or clonal T-cell populations that are frequently observed may reflect the accumulation of clonal (CD8-positive) T-cells. These clonal B-cell and T-cell populations recognize a more limited range of epitopes, increasing the patient's susceptibility to chronic infection [236, 239, 240]. An important question is to what extent this is applicable to the pathogenesis B-cell PTLD. Perhaps iatrogenic immunosuppression following transplantation favors accumulation of oligoclonal B-cells that may eventually result in EBV-negative PTLD due to mutation, selection and aberrant proliferation of a monoclonal B-cell. Simultaneously, suppression of T-cells could promote expansion of clonal populations in PTLD lesions.

Senile EBV-positive DLBCLs are predominantly of ABC origin which correlates with activation of NF-κB-related pathways [241]. LMP1 is positive in the majority of the cases (>90%) and may be accompanied by EBNA2 expression (25%-30% of the cases) corresponding to the latency II (LMP1+/EBNA2-) or latency III (LMP1+/EBNA2+) program. Expression of viral proteins is thought to be tolerated only in the context of immunodeficiency (HIV infection or organ transplantation) suggesting that at least part of the elderly LPD patients are considerably immunocompromised [206, 242]. Genetic alterations of *BCL-2*, *BCL-6* or *C-MYC* are rarely found in EBV-positive DLBCL of the elderly suggesting that chromosomal aberrations are dispensable in the presence of EBV [242, 243].

8.2.2.5. PTLDs

The focus of this chapter lies on PTLDs, an emerging problem in medicine. Iatrogenic immunosuppression following organ transplantation is together with AIDS the most prevalent form of acquired immunodeficiency [244].

PTLDs are most likely caused by a combination of different factors (age at transplantation, graft type, immunosuppression, EBV; *supra*, 3. Risk factors in PTLD) and as many of these are intercorrelated it is difficult to analyze the contribution of each factor separately. Blood transfusions could be regarded as a rare example of transplantation without immunosuppression, and have in some studies been associated with a higher risk for Hodgkin lymphoma. A possible explanation is that blood transfusions can be considered as a source of latently infected B-cells. Nevertheless, these results are questionable because of the variety of underlying diseases of the recipients that can theoretically also contribute to cancer development [61]. Immunosuppression without transplantation occurs in individuals with congenital or acquired (HIV, treatment with immunomodulatory agents) immunodeficiency (and high age), conditions that are also associated with a higher incidence of lymphoma. However, the genetic defect itself or chronic antigen stimulation (HIV infection, autoimmune disease, *Helicobacter pylori* infection) may also contribute to a higher risk for malignancy [61].

Different groups have attempted to generate a PTLD mouse model by (1) injecting primary EBV-positive human PTLD tumor cells or (2) *in vitro* transformed B-cells in severely combined immunodeficient (SCID) mice [245, 246], and (3) by generating mice that overexpress the EBV-protein LMP1 specifically in B-cells, resulting in the development of a PTLD-like lymphoproliferative disease [247]. When validated, such mouse models will represent valuable tools for molecular and preclinical studies on PTLD pathogenesis.

In this part of the chapter we try to shed light on the known parameters that drive PTLD and aim to suggest new directions for the development of novel therapeutics based on the current molecular insights in PTLD pathogenesis. The key pathogenic mechanisms are summarized in Figure 3.

9. Oncogenic Potential of EBV in PTLD

Since the discovery of EBV, evidence for a potential role of EBV in oncogenesis has accumulated (Table 4). *In vitro*, the oncogenic potential of EBV is demonstrated by the transformation of B-cells into latently infected lymphoblastoid cell lines (LCLs). LCLs express the EBV broad latency program (LMP1+/EBNA2+) and typically upregulate B-cell activation markers that are also expressed in B-cells upon antigenic or mitogenic stimulation [35]. Cell cycle activation by induction of cyclin-dependent kinases and upregulation of anti-apoptotic genes (*BIRC5* encoding survivin) are among the earliest events following *in vitro* EBV infection of human tonsillar B-cells [248]. Comparison of established LCLs with normal B-cells additionally revealed upregulation of spindle checkpoint-related genes (including *PLK1, AURKA/B, NUP37, CENPA, BUB1B, CDCA8*) which may compromise the stability of the host genome. Downregulation of pathways involved in T-cell/B-cell activation (*CD3D, CD4, CD3G, ZAP70, LCP2, ITK*) and decreased expression of MHC-II/TCR/BCR and cytokines (*CXCR4, CXCL1*) indicate that EBV infection may enable immune evasion of infected lymphoma cells [249]. Together these data show us that EBV simultaneously influences many different signaling pathways that favor survival and offer a selective advantage to the infected cell. *In vivo*, the impact of EBV in translated in the induction of transient proliferation and latent persistence in non-pathogenic memory B-cells.

When taking into account the gene expression changes observed in LCLs, it is remarkable that in infected individuals EBV is not primarily oncogenic and even minimizes the risk of cancer by pushing its host cell towards a resting state [129]. The finding that EBV-driven B-cell lymphoproliferations are mainly associated with (primary or secondary) immunodeficiency suggests that a proper host immune response is sufficient to protect from potentially fatal EBV driven malignancy. On the other hand not all immunosuppressed individuals develop lymphoproliferative disorders although they carry approximately 50 times more infected cells than healthy EBV carriers. Even in an immunosuppressed state, EBV-associated tumors are rare. Only when an infected naive B-cell fails at becoming a memory cell and when CTL function is disrupted due to e.g., immunosuppressive drugs, uncontrolled lymphoproliferation can occur. The same could happen with any B-cell other than a naive B-cell that becomes infected by EBV (the so-called bystander-infected cells, e.g., memory B-cells). Such clones of directly infected germinal center B-cells and memory cells have been found in acutely infected patients, but in a normal host they are eliminated by a CTL response [250]. In infectious mononucleosis (IM) up to 50% of memory B-cells can be EBV-infected but because they do not express broad latency and are not proliferating blasts IM does not result in malignancy [147].

Table 4. Arguments pro and contra an oncogenic role of EBV

Arguments pro
In vitro evidence demonstrates the oncogenic properties of EBV(-encoded proteins)
Transgenic mice overexpressing LMP1 in B-cells develop lymphomas
Injection of an EBV-transformed LCL in mice induces lymphomas
EBV naivety is a risk factor for PTLD development.
Preemptive infusion with EBV-specific CTLs decreases the risk for PTLD development
EBV-positive lymphoma arises earlier following transplantation than EBV-negative lymphoma
Clonal EBV in monoclonal tumors suggests EBV infection is early event in PTLD pathogenesis
Some lymphoma subtypes are invariably associated with EBV (endemic Burkitt lymphoma, nasal-type extranodal NK/T-cell lymphoma, primary CNS lymphoma in HIV-patients)
Arguments contra
Because EBV is a ubiquitous virus its presence in (immunodeficiency-related) lymphoma could be coincidental
Not all PTLDs are EBV-positive
EBV-postive lymphoma is still rare (even in immunocompromised individuals) despite the ubiquity of EBV

Abbreviations: CNS: central nervous system; CTL: cytotoxic T-lymphocyte; EBV: Epstein-Barr virus; HIV: human immunodeficiency virus; LCL: lymphoblastoid cell line; LMP: latency membrane protein; NK-cell: natural killer cell; PTLD: post-transplant lymphoproliferative disorder.

EBV-driven monoclonal B-cell PTLD has been mainly associated with latency type III, although the other latency profiles also occur, partly depending on the histogenic lymphoma subtype. More profound immunosuppression is linked to a higher latency pattern in which more viral proteins are expressed. Also, GCB lymphoma rather expresses latency I, while more elaborate latency patterns are associated with post-GC or ABC lymphoma [142]. The reason for this is not clear but may be related to opposing molecular pathways: GCB-derived lymphomas frequently rely on aberrant C-MYC signaling and studies have demonstrated that C-MYC expression is incompatible with LMP1 expression (*infra*, 12.1 Post-transplantation Burkitt lymphoma). It is generally accepted that LMP1 and EBNA2 are indispensable for oncogenesis [251, 252] so EBV-associated malignancies expressing latency I or II probably require additional genetic alterations or stimulating interactions with the microenvironment [35, 243].

It is not clear whether for a given PTLD all tumor cells express the same latency program. In a study by Vakiani *et al.* the number of LMP1- and EBNA2-positive cells varied, suggesting the expression of multiple latency types [253]. Heterogeneous expression of viral proteins may have important implications for immunotherapy and may explain the variable success of reduction of immunosuppression in treatment of EBV-positive PTLD (*supra*, 5. Treatment options for PTLD). Tumor cells expressing many viral proteins will be rapidly eliminated whereas those with a more limited expression pattern could escape.

Keeping in mind the ubiquity of EBV, the presence of EBV in PTLD could be a mere coincidence rather than it being the cause of disease. However, the occurrence of clonal EBV in monoclonal tumors suggests that EBV infection is an early event in lymphomagenesis [5]. Furthermore, EBV-positive M-PTLD arises significantly earlier following transplantation than EBV-negative cases indicating that EBV infection is a driver of disease onset [7].

9.1. EBV Lytic Infection in PTLD

In an immunocompetent host infected B-cells rarely undergo lytic infection. In contrast, dispersed lytically active tumor cells are frequently observed in EBV-associated PTLD (unpublished observation; [254]). Since the lytic cycle of EBV is associated with destruction of the host cell, lytic activity should be limited for the tumor to be viable. This is reflected by the occurrence of the two EBV types (*supra*, 8.1.3 Infectious life cycle of EBV). Type A EBV, which has less lytic potential than type B EBV, has been identified in the vast majority (92%) of a series of B-cell PTLDs whereas type B EBV seems to be more prevalent in HIV patients with late-onset EBV-associated lymphoma (*supra*, 8.2.2.1 Lymphoma in human immunodeficiency virus (HIV)-infected patients). This suggests that the degree and duration of immunodeficiency are associated with the EBV genotype [219]. The potential association between the graft type and the EBV strain is not yet explored but because post-transplantation the degree of immunosuppression depends on the graft, different grafts may be associated with a predilection for one the two EBV strains.

Independently of the strain the lytic program of EBV seems to be of importance during the early stages of B-cell transformation, in particular for immune evasion and angiogenesis. The viral *BCRF-1* gene encodes viral IL-10 that suppresses IFN-gamma synthesis and CTLs [255]. The viral BZLF-1 protein on the other hand has been associated with increased expression of VEGF (vascular endothelial growth factor) and IL-6, both involved in angiogenesis [256]. More evidence for the role of the lytic program in promoting EBV-driven lymphomagenesis is given by a recent animal study. Injection of lytic replication-competent EBV virus in a humanized mouse model (in which human fetal CD34-positive hematopoietic stem cells and thymus/liver tissue were transplanted) resulted in more frequent lymphoma development than injection of the lytic replication-defective variant [257]. *In vitro* studies have shown that B-cells transformed with lytically defective EBV produce markedly less proliferation-promoting factors (IL-6, IL-10, and viral IL-10) [258] indicating that the lytic EBV replication program is an important promotor of lymphomagenesis.

9.2. Pathogenesis of EBV-Negative PTLD and the Difference with EBV-Positive Cases

Although the majority of PTLDs (60%-80%) is associated with EBV infection, a significant part is negative for this virus. Currently, it is not clear whether these EBV-negative cases represent true PTLDs or whether they are coincidental cases of lymphoma that are indistinguishable from lymphoma in an immunocompetent host [259].

One possible explanation for the pathogenesis of EBV-negative PTLD is provided by the hit-and-run theory which states that after transformation EBV-infected B-cells may eventually lose (part of) the viral genome. This theory is based on loss of the EBV genome in a number of cells of the EBV-positive Burkitt lymphoma Akata cell line [260]. It is possible that after transformation, the viral episome becomes redundant for survival of the cell (due to the accumulation of genetic aberrations) and is lost as expression of viral proteins makes the infected cells a target for the immune system [143]. Until now the (little) evidence that supports the occurrence of hit-and-run EBV infection as a cause of malignancy is limited to *in vitro* studies [261].

Given the strong association between EBV and PTLD it is feasible that other infectious agents are implicated in the pathogenesis of EBV-negative PTLD. A possible candidate is HHV8 that is present in all primary effusion lymphomas and Castleman-associated lymphomas and is like EBV a gamma Herpesvirus that persistently infects B-cells. However, if HHV8 is found at all in PTLD, these cases are frequently associated with previous/simultaneous HHV-8-related disorders (Castleman's disease or Kaposi's sarcoma) which probably favored development of HHV-8-positive PTLD [262, 263].

A few studies have suggested a role for the Cytomegalovirus (CMV) as a risk factor for PTLD development. However as CMV does not infect B-cells it can only play an indirect role. A recent study strongly associated CMV with reactivation of EBV which could be attributed to the immunosuppressive effects of CMV [264]. Alternatively, CMV could contribute to PTLD onset via chronic antigen stimulation.

As in HIV-positive patients, chronic immune activation post-transplantation by the graft may account for (part of) EBV-negative PTLDs. This hypothesis is discussed more in detail in 11.2 Chronic antigen stimulation.

Finally, it is possible that EBV-negative PTLD is truly independent of infection, immune status or presence of a graft. Two small gene expression profiling (GEP) studies have been performed on PTLD cases in an attempt to elucidate the differences between EBV-positive and –negative cases. These studies yielded somewhat conflicting results. Craig *et al.* performed a microarray analysis on a group of 4 EBV-positive and 4 EBV-negative M-PTLDs and demonstrated segregation of these cases based on the EBV status. Antiviral immune responses (*IRF7*, *EBI2-3*, interferon-induced: *MX1*, *IFITM1*, *IFITM3*) and genes involved in the cell cycle (*CDC2*, *CKS2*, *CDKN3*) were upregulated in EBV-positive compared to EBV-negative M-PTLD. Components of the BCR and their downstream signaling molecules (*SYK*, *LYN*, *LCK*, *SH3BP5*, and *BLNK*) on the other hand were downregulated in EBV-positive compared to EBV-negative M-PTLD [265]. These results are reminiscent of the gene expression differences between *in vitro* EBV transformed LCL and normal B-cells (*supra*, 9. Oncogenic potential of EBV in PTLD).

One explanation for the decreased expression of BCR components is the activity of LMP2A, a viral EBV latency protein that takes over BCR signaling (*supra*, 8.1.3 Infectious life cycle of the Epstein-Barr virus). This mechanism of action also explains how some PTLDs that lack a BCR as a result of crippling Ig mutations can persist [259, 265].

The group of Vakiani *et al.* could not reproduce the segregation of EBV-positive and -negative tumors in their series of 12 PTLDs (1 IM-like lesion, 5 P-PTLD and 6 M-PTLD) but showed that PTLDs were clearly distinct from immunocompetent non-Hodgkin lymphomas [253]. Clearly, no consensus exists on the role of EBV and the molecular features of PTLD. Based on the results of gene expression profiling on our series of 33 post-transplant DLBCLs (72% EBV-positive), we were able to explain some of the inconsistencies [266]. First of all, we confirmed that EBV-positive post-transplant DLBCLs do differ from EBV-negative post-transplant DLBCLs. The major differentially expressed pathways involve innate immune responses induced by IFN (*IFIT, IFI, OAS, HERC5*), natural killer and CTLs (*KLRD1, NKG7*, perforin, granulysin) which were significantly overrepresented in EBV-positive post-transplant DLBCL compared to EBV-negative post-transplant DLBCL. In contrast to previous GEP studies on LCL (*supra*), cell cycle activation and upregulation of anti-apoptotic genes were not among the primary pathways associated with EBV-positive PTLD. This discrepancy may be explained by the absence of a microenvironment when studying *in vitro* EBV-induced transformation. The differences between the study of Craig *et al.* and ours are likely due to different methods and stringency in GEP analysis and the proportion of GCB and ABC lymphomas included in the study. In both studies, all EBV-positive M-PTLD were of ABC origin, however 3 of 4 EBV-negative M-PTLD were of GCB origin in the study of Craig *et al.* compared to 5 of 11 of the EBV-negative M-PTLD in our study.

A new finding we reported is the upregulation of genes involved in immunotolerance (*IDO-1, VSIG4, CD274*) in EBV-positive compared to EBV-negative post-transplant DLBCL. IDO-1 (indoleamine 2,3-dioxygenase 1) is involved in suppression of T-cells and induction of regulatory T-cells that modulate immune responses. Interestingly, IDO-1 upregulation was demonstrated in EBV-positive but not in EBV-negative gastric carcinoma [267] suggesting that its upregulation is specifically triggered by (the presence of) EBV and does not depend on the tissue environment. Immunohistochemical staining on our series of EBV-positive post-transplant DLBCL revealed that IDO-1 can be expressed by both tumor cells and dendritic cells indicative for reciprocal interactions between tumor cells and stroma.

Also VSIG4 and CD274 are negative regulators of T-cells. VSIG4 is a member of the B7 family of immune regulatory proteins and suppresses T-cell proliferation as well as IL-2 production [268]. CD274 is better known as programmed death ligand 1 (PDL-1) and blocks T-cell proliferation and cytokine production when it interacts with its receptor (PDCD1) expressed on T-cells. CD274 is known to be induced in EBV-positive PTLD (potentially by LMP1) [269].

Proteins involved in immunotolerance may be directly induced by EBV in the malignant cells or may be expressed in the surrounding stroma. Most likely both mechanisms occur. Importantly, the induction of immunotolerance may contribute to the early onset of EBV-positive compared to EBV-negative PTLD. Based on the central importance of inflammation as well as immunotolerance we hypothesize that EBV-positive PTLDs are dependent on the microenvironment and the oncogenic stimuli of EBV compared to EBV-negative PTLDs. Therefore, it is possible that the current treatment protocol for PTLD, which is based on RIS, rituximab, and chemotherapy (*supra*, 5. Treatment options for PTLD) is not sufficient to effectively treat EBV-associated PTLDs. New therapeutic approaches should focus more on modulation of the microenvironment (e.g., inhibition of IDO-1) and blocking of oncogenic EBV signaling (e.g., inhibition of LMP1).

Finally our study revealed that EBV-negative post-transplant DLBCL is biologically similar to EBV-negative DLBCL in immunocompetent individuals. This result is partly argued by the study of Vakiani *et al.* who stated that PTLDs differ from non-Hodgkin lymphomas in the general population. However, only 4/12 cases included in that GEP study were EBV-negative, suggesting that is was actually the different EBV-status that resulted in segregation of the lymphomas based on the immune status. Decreased T-cell signaling in biopsies from EBV-negative transplant compared to EBV-negative immunocompetent patients was the only significantly differentially expressed pathway we found and is very likely due to the immunosuppressive regimen administrated following transplantation. This difference underscores that the immunocompromised condition of PTLD patients should not be overlooked. The observation that some EBV-negative PTLDs may regress upon RIS suggests a role for immune responses in at least part of the EBV-negative lesions probably because effective anti-tumor immune responses may be established also when EBV is not involved. Furthermore, it is possible that despite the biological similarity with lymphoma in the general population EBV-negative post-transplant lymphoma disseminates more easily due to the weakened immune system of transplant recipients.

10. Pathogenesis of Early and Polymorphic PTLD

At an early stage, aberrant polyclonal B-cell proliferation (induced by EBV) may give rise to early or polymorphic PTLD (E- and P-PTLD) primarily resembling florid reactive infiltrations. Normally, no cytogenetic alterations are present in E-PTLD and although clonal genomic alterations are rare in P-PTLD, *BCL-6* is mutated in 50% of the cases and associated with aggressive disease [270]. A study that analyzed chromosomal imbalances in PTLD reported loss of 17q23-q25 in one of three polyclonal PTLDs whereas more alterations (gain of 1q31-q44, 5p, 10q23-q26 and loss of X) were detected in monoclonal P-PTLD (of note, all cases were EBV-positive and none of the imbalances was recurrent) [271]. Another study reported clonal lesions (rearrangement of 1q21.3 and a gain of the X chromosome) in 15% of a series of 13 P-PTLD [272]. These findings illustrate that P-PTLDs are premalignant lesions in which genetic aberrations start to accumulate. It is not known whether aberrant somatic hypermutation (SHM), which is involved in DLBCL, also plays a role in P-PTLD. One study comprising 5 P-PTLD found no aberrant SHM of *PIM-1*, *PAX-5*, *RhoH/TTF* or *C-MYC* [273] but these results do not exclude that other genes are affected.

11. Pathogenesis of Monomorphic PTLD

Similarly to the immunocompetent population, DLBCL is the most frequently occurring lymphoma subtype in transplant patients. Pathologic studies have confirmed that like DLBCL in immunocompetent hosts, post-transplant DLBCL may be of GCB or ABC/non-GCB origin [274]. The cell of origin is classically determined based on the Hans' immunostain algorithm that uses three markers (CD10, BCL6, MUM1) to distinguish GCB and non-GCB DLBCL

[275]. By adding two markers (GCET and FOXP1) Choi *et al.* refined the Hans' algorithm [276].

Genotypic analysis of somatic hypermutation (SHM) of the immunoglobulin variable chain (IgV) provides a complementary approach to immunophenotyping to more precisely determine whether a lymphoma derives from a naive pre-GC B-cell (unmutated IgV), a centroblast in the GC (ongoing IgV mutation with intraclonal heterogeneity) or a centrocyte/post-GC B-cell (stable IgV mutations). Using this method it has been demonstrated that the vast majority of PTLDs (75% of P-PTLD and 65% of DLBCL) carry IgV mutations indicating that mainly GC and post-GC B-cells give rise to PTLD, both EBV-positive and –negative cases [7].

Interestingly, EBV has been associated with hypermutation of IgV even in the absence of follicular dendritic cells, follicular T-helper cells or a functional B-cell receptor suggesting that EBV may rescue defective B-cells and possibly offers a selective advantage to infected B-cells [277].

A recurrent observation is that EBV-positive PTLDs seem to be more frequently of ABC/non-GCB origin, while for EBV-negative PTLDs such predilection is less outspoken [265, 266, 278]. The reason for this is unclear but could be related to the signaling pathways that are induced by EBV, among which NF-κB that is highly characteristic for lymphomas of ABC/non-GCB origin.

Since in the general population the cell of origin of DLBCL is strongly associated with prognosis (*supra*, 8.2.1 Lymphoma in immunocompetent individuals) an interesting question is whether this also applies to post-transplant DLBCL. However, the association of EBV with ABC/non-GCB PTLD complicates this issue.

11.1. Aberrant Somatic Hypermutation

Similarly to DLBCL in immunocompetent hosts aberrant somatic hypermutation (SHM) seems to be an important pathogenic mechanism in post-transplant DLBCL. Importantly, because primarily the 5' regulatory region is targeted aberrant SHM may alter the expression profile of the affected genes [7]. In a series of 18 post-transplant DLBCL aberrant SHM of *PIM-1*, *PAX-5*, *RhoH/TTF* and/or *C-MYC* was detected in nearly 40% of the cases, independently of the EBV status. The frequency was similar in AIDS-related DLBCL but lower than in DLBCL of immunocompetent patients [273].

11.2. Chronic Antigen Stimulation

In HIV-associated lymphoma antigen stimulation is an important cause of disease. Similarly, PTLD could result from chronic antigen stimulation provided by the graft, promoting cell proliferation and associated mutation of a selected clone. However because 50% of PTLD cases lack a functional B-cell receptor (BCR) due to the high rate of aberrant SHM (*supra*) antigen stimulation may play a role in only a fraction of the cases [7]. In normal conditions, B-cells with a crippled BCR die from apoptosis, but EBV can rescue such cells via signaling of LMP2A that mimics a functional BCR and/or via BCL-2 upregulation by LMP1 (*supra*). In EBV-negative PTLDs with a crippled BCR, other mechanisms such as inactivation of pro-apoptotic *DAP-K* (*infra*, 11.5 Epigenetic alterations in PTLD) may contribute to cell survival [279]. In a study involving 30 post-transplant DLBCL with a functional BCR, 17 cases (57%) were EBV-negative which is more than expected when taking into account the strong association between EBV and PTLD. It is important to note that the majority of these EBV-negative cases (71%) had centroblastic morphology indicating that they are of germinal center (GC) origin [279]. Based on these findings we hypothesize that chronic antigen stimulation predisposes to the development of (part of) EBV-negative PTLDs that are primarily of GC origin possibly because mainly naïve B-cells are persistently triggered by graft antigens.

The observation that only a subgroup of PTLDs with a functional BCR appears to select for mutations that enhance antigen binding affinity and that recurrent variation of the IgV chain is rare has been put forward as an argument to conclude that antigen stimulation is not a major driver of PTLD [279]. However, in our view the lack of productive affinity maturation in PTLD does not exclude a potential role for chronic antigen stimulation as this process could be deregulated in the progression to malignancy. Also the finding that 90% of post-SOT PTLDs arise from host lymphocytes strongly suggests a role for B-cell stimulation by the graft (*supra*). Despite the large number of PTLDs with a dysfunctional BCR, it is not unlikely that chronic immune triggering of the solid graft plays a role in the initial stages of PTLD development.

11.3. Genetic Alterations

Despite the strong association between EBV and post-transplant lymphoma, infection by the oncogenic virus is probably not sufficient to cause malignancy, which requires additional (epi)genetic alterations. The analysis of genetic lesions in monoclonal PTLD has been largely limited to oncogenes that are known to be involved in non-Hodgkin lymphomas in the general population (*BCL-2*, *BCL-6*, *C-MYC*, *TP53*) [270, 280]. Because of the rarity of PTLD, so far few studies have reported on the genomic aberrations that underlie this disease. Array-comparative genomic hybridization (array-CGH) and a single nucleotide polymorphism (SNP)-based array experiment have demonstrated that post-transplant DLBCL has genomic gains (8q24 containing *C-MYC*, 3q27 containing *BCL-6*, 18q21 containing *BCL-2*, 7q containing *CDK6*) and losses (17p13 containing *TP53*) in common with DLBCL arising in immunocompetent individuals suggesting that these disorders share pathogenetic mechanisms. Besides these common aberrations, post-transplant DLBCL also bears more distinctive alterations (5p gain and 4q, 17q, Xp losses) [271, 272].

Overall PTLD seems to be characterized by a lower frequency of unbalanced genomic aberrations (51% of PTLDs in a study by Poirel *et al* [271]) than lymphoma in the immunocompetent population. A possible explanation is the mutator phenotype which is induced when loss of a gene involved in DNA mismatch repair accelerates the accumulation of mutations in numerous other genes (mainly in microsatellite sequences) resulting in microsatellite-instability (MSI, genetic hypermutability). Although mice with a deficiency in mismatch repair genes frequently develop lymphomas [281], MSI seems to be restricted to immunodeficiency-related lymphomas. The neoantigens that are formed as a result of MSI have been associated with tumor-infiltrating lymphocytes suggesting that MSI lymphomas are more immunogenic [282]. It is likely that such immunogenic lymphomas are only tolerated in an immunocompromised host, accounting for the lack of MSI lymphomas in immunocompetent individuals.

MSI affects only a fraction of PTLDs (in a series of 111 PTLDs 8% had MSI [283]) but may play an important role in disease onset, progression and also response to chemotherapy. It is likely that MSI results in increased chemosensitivity because of defective repair of chemotherapy-induced genetic lesions. Importantly, the presence of MSI seems unrelated to the EBV-status of PTLD [283].

An alternative explanation for the seemingly low rate of chromosomal aberrations in PTLD is the involvement of balanced genomic alterations and epigenetic gene silencing, events that are not detected by array-CGH. This is illustrated by cytogenetic analysis with trypsin-Giemsa banding of 36 PTLDs that demonstrated cytogenetic abnormalities in 72% of the monomorphic cases [272].

A commonly occurring phenomenon in (hematological) cancers is loss of heterozygosity (LOH), i.e., loss of one of the parental alleles present in the individual's normal cells. Inactivation of the remaining allele (e.g., encoding a tumor suppressor) may eventually contribute to cancer development. Interestingly, in the study of Rinaldi *et al.* LOH was reported in PTLD but did not always correlate with loss of DNA whereas in DLBCL of immunocompetent hosts loss of DNA with no LOH was frequent [284]. Theoretically, loss of one allele and subsequent duplication of the remaining one could account for LOH without loss of DNA but this is unlikely to happen. Uniparental disomy (UD) also known as copy-neutral LOH provides a potential mechanism and occurs when a person receives two copies of (part of) a chromosome from one parent and none from the other. If by coincidence both alleles are mutated this could result in inactivation of the encoded protein.

Whereas previously no clear association between the complexity of genomic aberrations and the EBV-status was shown [271] a study by Rinaldo *et al.* confirmed that EBV-positive post-transplant DLBCL is associated with less recurrent genetic lesions than EBV-negative cases. In particular, EBV-negative post-transplant DLBCL was associated with gains of 7p, 7q and 11q24-q25 and del(4q25-q35) [285]. Cytogenetic analysis on the other hand revealed that EBV-positive post-transplant DLBCL frequently harbor trisomies of chromosomes 9 and 11 [272].

Comparison of DLBCL in post-transplant and immunocompetent cases showed lack of del(13q14.3) in post-transplant cases and more frequent gains of 18q, LOH at 6q21-q22 and 6p21.32-21.33 in immunocompetent cases [285]. Curiously, copy-neutral LOH of the MHCII locus at 6p did not occur in post-transplant DLBCL in contrast to DLBCL in immunocompetent patients. Decreased expression or absence of MHCII is a relatively common event in DLBCL that results in reduced infiltration and activation of T-cells contributing to immune escape [286]. It is possible that due to iatrogenic immunodeficiency post-transplantation downregulation of MHCII is not required [285].

Interestingly, in both post-transplant and HIV-associated DLBCL deletions targeted genes overlapping fragile sites (i.e., regions of genomic instability often associated with double-stranded DNA breaks) more frequently than in DLBCL of immunocompetent patients, be it at other sites (the del(2p16.1) containing FRA2E in post-transplant and deletion of FHIT overlapping with FRA3B in HIV-associated DLBCL). This higher genomic instability in immunodeficiency-associated DLBCL could be due to integration of viral DNA [176, 285]. FRA2E is very similar to an EBV insertion site discovered in a Burkitt lymphom cell line [285, 287] and contains *FANCL* (encoding an ubiquitine ligase important in DNA repair) and

VRK2 (encoding a negative regulator of the MAPK pathway) [288]. Although EBV is thought to be maintained as an episome (*supra*, 8.1.3 Infectious life cycle of EBV) these data suggest that integration in the host genome may be more frequent than is generally assumed.

11.4. Polymorphisms in the EBV and the Host Genome

Given the ubiquity of EBV it is actually surprising that EBV-associated malignancies are relatively uncommon, even in immunocompromised individuals. In addition, it is not clear why some transplant patients develop PTLD and others are never affected. Part of the solution to these questions probably lies in the genetic variations between individuals and in the EBV genome.

Human Leukocyte Antigen (HLA) matching is an important factor for successful organ transplantation. Apart from their role in rejection, particular HLA loci have been implicated in PTLD. Intriguingly, specific HLA loci may predispose to PTLD (e.g., HLA-A26, B-38) while others may be protective (e.g., HLA-A1, B8, DR3). The central role of HLA molecules in immune response triggering especially via interaction with CLTs and NK-cells may explain the association with PTLD development. Because of the wide variety of HLA loci, (EBV) antigens are presented differently by specific HLA molecules resulting in a more or less efficient CLT induction (targeting EBV-positive PTLD). Notably, HLA class I proteins serve as co-receptors for EBV infection of B-cells (*supra*, 8.1.3 Infectious life cycle of EBV). Therefore, different HLA loci may more or less efficiently mediate entry of EBV.

An interesting observation is that apart from recipient haplotypes also certain donor haplotypes are associated with PTLD. The most feasible explanation is that the latter are implicated in donor-derived PTLD [289].

Insight in the association of particular HLA haplotypes with PTLD may be useful in the clinic, and especially in the context of organ transplantation HLA specificities are readily available. Because it is not yet clear how different HLA loci cooperate to influence the risk for PTLD development and because most data are derived from small case series [289, 290] the prognostic use of HLA typing is currently limited.

Intricate interactions between cytokines form a dynamic network that modulates immune responses and because polymorphisms in cytokine-encoding genes may considerably alter the signaling properties of the affected cytokines such genetic variations may have important implications. Of the cytokines and their receptors that have been genotyped a few have been associated with PTLD. Polymorphisms resulting in decreased IFN-gamma synthesis [291] or increased levels of TNF-alpha [292] have been identified that may predispose transplant recipients to PTLD. Theoretically, decreased IFN-gamma levels may impair CTL activation whereas increased TNF-alpha can promote tumor development [293]. Conversely, certain IL-1RN and IL-1beta variants that induce more severe inflammation (targeting EBV) [294] may be protective against PTLD.

When interpreting the association between particular polymorphisms and PTLD it is important to take into account that the association may differ for different grafts and PTLD subtypes. Therefore, the potential importance of a polymorphism should always be evaluated in the context of the individual patient. In time, cytokine genotyping of validated polymorphisms may acquire a role in the identification of transplant recipients at high risk for

PTLD development in combination with other parameters for risk assessment (*supra*, 3. Risk factors in PTLD).

Although EBV is considered to be genetically stable, polymorphisms in viral genes have been described that affect the signaling properties and immune recognition of the encoded proteins.

Variations in the gene encoding LMP1 have been associated with differential induction of NF-κB [295] and can affect the EBV viral load in peripheral blood [296].

EBNA1 was originally thought to be immunologically silent (*supra*, 8.1.3 Infectious life cycle of EBV), however a recent study demonstrated EBNA1-specific CLTs in EBV-positive PTLD patients [297]. The immunogenicity of EBNA1 was correlated with a polymorphism that greatly enhanced T-cell recognition. Importantly, HLA alleles influenced the magnitude of the response.

Put together, these findings demonstrate considerable genetic variability between individuals as well as in the EBV genome. Although the impact of each individual variant on PTLD development is probably limited, the interaction between all variants may substantially influence the course of disease.

11.5. Epigenetic Aberrations

The role of aberrant epigenetic silencing of tumor suppressors or activation of proto-oncogenes in the development of lymphoma is well-known and although little data is available a few studies highlight a role for epigenetic modifications in PTLD. The *DAP-K* (death-associated protein kinase) gene is epigenetically inactivated in 90% of the PTLDs, which potentially contributes to survival of lymphoma cells lacking a functional BCR [279]. Silencing of DAP-K may (partly) cancel out induction of apoptosis triggered by aberrant C-MYC signaling (*infra*, 12.1 Post-transplantation Burkitt lymphoma) [7]. Promotor hypermethylation of *MGMT* (O6-methylguanine-DNA methyltransferase) is also frequent in PTLD and results in reduced mismatch repair [298]. Like mismatch repair knock-out mice, also inactivation of *MGMT* promotes lymphomagenesis in mice (*supra*, 11.3 Genetic alterations) [299].

Interestingly, EBV infection may alter the epigenetic patterns of the host genome. During latency the majority of the promotors of the EBV episome are silenced via methylation for which EBV harnesses the host cells epigenetic machinery. Remarkably, EBV proteins may also indirectly alter methylation of cellular genes. Shortly after infection LMP1 downregulates DNMT1 while DNMT3A is upregulated. These changes in expression of DNA methylating enzymes have been associated with clustered methylation changes of the host genome [300]. These findings illustrate the intimate relationship between EBV and its host cell and the far-reaching implications of EBV infection on B-cell biology.

11.6. Microenvironment

The tumor microenvironment consists of the collection of stromal and immune cells that make up the cellular environment in which the tumor cells reside and has been shown to significantly influence prognosis in different tumor types [301, 302]. Because of iatrogenic immune suppression following transplantation one could expect that infiltration of reactive stroma in PTLD lesions is very limited or absent, however we have shown that substantial immune responses can still be mounted in EBV-positive PTLD patients (*supra*, 9.2 Pathogenesis of EBV-negative PTLD and the difference with EBV-positive cases).

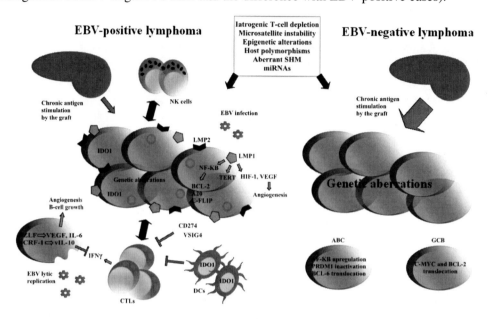

Figure 3. Proposed common and distinct pathogenetic mechanisms in EBV-positive and -negative lymphoma.

The pathogenesis of EBV-positive and -negative lymphoma is marked by a number of common as well as distinct pathogenetic mechanisms. Mechanisms that contribute to both EBV-positive and -negative lymphoma are shown in the box and involve iatrogenic T-cell suppression (which applies in particular to transplant recipients), microsatellite instability (resulting in accumulation of mutations), epigenetic alterations (mainly hypermethylation), host polymorphisms (in particular in genes encoding proteins involved in immunity), aberrant somatic hypermutation (SHM, resulting in accumulation of point mutations) and aberrant up- or downregulation of host miRNAs (which may substantially impact gene expression). The main distinctive features of EBV-positive and -negative lymphomas are the EBV status and the associated microenvironment. EBV infection is one of the earliest events in the pathogenesis of EBV-positive lymphoma. Two key proteins that are expressed in the EBV growth program (latency III) are LMP1 and LMP2. LMP1 is analogous to CD40 and promotes cell transformation by inducing NF-κB, that in turn upregulates BCL-2, A20 and C-FLIP, all involved in blocking apoptosis. LMP1 also induces TERT, an enzyme that is crucial for maintenance of the chromosome telomeres. Upregulation of HIF-1 and VEGF promote angiogenesis. LMP2 mimics a chronically active B-cell receptor (BCR) and prevents BCR-mediated activation of EBV lytic replication. LMP2 also provides the necessary survival signals which can compensate for the loss of a functional BCR. The expression of these (and other) EBV proteins attracts cytotoxic T-lymphocytes (CTLs) and natural killer (NK) cells to the site of the tumor however the question remains whether effective anti-tumor responses can be produced as also tolerant immune responses are induced. IDO1 (expressed in tumor cells as well as dendritic cells, DCs), CD274 and VSIG4 all suppress T-cells and may substantially impair the activity of CTLs. A minority of the EBV-positive cells actively produce viral particles and promote lymphoma growth by expression of IL-6 and VEGF. Also viral IL-10 is expressed and antagonizes IFN-gamma contributing to suppression of anti-tumor immune responses. In contrast to EBV-positive lymphoma, anti-tumor responses seem to be less prominent in EBV-negative lymphoma where chronic antigen stimulation by the graft (in transplant patients) and accumulating genetic alterations are presumably the main drivers of malignancy. EBV-positive lymphoma is predominantly of activated B-cell origin in contrast to EBV-negative lymphoma that may be of activated or germinal center B-cell (ABC or GCB) origin. Importantly, the cell of origin is associated with distinct genetic alterations.

An important question that arises is what the exact role of EBV is in inducing the responses observed in lesions of EBV-positive PTLD. An early study of T-cell infiltration in EBV-positive PTLD suggested that the observed lymphocyte infiltration represents a general response to iatrogenic immunosuppression rather than to EBV [303]. However the significant gene expression differences between EBV-positive and -negative post-transplant DLBCLs that our microarray study revealed indicate that the relationship between PTLD and the immune system is far more complex. Most likely, the observed immune responses are caused by the combined effect of the immunosuppressive regimen and EBV.

The first indication that tumor-infiltrating immune cells could influence prognosis of PTLD patients came from the analysis of CTLs and regulatory T-cells (Treg cells) in a series of 31 monomorphic PTLDs (30 DLBCLs and 1 Burkitt lymphoma). High counts of both CD3-positive T-cells and TIA-1-positive CTLs were associated with a favorable prognosis. Over 75% of the cases included in this study were EBV-positive (by EBER ISH). Unfortunately the EBV-status was not taken into account in the quantification of lymphocyte infiltration [303].

Treg cells are important modulators of the immune system and prevent excessive immune activation. Independently of the EBV-status, the infiltration of Treg cells is very limited in PTLD [303]. This may be attributed to the obstruction of Treg cell development by immunosuppressive agents. Analysis of the normal intestinal mucosa showed that liver transplant patients on a long-term combination regimen had significantly lower levels of Treg cells compared to healthy controls [304]. Although the scarcity of Treg cells in PTLD lesions may impede suppression of anti-tumor immune responses, also inhibition of B-cell proliferation by these cells is alleviated potentially contributing to PTLD development [303].

Apart from extensive expression of proinflammatory cytokines, EBV-positive post-transplant DLBCL is characterized by notable tolerogenic immune responses (*supra*, 9.2 Pathogenesis of EBV-negative PTLD and the difference with EBV-positive cases). Furthermore EBV-encoded proteins may also contribute to local immune suppression. *In vitro* experiments showed that recombinant LMP1 peptide sequences strongly inhibit CTLs and NK-cells. Interestingly, LMP1 has been detected in B-cell lymphoma cell line-derived exosomes providing a mechanism for LMP1 secretion in the microenvironment [305]. These findings raise the question whether the inflammatory infiltrates in PTLD lesions are (partially) functionally impaired but currently this issue remains unresolved.

12. The Role of EBV in Less Common Monomorphic PTLD Subtypes

Except for DLBCL, other B-cell lymphoma variants have been described in transplant patients, be it less frequently. Also PTLDs of T-cell origin occur, but the number of reported cases is very limited. In the last part of this chapter, we discuss the role of EBV in the pathogenesis of post-transplant Burkitt lymphoma, plasmablastic lymphoma, Hodgkin (like) lymphoma and T-cell PTLD.

12.1. Post-Transplant Burkitt Lymphoma

Burkitt lymphoma (BL) is a highly aggressive GC-derived lymphoma characterized by a high mitotic rate and numerous tingible body macrophages (loaded with debris from apoptotic cells). Three clinical variants of BL are recognized: endemic BL (with a high prevalence in equatorial Africa), sporadic BL (prevalent in Western countries) and immunodeficiency-associated BL (primarily affecting HIV-infected patients, but also reported in transplant recipients). A common hallmark of BLs is the presence of translocations involving *C-MYC* (mainly with *IgH*: t(8;14)(q24;q32)) which are also found in PTLDs with Burkitt-like morphology [272].

The association with EBV is different for the three BL subtypes and is strongest in the endemic variant (nearly 100% EBV-positive), followed by the immunodeficiency-associated variant (30%-80% EBV-positive) and sporadic BL (15%-20% EBV-positive) [306, 307]. Notably, EBV-positive Burkitt lymphoma is the tumor showing the most limited expression of viral genes (only EBNA1, EBERs and a particular set of miRNAs) and almost completely lacks the proteins that are normally required for oncogenesis [308]. A potential explanation lies in presence of the *C-MYC* translocation which promotes apoptosis via ARF-mediated upregulation of TP53 [309] suggesting that EBV primarily plays an anti-apoptotic role in Burkitt lymphoma. Indeed, both EBNA1 and the EBERs have the potential to counter apoptosis [310, 311], to promote cell survival and to maintain the germinal center phenotype by various mechanisms (reviewed in [243]). The consistent absence of LMP1 in EBV-positive Burkitt lymphomas may be due to its signaling properties: LMP1 induces NF-κB, which in turn suppresses C-MYC indicating that LMP1 expression is incompatible with C-MYC-driven lymphomagenesis [312, 313].

12.2. Post-Transplant Plasmablastic Lymphoma

Plasmablastic lymphoma (PBL) is an aggressive terminally differentiated variant of DLBCL that has many morphological and immunophenotypic characteristics in common with a reactive/non-neoplastic plasmablast (a B-cell in the initial stages of plasma cell differentiation). PBL typically arises in the oral cavity of HIV-positive patients but has also been reported in transplant recipients [8, 314]. In our meta-analysis we summarized the characteristics of 302 PBLs of which 35 (12 cases from our center) occurred in transplant patients (Morscio *et al.*, accepted by AJSP 2014). Overall, 67% of the 35 post-transplant PBL were positive for EBV (by EBER ISH or LMP1 staining) which (based on our series) most commonly expressed latency program II. The relative rarity of the latency I program is rather unexpected since underlying *C-MYC* translocations have been strongly associated with PBL pathogenesis (in particular in HIV patients, [315]). If, like for EBV-positive Burkitt lymphoma, C-MYC expression is incompatible with LMP1 signaling (*supra*, 12.1 Post-transplantation Burkitt lymphoma), we would expect latency I (in which LMP1 is not expressed) to be the predominant program in EBV-positive PBL. A possible explanation could be that, in contrast to HIV-related PBL, *C-MYC* translocations play a minor role in post-transplant PBL. Indeed, in our meta-analysis we documented *C-MYC* translocations in only 25% of post-transplant PBL compared to 73% of HIV-related PBL.

12.3. Post-Transplant Hodgkin Lymphoma-Like and Classic Hodgkin-Type Lymphoma

Because of their polymorphous histology, PTLDs resembling Hodgkin lymphoma are among the most difficult M-PTLDs to diagnose (*supra*, 2. PTLD histology). Nearly all cases are positive for EBV and typically express LMP1 [4, 316]. Because of their rarity, the molecular pathogenesis of Hodgkin-like lesions is largely unknown. Studies are further complicated by the overlapping features between lesions resembling HL and polymorphic PTLD since large cells reminiscent of Reed-Sternberg cells (the hallmark cells of classic HL) may also be observed in some P-PTLDs [13]. Rare case reports describing progression of P-PTLD to classic Hodgkin lymphoma (characterized by Hodgkin and RS cells) [317, 318] raise the suspicion that RS-like cells in polymorphic PTLD lesions may eventually become tumor cells, most likely promoted by EBV.

12.4. Post-Transplant T-Cell Lymphoma

Mature T-cell lymphomas arise from post-thymic T-cells and are divided into $\alpha\beta$ (>95%) and $\gamma\delta$ (<5%) T-cell lymphomas based on the T-cell receptor structure. The vast majority of peripheral T-cells express a T-cell receptor composed of $\alpha\beta$ chains. $\gamma\delta$ T-cells belong to the innate immune system and are found mainly in the splenic red pulp and epithelial sites and rarely in lymph nodes [319]. Currently, the WHO discriminates 21 different mature T-cell and NK-cell neoplasms (including 3 provisional categories), many of which have also been reported in transplant patients [6, 9] (Table 1). Overall, T-cell PTLD is rare, accounting for 15% of PTLDs in Western countries [6].

T-cell PTLD predominantly arises extranodally and most commonly involves bone (marrow) (25%), skin (24%), liver (24%), spleen (20%), lung/pleura (14%), peripheral blood (14%) and gastro-intestinal tract (13%). In contrast to B-cell PTLD, the CNS is rarely involved (5%) [6]. PTLDs of T-cell origin generally arise late after transplantation (median 72 months); a minority of cases (10%) arises within the year following transplantation compared to 38% of monomorphic B-cell PTLD [6, 71].

Only one third of T-cell PTLDs is associated with EBV, mainly extranodal nasal-type NK/T-cell lymphomas (ENKTCL, 100% EBV-related) and PTCL, NOS (39% EBV-related). ENKTCL primarily affects the nose and is characterized by necrosis and extensive infiltration of inflammatory cells suggesting an important role for the microenvironment. This is supported by *in vitro* culture of NK-cells which are heavily dependent on IL-2. Notably, LMP1 expression is associated with a reduced need for IL-2 [320] pointing to an indirect role of LMP1 in ENKTCL pathogenesis by sensitizing EBV-infected NK-cells to the growth-promoting effects of IL-2 [243].

In contrast to B-cell PTLD, EBV-positive T-cell PTLDs do not arise earlier post-transplantation than EBV-negative T-cell PTLD [6, 9]. Gene expression profiling revealed upregulation of cell cycle-related pathways and NF-κB in EBV-positive ENKTCL [321], strikingly similar to EBV-positive B-cell lymphomas.

It has been postulated that EBV-negative T-cell PTLDs arise as a result of aberrant T-cell responses against a limited number of EBV-infected B-cells [322]. This hypothesis is illustrated by a patient from our T-cell PTLD series in whom a clonal EBV-positive B-immunoblast population was detected [6].

Very few cytogenetic studies of small series of T-cell PTLD are currently available significantly limiting our insight in disease onset and progression. Like B-cell PTLDs T-cell PTLDs probably have genetic features in common with their counterpart in the general population [272].

Conclusion

PTLDs comprise a heterogeneous spectrum of disorders that affect a rising number of transplant patients. Although malignant PTLDs have many morphological and cytogenetic features in common with lymphoma in the general population, the distinct immune status of transplant patients and the involvement of EBV represent important differences.

Several observations point towards the fact that EBV-positive post-transplant lymphomas are different from EBV-negative post-transplant lymphomas. In EBV-positive cases (tolerant) immune responses play an important role and genomic aberrations are less complex in comparison with EBV-negative PTLD lymphoma. Restoration of the immune system (by reduction of immunosuppression, infusion of cytotoxic T-lymphocytes) frequently elicits a good therapeutic response as opposed to EBV-negative PTLD. The latter in contrast may be more 'autonomous' with aggressive progression depending less on the microenvironement and more on accumulated genetic alterations.

The prognostic significance of EBV is currently not clearly proven as in many studies EBV-positive and –negative PTLDs are not discriminated and because currently EBV-positive and –negative lymphomas are treated with essentially the same protocols. The data presented here suggest a positive prognostic significance of EBV on response to reduction of immunosuppression, rituximab and chemotherapy but larger studies are necessary to further prove these findings.

The pathogenic differences between EBV-positive and –negative PTLDs represent attractive opportunities for the development of targeted therapies which may markedly improve the outcome of PTLD patients. An important caveat however is that new therapeutic approaches should allow preservation of the graft - a problem that is not encountered in lymphoma of the general population.

Glossary

Acquired immunodeficiency

Secondary immunodeficiency that is not caused by a genetic immune system defect, but by medical treatment (iatrogenic immunosuppression) or another external cause (e.g., human immunodeficiency virus infection). Iatrogenic suppression of immune responses is applied following transplantation to prevent immune-mediated graft rejection. Both iatrogenic and HIV-related immunodeficiency (like primary immunodeficiency) are associated with a higher incidence of malignancy, frequently EBV-driven lymphoma.

Primary immunodeficiency
Immunodeficiency caused by a *de novo* or inherited defect in the immune system. Diseases that cause primary immunodeficiency are rare, but are -like acquired immunodeficiency- associated with a higher incidence of malignancy, frequently EBV-associated lymphoma.

RIS
Reduction of immunosuppression, i.e., reduction of the dose of immunosuppressive drugs administered to transplant recipients. In most cases RIS is the first intervention that is performed in patients diagnosed with PTLD in an attempt to restore (tumor-specific) immune responses. Generally, EBV-positive PTLDs respond better to RIS than EBV-negative PTLDs underscoring the central role of the microenvironment in the former.

CHOP
Chemotherapeutic regimen composed of cyclophosphamide (an alkylating agent), adriamycin (or hydroxydaunorubicin, a DNA-intercalating antracycline), vincristin (or oncovine, a vinca alkaloid that inhibits mitosis) and prednisone (an immunosuppressive corticosteroid drug). CHOP is the most commonly used cocktail for the treatment of non-Hodgkin lymphoma (in immunocompetent as well as immunodeficient patients) and is administered in a two-week or three-week interval (CHOP-14 and CHOP-21 respectively) As first-line therapy, CHOP is frequently combined with rituximab (an anti-CD20 antibody, R-CHOP).

Rituximab
A chimeric monoclonal antibody targeting CD20, a membrane protein expressed during nearly all stages of B-cell development. Rituximab is commonly combined with CHOP chemotherapy for the treatment of non-Hodgkin lymphoma. Rituximab kills CD20-positive B-cells by (1) antibody-dependent cellular cytotoxicity, (2) inducing apoptosis, (3) causing downregulation of the B-cell receptor. Rituximab treatment is associated with limited toxicity, however resistance can be induced by downregulation of CD20 on lymphoma cells.

EBV viral load
Also known as the viral titer is the amount of EBV DNA copies in the peripheral blood of EBV-infected individuals and is used as a means to estimate the severity of EBV disease. In transplant patients, the EBV viral load is closely monitored to predict the onset of PTLD. However, the reliability of the viral load in PTLD risk assessment is highly debated.

EBV latency
The stage in the viral life cycle in which no virions are produced (as opposed to the lytic stage). During viral latency of EBV, three associated patterns of viral protein expression (so called latency programs) may be expressed. During infection of the B-cell, these latency programs guide the B-cell through the germinal center reaction pushing it towards the resting memory cell stage. Different latency proteins are implicated in EBV-driven lymphomagenesis demonstrated by the expression of a particular latency program in different lymphoma subtypes.

Microenvironment
The environment composed of non-neoplastic stroma and immune cells in which the tumor cells reside. Whereas previously only the neoplastic cells were the focus of most research, recent studies have shown that the microenvironment is in fact an important component of the tumor that may considerably influence prognosis.

Summary Points List

- Post-transplant lymphoproliferative disorder (PTLD) is a heterogeneous and potentially fatal condition that affects an increasing number of transplant recipients. Although numerous risk factors have been described, it is currently not possible to accurately predict which transplant recipient will eventually develop PTLD and after what time interval following transplantation.
- Data and results from many studies on PTLD are obscured because EBV-positive and -negative cases are not discriminated. However, biological as well as clinical differences between EBV-positive and -negative PTLDs suggest that these are different entities that should be analyzed and treated separately.
- EBV-positive PTLD is -in contrast to EBV-negative PTLD- characterized by intricate interactions with the surrounding stroma demonstrating that (1) despite the immunocompromised condition post-transplantation immune responses can still be established and (2) that the microenvironment plays a central role in the pathogenesis of EBV-positive PTLD.
- EBV-negative PTLD is biologically similar to EBV-negative lymphoma occurring in the general population, however the different immune status of the host should be taken into account in the treatment plan.
- The biological differences between EBV-positive and -negative PTLD may be exploited in the development of new targeted therapies. Modulation of the microenvironment could represent an attractive approach for treatment of EBV-positive cases. However caution is required as novel therapeutics (that alter immune responses) should be compatible with preservation of the graft in transplant recipients.
- Currently, the prognostic impact of EBV is not clear, but several data points towards a positive prognostic significance of the presence of EBV on the outcome of lymphoma patients.

Future Issue List

- Currently, EBV-positive and -negative PTLD cases are frequently pooled in most studies. Based on the data presented in this chapter, EBV-positive and -negative PTLDs should be distinguished in future studies in order to define further the molecular-genetic differences between both disorders.
- We put forward EBV as a predictor of good prognosis, however the impact of EBV on therapy response and outcome of PTLD patients has to be confirmed in larger

studies. In addition, a PTLD-adjusted staging system that takes into account the particular characteristics of the PTLD patient population should be established and validated. Future studies have to determine whether the EBV status should be included in such a staging system.

- The identification of EBV-positive and -negative PTLD as two separate entities should be the basis for the development of more targeted treatment modalities. Treatment of EBV-positive PTLD should aim at modulation of immune responses (e.g., IDO-1 blockers) whereas for EBV-negative PTLD, the treatment should target the neoplastic cells.

References

[1] Kuper H, Adami HO,Trichopoulos D: Infections as a major preventable cause of human cancer. *J. Intern. Med.* 2000, 248:171-183.

[2] Murray JE, Wilson RE, Tilney NL, Merrill JP, Cooper WC, Birtch AG, Carpenter CB, Hager EB, Dammin GJ,Harrison JH: Five years' experience in renal transplantation with immunosuppressive drugs: survival, function, complications, and the role of lymphocyte depletion by thoracic duct fistula. *Ann. Surg.* 1968, 168:416-435.

[3] Mucha K, Foroncewicz B, Ziarkiewicz-Wroblewska B, Krawczyk M, Lerut J,Paczek L: Post-transplant lymphoproliferative disorder in view of the new WHO classification: a more rational approach to a protean disease? *Nephrol. Dial. Transplant.* 2010, 25:2089-2098.

[4] Swerdlow SH, Campo E, Harris NL, Jaffe ES, PIleri SA, Stein H, THiele J, Vardiman JM: *WHO Classification of Tumours of Haematopoietic and Lymphoid Tissues.* New York: IARC Press; 2008.

[5] Tran H, Nourse J, Hall S, Green M, Griffiths L,Gandhi MK: Immunodeficiency-associated lymphomas. *Blood Rev.* 2008, 22:261-281.

[6] Herreman A, Dierickx D, Morscio J, Camps J, Bittoun E, Verhoef G, De Wolf-Peeters C, Sagaert X,Tousseyn T: Clinicopathological characteristics of posttransplant lymphoproliferative disorders of T-cell origin: single-center series of nine cases and meta-analysis of 147 reported cases. *Leuk Lymphoma* 2013, 54:2190-2199.

[7] Capello D, Rossi D,Gaidano G: Post-transplant lymphoproliferative disorders: molecular basis of disease histogenesis and pathogenesis. *Hematol. Oncol.* 2005, 23:61-67.

[8] Benitez CE, Rey P, Zoroquiain P, Martinez J, Ramirez P, Arrese M, Perez-Ayuso RM,Valbuena JR: Early-onset EBV-positive post-transplant plasmablastic lymphoma arising in a liver allograft: a case report and literature review. *Int. J. Surg. Pathol.* 2013, 21:404-410.

[9] Swerdlow SH: T-cell and NK-cell posttransplantation lymphoproliferative disorders. *Am. J. Clin. Pathol.* 2007, 127:887-895.

[10] Tiede C, Maecker-Kolhoff B, Klein C, Kreipe H,Hussein K: Risk factors and prognosis in T-cell posttransplantation lymphoproliferative diseases: reevaluation of 163 cases. *Transplantation* 2013, 95:479-488.

[11] Semakula B, Rittenbach JV,Wang J: Hodgkin lymphoma-like posttransplantation lymphoproliferative disorder. *Arch. Pathol. Lab. Med.* 2006, 130:558-560.

[12] Ranganathan S, Webber S, Ahuja S,Jaffe R: Hodgkin-like posttransplant lymphoproliferative disorder in children: does it differ from posttransplant Hodgkin lymphoma? *Pediatr. Dev. Pathol.* 2004, 7:348-360.

[13] Pitman SD, Huang Q, Zuppan CW, Rowsell EH, Cao JD, Berdeja JG, Weiss LM,Wang J: Hodgkin lymphoma-like posttransplant lymphoproliferative disorder (HL-like PTLD) simulates monomorphic B-cell PTLD both clinically and pathologically. *Am. J. Surg. Pathol.* 2006, 30:470-476.

[14] Durandy A: Anti-B cell and anti-cytokine therapy for the treatment of post-transplant lymphoproliferative disorder: past, present, and future. *Transpl. Infect. Dis.* 2001, 3:104-107.

[15] Johnson LR, Nalesnik MA,Swerdlow SH: Impact of Epstein-Barr virus in monomorphic B-cell posttransplant lymphoproliferative disorders: a histogenetic study. *Am. J. Surg. Pathol.* 2006, 30:1604-1612.

[16] Allen U, Preiksaitis J,Practice ASTIDCo: Epstein-barr virus and posttransplant lymphoproliferative disorder in solid organ transplant recipients. *Am. J. Transplant.* 2009, 9 Suppl 4:S87-96.

[17] Cohen JI: Epstein-Barr virus infection. *N. Engl. J. Med.* 2000, 343:481-492.

[18] LaCasce AS: Post-transplant lymphoproliferative disorders. *Oncologist* 2006, 11:674-680.

[19] Curtis RE, Travis LB, Rowlings PA, Socie G, Kingma DW, Banks PM, Jaffe ES, Sale GE, Horowitz MM, Witherspoon RP, Shriner DA, Weisdorf DJ, Kolb HJ, Sullivan KM, Sobocinski KA, Gale RP, Hoover RN, Fraumeni JF, Jr.,Deeg HJ: Risk of lymphoproliferative disorders after bone marrow transplantation: a multi-institutional study. *Blood* 1999, 94:2208-2216.

[20] Lucas KG, Small TN, Heller G, Dupont B,O'Reilly RJ: The development of cellular immunity to Epstein-Barr virus after allogeneic bone marrow transplantation. *Blood* 1996, 87:2594-2603.

[21] Dharnidharka VR: Epidemiology of PTLD. In Post-transplant lymphoproliferative disorders. Edited by Dharnidharka VR, Green, M., Webber, S.A., Editor. New York: *Springer*; 2010:

[22] Ibrahim HA,Naresh KN: Posttransplant lymphoproliferative disorders. *Adv. Hematol.* 2012, 2012:230173.

[23] Murukesan V,Mukherjee S: Managing post-transplant lymphoproliferative disorders in solid-organ transplant recipients: a review of immunosuppressant regimens. Drugs 2012, 72:1631-1643.

[24] Nourse JP, Jones K,Gandhi MK: Epstein-Barr Virus-related post-transplant lymphoproliferative disorders: pathogenetic insights for targeted therapy. *Am. J. Transplant.* 2011, 11:888-895.

[25] Eckrich MJ, Frangoul H, Knight J, Mosse C,Domm J: A case of pediatric PTLD following autologous stem cell transplantation and review of the literature. *Pediatr. Transplant.* 2012, 16:E15-18.

[26] Cohena Y,Nagler A: Hematopoietic stem-cell transplantation using umbilical-cord blood. *Leuk Lymphoma* 2003, 44:1287-1299.

[27] Gong JZ, Bayerl MG, Sandhaus LM, Sebastian S, Rehder CW, Routbort M, Lagoo AS, Szabolcs P, Chiu J, Comito M, Buckley PJ: Posttransplant lymphoproliferative disorder after umbilical cord blood transplantation in children. *Am. J. Surg.* Pathol 2006, 30:328-336.

[28] Shapiro RS, McClain K, Frizzera G, Gajl-Peczalska KJ, Kersey JH, Blazar BR, Arthur DC, Patton DF, Greenberg JS, Burke B, et al.: Epstein-Barr virus associated B cell lymphoproliferative disorders following bone marrow transplantation. Blood 1988, 71:1234-1243.

[29] Zutter MM, Martin PJ, Sale GE, Shulman HM, Fisher L, Thomas ED, Durnam DM: Epstein-Barr virus lymphoproliferation after bone marrow transplantation. *Blood* 1988, 72:520-529.

[30] Caillard S, Lamy FX, Quelen C, Dantal J, Lebranchu Y, Lang P, Velten M, Moulin B, French Transplant C: Epidemiology of posttransplant lymphoproliferative disorders in adult kidney and kidney pancreas recipients: report of the French registry and analysis of subgroups of lymphomas. *Am. J. Transplant.* 2012, 12:682-693.

[31] Landgren O, Gilbert ES, Rizzo JD, Socie G, Banks PM, Sobocinski KA, Horowitz MM, Jaffe ES, Kingma DW, Travis LB, Flowers ME, Martin PJ, Deeg HJ, Curtis RE: Risk factors for lymphoproliferative disorders after allogeneic hematopoietic cell transplantation. *Blood* 2009, 113:4992-5001.

[32] Opelz G, Dohler B: Impact of HLA mismatching on incidence of posttransplant non-hodgkin lymphoma after kidney transplantation. *Transplantation* 2010, 89:567-572.

[33] Styczynski J, Gil L, Tridello G, Ljungman P, Donnelly JP, van der Velden W, Omar H, Martino R, Halkes C, Faraci M, Theunissen K, Kalwak K, Hubacek P, Sica S, Nozzoli C, Fagioli F, Matthes S, Diaz MA, Migliavacca M, Balduzzi A, Tomaszewska A, Camara Rde L, van Biezen A, Hoek J, Iacobelli S, Einsele H, Cesaro S, Infectious Diseases Working Party of the European Group for B, Marrow T: Response to rituximab-based therapy and risk factor analysis in epstein barr virus-related lymphoproliferative disorder after hematopoietic stem cell transplant in children and adults: a study from the Infectious Diseases Working Party of the European Group for Blood and Marrow Transplantation. *Clin. Infect. Dis.* 2013, 57:794-802.

[34] Chadburn A, Suciu-Foca N, Cesarman E, Reed E, Michler RE, Knowles DM: Post-transplantation lymphoproliferative disorders arising in solid organ transplant recipients are usually of recipient origin. *Am. J. Pathol.* 1995, 147:1862-1870.

[35] Hopwood P, Crawford DH: The role of EBV in post-transplant malignancies: a review. *J. Clin. Pathol.* 2000, 53:248-254.

[36] Capello D, Rasi S, Oreste P, Veronese S, Cerri M, Ravelli E, Rossi D, Minola E, Colosimo A, Gambacorta M, Muti G, Morra E, Gaidano G: Molecular characterization of post-transplant lymphoproliferative disorders of donor origin occurring in liver transplant recipients. *J. Pathol.* 2009, 218:478-486.

[37] Olagne J, Caillard S, Gaub MP, Chenard MP, Moulin B: Post-transplant lymphoproliferative disorders: determination of donor/recipient origin in a large cohort of kidney recipients. *Am. J. Transplant.* 2011, 11:1260-1269.

[38] Weissmann DJ, Ferry JA, Harris NL, Louis DN, Delmonico F, Spiro I: Posttransplantation lymphoproliferative disorders in solid organ recipients are predominantly aggressive tumors of host origin. *Am. J. Clin. Pathol.* 1995, 103:748-755.

[39] Green M, Soltys K, Rowe DT, Webber SA,Mazareigos G: Chronic high Epstein-Barr viral load carriage in pediatric liver transplant recipients. *Pediatr. Transplant.* 2009, 13:319-323.

[40] Schaffer K, Hassan J, Staines A, Coughlan S, Holder P, Tuite G, McCormick AP, Traynor O, Hall WW,Connell J: Surveillance of Epstein-Barr virus loads in adult liver transplantation: associations with age, sex, posttransplant times, and transplant indications. *Liver Transpl.* 2011, 17:1420-1426.

[41] Holman CJ, Karger AB, Mullan BD, Brundage RC,Balfour HH, Jr.: Quantitative Epstein-Barr virus shedding and its correlation with the risk of post-transplant lymphoproliferative disorder. *Clin. Transplant.* 2012, 26:741-747.

[42] Yang J, Tao Q, Flinn IW, Murray PG, Post LE, Ma H, Piantadosi S, Caligiuri MA,Ambinder RF: Characterization of Epstein-Barr virus-infected B cells in patients with posttransplantation lymphoproliferative disease: disappearance after rituximab therapy does not predict clinical response. *Blood* 2000, 96:4055-4063.

[43] Rowe DT, Webber S, Schauer EM, Reyes J,Green M: Epstein-Barr virus load monitoring: its role in the prevention and management of post-transplant lymphoproliferative disease. *Transpl. Infect. Dis.* 2001, 3:79-87.

[44] Wadowsky RM, Laus S, Green M, Webber SA,Rowe D: Measurement of Epstein-Barr virus DNA loads in whole blood and plasma by TaqMan PCR and in peripheral blood lymphocytes by competitive PCR. *J. Clin. Microbiol.* 2003, 41:5245-5249.

[45] Hakim H, Gibson C, Pan J, Srivastava K, Gu Z, Bankowski MJ,Hayden RT: Comparison of various blood compartments and reporting units for the detection and quantification of Epstein-Barr virus in peripheral blood. *J. Clin. Microbiol.* 2007, 45:2151-2155.

[46] Wagner HJ, Wessel M, Jabs W, Smets F, Fischer L, Offner G,Bucsky P: Patients at risk for development of posttransplant lymphoproliferative disorder: plasma versus peripheral blood mononuclear cells as material for quantification of Epstein-Barr viral load by using real-time quantitative polymerase chain reaction. *Transplantation* 2001, 72:1012-1019.

[47] Stevens SJ, Verschuuren EA, Verkuujlen SA, Van Den Brule AJ, Meijer CJ,Middeldorp JM: Role of Epstein-Barr virus DNA load monitoring in prevention and early detection of post-transplant lymphoproliferative disease. *Leuk. Lymphoma* 2002, 43:831-840.

[48] Weinstock DM, Ambrossi GG, Brennan C, Kiehn TE,Jakubowski A: Preemptive diagnosis and treatment of Epstein-Barr virus-associated post transplant lymphoproliferative disorder after hematopoietic stem cell transplant: an approach in development. *Bone Marrow Transplant.* 2006, 37:539-546.

[49] Tsai DE, Douglas L, Andreadis C, Vogl DT, Arnoldi S, Kotloff R, Svoboda J, Bloom RD, Olthoff KM, Brozena SC, Schuster SJ, Stadtmauer EA, Robertson ES, Wasik MA,Ahya VN: EBV PCR in the diagnosis and monitoring of posttransplant lymphoproliferative disorder: results of a two-arm prospective trial. *Am. J. Transplant.* 2008, 8:1016-1024.

[50] Gartner BC, Fischinger J, Schafer H, Einsele H, Roemer K,Muller-Lantzsch N: Epstein-Barr viral load as a tool to diagnose and monitor post-transplant lymphoproliferative disease. *Recent Results Cancer Res.* 2002, 159:49-54.

[51] Gil L, Styczynski J, Komarnicki M: Strategy of pre-emptive management of Epstein-Barr virus post-transplant lymphoproliferative disorder after stem cell transplantation: results of European transplant centers survey. *Contemp. Oncol.* (Pozn) 2012, 16:338-340.

[52] Omar H, Hagglund H, Gustafsson-Jernberg A, LeBlanc K, Mattsson J, Remberger M, Ringden O, Sparrelid E, Sundin M, Winiarski J, Yun Z, Ljungman P: Targeted monitoring of patients at high risk of post-transplant lymphoproliferative disease by quantitative Epstein-Barr virus polymerase chain reaction. *Transpl. Infect. Dis.* 2009, 11:393-399.

[53] Bakker NA, Verschuuren EA, Erasmus ME, Hepkema BG, Veeger NJ, Kallenberg CG, van der Bij W: Epstein-Barr virus-DNA load monitoring late after lung transplantation: a surrogate marker of the degree of immunosuppression and a safe guide to reduce immunosuppression. *Transplantation* 2007, 83:433-438.

[54] Fox CP, Burns D, Parker AN, Peggs KS, Harvey CM, Natarajan S, Marks DI, Jackson B, Chakupurakal G, Dennis M, Lim Z, Cook G, Carpenter B, Pettitt AR, Mathew S, Connelly-Smith L, Yin JA, Viskaduraki M, Chakraverty R, Orchard K, Shaw BE, Byrne JL, Brookes C, Craddock CF, Chaganti S: EBV-associated post-transplant lymphoproliferative disorder following in vivo T-cell-depleted allogeneic transplantation: clinical features, viral load correlates and prognostic factors in the rituximab era. *Bone Marrow Transplant.* 2013.

[55] Smets F, Latinne D, Bazin H, Reding R, Otte JB, Buts JP, Sokal EM: Ratio between Epstein-Barr viral load and anti-Epstein-Barr virus specific T-cell response as a predictive marker of posttransplant lymphoproliferative disease. *Transplantation* 2002, 73:1603-1610.

[56] Lee TC, Goss JA, Rooney CM, Heslop HE, Barshes NR, Caldwell YM, Gee AP, Scott JD, Savoldo B: Quantification of a low cellular immune response to aid in identification of pediatric liver transplant recipients at high-risk for EBV infection. *Clin. Transplant.* 2006, 20:689-694.

[57] Green M, Michaels MG: Epstein-Barr virus infection and posttransplant lymphoproliferative disorder. *Am. J. Transplant.* 2013, 13 Suppl 3:41-54; quiz 54.

[58] Manez R, Breinig MC, Linden P, Wilson J, Torre-Cisneros J, Kusne S, Dummer S, Ho M: Posttransplant lymphoproliferative disease in primary Epstein-Barr virus infection after liver transplantation: the role of cytomegalovirus disease. *J. Infect. Dis.* 1997, 176:1462-1467.

[59] Hiwarkar P, Gaspar HB, Gilmour K, Jagani M, Chiesa R, Bennett-Rees N, Breuer J, Rao K, Cale C, Goulden N, Davies G, Amrolia P, Veys P, Qasim W: Impact of viral reactivations in the era of pre-emptive antiviral drug therapy following allogeneic haematopoietic SCT in paediatric recipients. *Bone Marrow Transplant.* 2013, 48:803-808.

[60] Humar A, Malkan G, Moussa G, Greig P, Levy G, Mazzulli T: Human herpesvirus-6 is associated with cytomegalovirus reactivation in liver transplant recipients. *J. Infect. Dis.* 2000, 181:1450-1453.

[61] Birkeland SA, Hamilton-Dutoit S: Is posttransplant lymphoproliferative disorder (PTLD) caused by any specific immunosuppressive drug or by the transplantation per se? *Transplantation* 2003, 76:984-988.

[62] Cao S, Cox KL, Berquist W, Hayashi M, Concepcion W, Hammes GB, Ojogho OK, So SK, Frerker M, Castillo RO, Monge H,Esquivel CO: Long-term outcomes in pediatric liver recipients: comparison between cyclosporin A and tacrolimus. *Pediatr. Transplant.* 1999, 3:22-26.

[63] Schubert S, Renner C, Hammer M, Abdul-Khaliq H, Lehmkuhl HB, Berger F, Hetzer R,Reinke P: Relationship of immunosuppression to Epstein-Barr viral load and lymphoproliferative disease in pediatric heart transplant patients. *J. Heart Lung Transplant.* 2008, 27:100-105.

[64] Durrbach A, Pestana JM, Pearson T, Vincenti F, Garcia VD, Campistol J, Rial Mdel C, Florman S, Block A, Di Russo G, Xing J, Garg P,Grinyo J: A phase III study of belatacept versus cyclosporine in kidney transplants from extended criteria donors (BENEFIT-EXT study). *Am. J. Transplant.* 2010, 10:547-557.

[65] Grinyo J, Charpentier B, Pestana JM, Vanrenterghem Y, Vincenti F, Reyes-Acevedo R, Apanovitch AM, Gujrathi S, Agarwal M, Thomas D,Larsen CP: An integrated safety profile analysis of belatacept in kidney transplant recipients. *Transplantation* 2010, 90:1521-1527.

[66] Vincenti F, Charpentier B, Vanrenterghem Y, Rostaing L, Bresnahan B, Darji P, Massari P, Mondragon-Ramirez GA, Agarwal M, Di Russo G, Lin CS, Garg P,Larsen CP: A phase III study of belatacept-based immunosuppression regimens versus cyclosporine in renal transplant recipients (BENEFIT study). *Am. J. Transplant.* 2010, 10:535-546.

[67] Thompson MP,Kurzrock R: Epstein-Barr virus and cancer. *Clin. Cancer Res.* 2004, 10:803-821.

[68] Dierickx D, Tousseyn T, Requile A, Verscuren R, Sagaert X, Morscio J, Wlodarska I, Herreman A, Kuypers D, Van Cleemput J, Nevens F, Dupont L, Uyttebroeck A, Pirenne J, De Wolf-Peeters C, Verhoef G, Brepoels L,Gheysens O: The accuracy of positron emission tomography in the detection of posttransplant lymphoproliferative disorder. *Haematologica* 2013, 98:771-775.

[69] Graf N, Herrmann K, Numberger B, Zwisler D, Aichler M, Feuchtinger A, Schuster T, Wester HJ, Senekowitsch-Schmidtke R, Peschel C, Schwaiger M, Keller U, Dechow T,Buck AK: [18F]FLT is superior to [18F]FDG for predicting early response to antiproliferative treatment in high-grade lymphoma in a dose-dependent manner. *Eur. J. Nucl. Med. Mol. Imaging* 2013, 40:34-43.

[70] Murphy SB: Classification, staging and end results of treatment of childhood non-Hodgkin's lymphomas: dissimilarities from lymphomas in adults. *Semin. Oncol.* 1980, 7:332-339.

[71] Dierickx D, Tousseyn T, Sagaert X, Fieuws S, Wlodarska I, Morscio J, Brepoels L, Kuypers D, Vanhaecke J, Nevens F, Verleden G, Van Damme-Lombaerts R, Renard M, Pirenne J, De Wolf-Peeters C,Verhoef G: Single-center analysis of biopsy-confirmed posttransplant lymphoproliferative disorder: incidence, clinicopathological characteristics and prognostic factors. *Leuk Lymphoma* 2013, 54:2433-2440.

[72] Ghobrial IM, Habermann TM, Ristow KM, Ansell SM, Macon W, Geyer SM,McGregor CG: Prognostic factors in patients with post-transplant lymphoproliferative disorders (PTLD) in the rituximab era. *Leuk Lymphoma* 2005, 46:191-196.

[73] A predictive model for aggressive non-Hodgkin's lymphoma. The International Non-Hodgkin's Lymphoma Prognostic Factors Project. *N. Engl. J. Med.* 1993, 329:987-994.

[74] Choquet S, Oertel S, LeBlond V, Riess H, Varoqueaux N, Dorken B,Trappe R: Rituximab in the management of post-transplantation lymphoproliferative disorder after solid organ transplantation: proceed with caution. *Ann. Hematol.* 2007, 86:599-607.

[75] Leblond V, Dhedin N, Mamzer Bruneel MF, Choquet S, Hermine O, Porcher R, Nguyen Quoc S, Davi F, Charlotte F, Dorent R, Barrou B, Vernant JP, Raphael M,Levy V: Identification of prognostic factors in 61 patients with posttransplantation lymphoproliferative disorders. *J. Clin. Oncol.* 2001, 19:772-778.

[76] Dierickx D, Tousseyn T, De Wolf-Peeters C, Pirenne J,Verhoef G: Management of posttransplant lymphoproliferative disorders following solid organ transplant: an update. *Leuk Lymphoma* 2011, 52:950-961.

[77] Green M: Management of Epstein-Barr virus-induced post-transplant lymphoproliferative disease in recipients of solid organ transplantation. *Am. J. Transplant.* 2001, 1:103-108.

[78] Swinnen LJ, LeBlanc M, Grogan TM, Gordon LI, Stiff PJ, Miller AM, Kasamon Y, Miller TP,Fisher RI: Prospective study of sequential reduction in immunosuppression, interferon alpha-2B, and chemotherapy for posttransplantation lymphoproliferative disorder. *Transplantation* 2008, 86:215-222.

[79] Trappe R, Oertel S, Leblond V, Mollee P, Sender M, Reinke P, Neuhaus R, Lehmkuhl H, Horst HA, Salles G, Morschhauser F, Jaccard A, Lamy T, Leithauser M, Zimmermann H, Anagnostopoulos I, Raphael M, Riess H, Choquet S, German PSG,European PN: Sequential treatment with rituximab followed by CHOP chemotherapy in adult B-cell post-transplant lymphoproliferative disorder (PTLD): the prospective international multicentre phase 2 PTLD-1 trial. *Lancet Oncol.* 2012, 13:196-206.

[80] Mamzer-Bruneel MF, Lome C, Morelon E, Levy V, Bourquelot P, Jacobs F, Gessain A, Mac Intyre E, Brousse N, Kreis H,Hermine O: Durable remission after aggressive chemotherapy for very late post-kidney transplant lymphoproliferation: A report of 16 cases observed in a single center. *J. Clin. Oncol.* 2000, 18:3622-3632.

[81] Swinnen LJ, Mullen GM, Carr TJ, Costanzo MR,Fisher RI: Aggressive treatment for postcardiac transplant lymphoproliferation. *Blood* 1995, 86:3333-3340.

[82] Choquet S, Trappe R, Leblond V, Jager U, Davi F,Oertel S: CHOP-21 for the treatment of post-transplant lymphoproliferative disorders (PTLD) following solid organ transplantation. *Haematologica* 2007, 92:273-274.

[83] Ghobrial IM, Habermann TM, Macon WR, Ristow KM, Larson TS, Walker RC, Ansell SM, Gores GJ, Stegall MD,McGregor CG: Differences between early and late posttransplant lymphoproliferative disorders in solid organ transplant patients: are they two different diseases? *Transplantation* 2005, 79:244-247.

[84] Oertel SH, Verschuuren E, Reinke P, Zeidler K, Papp-Vary M, Babel N, Trappe RU, Jonas S, Hummel M, Anagnostopoulos I, Dorken B,Riess HB: Effect of anti-CD 20 antibody rituximab in patients with post-transplant lymphoproliferative disorder (PTLD). *Am. J. Transplant.* 2005, 5:2901-2906.

[85] Gonzalez-Barca E, Domingo-Domenech E, Capote FJ, Gomez-Codina J, Salar A, Bailen A, Ribera JM, Lopez A, Briones J, Munoz A, Encuentra M, de Sevilla AF,

Gel/Tamo, Gelcab,Gotel: Prospective phase II trial of extended treatment with rituximab in patients with B-cell post-transplant lymphoproliferative disease. *Haematologica* 2007, 92:1489-1494.

[86] Choquet S, Leblond V, Herbrecht R, Socie G, Stoppa AM, Vandenberghe P, Fischer A, Morschhauser F, Salles G, Feremans W, Vilmer E, Peraldi MN, Lang P, Lebranchu Y, Oksenhendler E, Garnier JL, Lamy T, Jaccard A, Ferrant A, Offner F, Hermine O, Moreau A, Fafi-Kremer S, Morand P, Chatenoud L, Berriot-Varoqueaux N, Bergougnoux L,Milpied N: Efficacy and safety of rituximab in B-cell post-transplantation lymphoproliferative disorders: results of a prospective multicenter phase 2 study. *Blood* 2006, 107:3053-3057.

[87] Milpied N, Vasseur B, Parquet N, Garnier JL, Antoine C, Quartier P, Carret AS, Bouscary D, Faye A, Bourbigot B, Reguerre Y, Stoppa AM, Bourquard P, Hurault de Ligny B, Dubief F, Mathieu-Boue A,Leblond V: Humanized anti-CD20 monoclonal antibody (Rituximab) in post transplant B-lymphoproliferative disorder: a retrospective analysis on 32 patients. *Ann. Oncol.* 2000, 11 Suppl 1:113-116.

[88] Cartron G, Trappe RU, Solal-Celigny P,Hallek M: Interindividual variability of response to rituximab: from biological origins to individualized therapies. *Clin. Cancer Res.* 2011, 17:19-30.

[89] Elstrom RL, Andreadis C, Aqui NA, Ahya VN, Bloom RD, Brozena SC, Olthoff KM, Schuster SJ, Nasta SD, Stadtmauer EA,Tsai DE: Treatment of PTLD with rituximab or chemotherapy. *Am. J. Transplant.* 2006, 6:569-576.

[90] Perrine SP, Hermine O, Small T, Suarez F, O'Reilly R, Boulad F, Fingeroth J, Askin M, Levy A, Mentzer SJ, Di Nicola M, Gianni AM, Klein C, Horwitz S,Faller DV: A phase 1/2 trial of arginine butyrate and ganciclovir in patients with Epstein-Barr virus-associated lymphoid malignancies. *Blood* 2007, 109:2571-2578.

[91] Shirley CM, Chen J, Shamay M, Li H, Zahnow CA, Hayward SD,Ambinder RF: Bortezomib induction of C/EBPbeta mediates Epstein-Barr virus lytic activation in Burkitt lymphoma. *Blood* 2011, 117:6297-6303.

[92] Comoli P, Basso S, Labirio M, Baldanti F, Maccario R,Locatelli F: T cell therapy of Epstein-Barr virus and adenovirus infections after hemopoietic stem cell transplant. *Blood Cells Mol. Dis.* 2008, 40:68-70.

[93] Savoldo B, Goss JA, Hammer MM, Zhang L, Lopez T, Gee AP, Lin YF, Quiros-Tejeira RE, Reinke P, Schubert S, Gottschalk S, Finegold MJ, Brenner MK, Rooney CM,Heslop HE: Treatment of solid organ transplant recipients with autologous Epstein Barr virus-specific cytotoxic T lymphocytes (CTLs). *Blood* 2006, 108:2942-2949.

[94] Haque T, Wilkie GM, Jones MM, Higgins CD, Urquhart G, Wingate P, Burns D, McAulay K, Turner M, Bellamy C, Amlot PL, Kelly D, MacGilchrist A, Gandhi MK, Swerdlow AJ,Crawford DH: Allogeneic cytotoxic T-cell therapy for EBV-positive posttransplantation lymphoproliferative disease: results of a phase 2 multicenter clinical trial. *Blood* 2007, 110:1123-1131.

[95] Davis CL, Wood BL, Sabath DE, Joseph JS, Stehman-Breen C,Broudy VC: Interferon-alpha treatment of posttransplant lymphoproliferative disorder in recipients of solid organ transplants. *Transplantation* 1998, 66:1770-1779.

[96] Tosato G, Tanner J, Jones KD, Revel M,Pike SE: Identification of interleukin-6 as an autocrine growth factor for Epstein-Barr virus-immortalized B cells. *J. Virol.* 1990, 64:3033-3041.

[97] Hinrichs C, Wendland S, Zimmermann H, Eurich D, Neuhaus R, Schlattmann P, Babel N, Riess H, Gartner B, Anagnostopoulos I, Reinke P,Trappe RU: IL-6 and IL-10 in post-transplant lymphoproliferative disorders development and maintenance: a longitudinal study of cytokine plasma levels and T-cell subsets in 38 patients undergoing treatment. *Transpl. Int.* 2011, 24:892-903.

[98] Haddad E, Paczesny S, Leblond V, Seigneurin JM, Stern M, Achkar A, Bauwens M, Delwail V, Debray D, Duvoux C, Hubert P, Hurault de Ligny B, Wijdenes J, Durandy A,Fischer A: Treatment of B-lymphoproliferative disorder with a monoclonal anti-interleukin-6 antibody in 12 patients: a multicenter phase 1-2 clinical trial. *Blood* 2001, 97:1590-1597.

[99] Benkerrou M, Jais JP, Leblond V, Durandy A, Sutton L, Bordigoni P, Garnier JL, Le Bidois J, Le Deist F, Blanche S,Fischer A: Anti-B-cell monoclonal antibody treatment of severe posttransplant B-lymphoproliferative disorder: prognostic factors and long-term outcome. *Blood* 1998, 92:3137-3147.

[100] Fischer A, Blanche S, Le Bidois J, Bordigoni P, Garnier JL, Niaudet P, Morinet F, Le Deist F, Fischer AM, Griscelli C,et al.: Anti-B-cell monoclonal antibodies in the treatment of severe B-cell lymphoproliferative syndrome following bone marrow and organ transplantation. *N. Engl. J. Med.* 1991, 324:1451-1456.

[101] Tsai DE, Aqui NA, Vogl DT, Bloom RD, Schuster SJ, Nasta SD,Wasik MA: Successful treatment of T-cell post-transplant lymphoproliferative disorder with the retinoid analog bexarotene. *Am. J. Transplant.* 2005, 5:2070-2073.

[102] Sokolowska-Wojdylo M, Lugowska-Umer H,Maciejewska-Radomska A: Oral retinoids and rexinoids in cutaneous T-cell lymphomas. *Postepy Dermatol. Alergol.* 2013, 30:19-29.

[103] Faull RJ, Hollett P,McDonald SP: Lymphoproliferative disease after renal transplantation in Australia and New Zealand. *Transplantation* 2005, 80:193-197.

[104] Caillard S, Lelong C, Pessione F, Moulin B,French PWG: Post-transplant lymphoproliferative disorders occurring after renal transplantation in adults: report of 230 cases from the French Registry. *Am. J. Transplant.* 2006, 6:2735-2742.

[105] Kremers WK, Devarbhavi HC, Wiesner RH, Krom RA, Macon WR,Habermann TM: Post-transplant lymphoproliferative disorders following liver transplantation: incidence, risk factors and survival. *Am. J. Transplant.* 2006, 6:1017-1024.

[106] Opelz G,Dohler B: Lymphomas after solid organ transplantation: a collaborative transplant study report. *Am. J. Transplant.* 2004, 4:222-230.

[107] Jain A, Nalesnik M, Reyes J, Pokharna R, Mazariegos G, Green M, Eghtesad B, Marsh W, Cacciarelli T, Fontes P, Abu-Elmagd K, Sindhi R, Demetris J,Fung J: Posttransplant lymphoproliferative disorders in liver transplantation: a 20-year experience. *Ann. Surg.* 2002, 236:429-436; discussion 436-427.

[108] Buell JF, Gross TG, Hanaway MJ, Trofe J, Roy-Chaudhury P, First MR,Woodle ES: Posttransplant lymphoproliferative disorder: significance of central nervous system involvement. *Transplant. Proc.* 2005, 37:954-955.

[109] Schneck SA,Penn I: Cerebral neoplasms associated with renal transplantation. *Arch. Neurol.* 1970, 22:226-233.

[110] Castellano-Sanchez AA, Li S, Qian J, Lagoo A, Weir E,Brat DJ: Primary central nervous system posttransplant lymphoproliferative disorders. *Am. J. Clin. Pathol.* 2004, 121:246-253.

[111] Evens AM, Roy R, Sterrenberg D, Moll MZ, Chadburn A,Gordon LI: Post-transplantation lymphoproliferative disorders: diagnosis, prognosis, and current approaches to therapy. *Curr. Oncol. Rep.* 2010, 12:383-394.

[112] Maecker B, Jack T, Zimmermann M, Abdul-Khaliq H, Burdelski M, Fuchs A, Hoyer P, Koepf S, Kraemer U, Laube GF, Muller-Wiefel DE, Netz H, Pohl M, Toenshoff B, Wagner HJ, Wallot M, Welte K, Melter M, Offner G,Klein C: CNS or bone marrow involvement as risk factors for poor survival in post-transplantation lymphoproliferative disorders in children after solid organ transplantation. *J. Clin. Oncol.* 2007, 25:4902-4908.

[113] Lake W, Chang JE, Kennedy T, Morgan A, Salamat S,Baskaya MK: A case series of primary central nervous system posttransplantation lymphoproliferative disorder: imaging and clinical characteristics. *Neurosurgery* 2013, 72:960-970; discussion 970.

[114] Khedmat H,Taheri S: Post-transplantation lymphoproliferative disorders (PTLD) localized in the central nervous system: report from an international survey on PTLD. *Saudi J. Kidney Dis. Transpl.* 2013, 24:235-242.

[115] Sokal EM, Hoppenbrouwers K, Vandermeulen C, Moutschen M, Leonard P, Moreels A, Haumont M, Bollen A, Smets F,Denis M: Recombinant gp350 vaccine for infectious mononucleosis: a phase 2, randomized, double-blind, placebo-controlled trial to evaluate the safety, immunogenicity, and efficacy of an Epstein-Barr virus vaccine in healthy young adults. *J. Infect. Dis.* 2007, 196:1749-1753.

[116] Hui EP, Taylor GS, Jia H, Ma BB, Chan SL, Ho R, Wong WL, Wilson S, Johnson BF, Edwards C, Stocken DD, Rickinson AB, Steven NM,Chan AT: Phase I trial of recombinant modified vaccinia ankara encoding Epstein-Barr viral tumor antigens in nasopharyngeal carcinoma patients. *Cancer Res.* 2013, 73:1676-1688.

[117] Diekmann J, Adamopoulou E, Beck O, Rauser G, Lurati S, Tenzer S, Einsele H, Rammensee HG, Schild H,Topp MS: Processing of two latent membrane protein 1 MHC class I epitopes requires tripeptidyl peptidase II involvement. *J. Immunol.* 2009, 183:1587-1597.

[118] Cohen JI, Mocarski ES, Raab-Traub N, Corey L,Nabel GJ: The need and challenges for development of an Epstein-Barr virus vaccine. *Vaccine* 2013, 31 Suppl 2:B194-196.

[119] Heslop HE, Slobod KS, Pule MA, Hale GA, Rousseau A, Smith CA, Bollard CM, Liu H, Wu MF, Rochester RJ, Amrolia PJ, Hurwitz JL, Brenner MK,Rooney CM: Long-term outcome of EBV-specific T-cell infusions to prevent or treat EBV-related lymphoproliferative disease in transplant recipients. *Blood* 2010, 115:925-935.

[120] McKnight JL, Cen H, Riddler SA, Breinig MC, Williams PA, Ho M,Joseph PS: EBV gene expression, EBNA antibody responses and EBV+ peripheral blood lymphocytes in post-transplant lymphoproliferative disease. *Leuk Lymphoma* 1994, 15:9-16.

[121] Kenagy DN, Schlesinger Y, Weck K, Ritter JH, Gaudreault-Keener MM,Storch GA: Epstein-Barr virus DNA in peripheral blood leukocytes of patients with posttransplant lymphoproliferative disease. *Transplantation* 1995, 60:547-554.

[122] Shapiro-Shelef M,Calame K: Regulation of plasma-cell development. *Nat. Rev. Immunol.* 2005, 5:230-242.

[123] Ranuncolo SM, Polo JM, Dierov J, Singer M, Kuo T, Greally J, Green R, Carroll M,Melnick A: Bcl-6 mediates the germinal center B cell phenotype and lymphomagenesis through transcriptional repression of the DNA-damage sensor ATR. *Nat. Immunol.* 2007, 8:705-714.

[124] Liu YJ,Arpin C: Germinal center development. *Immunol. Rev.* 1997, 156:111-126.
[125] Thorley-Lawson DA: Epstein-Barr virus: exploiting the immune system. *Nat. Rev. Immunol.* 2001, 1:75-82.
[126] Pasqualucci L, Neumeister P, Goossens T, Nanjangud G, Chaganti RS, Kuppers R,Dalla-Favera R: Hypermutation of multiple proto-oncogenes in B-cell diffuse large-cell lymphomas. *Nature* 2001, 412:341-346.
[127] Sagardoy A, Martinez-Ferrandis JI, Roa S, Bunting KL, Aznar MA, Elemento O, Shaknovich R, Fontan L, Fresquet V, Perez-Roger I, Robles EF, De Smedt L, Sagaert X, Melnick A,Martinez-Climent JA: Downregulation of FOXP1 is required during germinal center B-cell function. *Blood* 2013, 121:4311-4320.
[128] Epstein MA, Achong BG,Barr YM: Virus Particles in Cultured Lymphoblasts from Burkitt's Lymphoma. *Lancet* 1964, 1:702-703.
[129] Thorley-Lawson DA: EBV the prototypical human tumor virus--just how bad is it? *J. Allergy Clin. Immunol.* 2005, 116:251-261; quiz 262.
[130] Laichalk LL, Hochberg D, Babcock GJ, Freeman RB,Thorley-Lawson DA: The dispersal of mucosal memory B cells: evidence from persistent EBV infection. *Immunity* 2002, 16:745-754.
[131] Chen MR: Epstein-barr virus, the immune system, and associated diseases. *Front Microbiol.*2011, 2:5.
[132] Furukawa M, Sakashita H, Kato C,Umeda R: Epstein-Barr virus infection of epithelial cells derived from primary cultures of adenoidal tissue. *Eur. Arch. Otorhinolaryngol.* 1990, 247:109-113.
[133] Young LS,Rickinson AB: Epstein-Barr virus: 40 years on. *Nat. Rev. Cancer* 2004, 4:757-768.
[134] Lemon SM, Hutt LM, Shaw JE, Li JL,Pagano JS: Replication of EBV in epithelial cells during infectious mononucleosis. *Nature* 1977, 268:268-270.
[135] Sixbey JW, Nedrud JG, Raab-Traub N, Hanes RA,Pagano JS: Epstein-Barr virus replication in oropharyngeal epithelial cells. *N. Engl. J. Med.* 1984, 310:1225-1230.
[136] Kobayashi R, Takeuchi H, Sasaki M, Hasegawa M,Hirai K: Detection of Epstein-Barr virus infection in the epithelial cells and lymphocytes of non-neoplastic tonsils by in situ hybridization and in situ PCR. *Arch. Virol.* 1998, 143:803-813.
[137] Niedobitek G, Agathanggelou A, Steven N,Young LS: Epstein-Barr virus (EBV) in infectious mononucleosis: detection of the virus in tonsillar B lymphocytes but not in desquamated oropharyngeal epithelial cells. *Mol. Pathol.* 2000, 53:37-42.
[138] Hudnall SD, Ge Y, Wei L, Yang NP, Wang HQ,Chen T: Distribution and phenotype of Epstein-Barr virus-infected cells in human pharyngeal tonsils. *Mod. Pathol.* 2005, 18:519-527.
[139] Karajannis MA, Hummel M, Anagnostopoulos I,Stein H: Strict lymphotropism of Epstein-Barr virus during acute infectious mononucleosis in nonimmunocompromised individuals. *Blood* 1997, 89:2856-2862.
[140] Tugizov SM, Berline JW,Palefsky JM: Epstein-Barr virus infection of polarized tongue and nasopharyngeal epithelial cells. *Nat. Med.* 2003, 9:307-314.
[141] Pegtel DM, Middeldorp J,Thorley-Lawson DA: Epstein-Barr virus infection in ex vivo tonsil epithelial cell cultures of asymptomatic carriers. *J. Virol.* 2004, 78:12613-12624.
[142] da Silva SR,de Oliveira DE: HIV, EBV and KSHV: viral cooperation in the pathogenesis of human malignancies. *Cancer Lett.* 2011, 305:175-185.

[143] Ambinder RF: Gammaherpesviruses and "Hit-and-Run" oncogenesis. *Am. J. Pathol.* 2000, 156:1-3.

[144] Rezk SA,Weiss LM: Epstein-Barr virus-associated lymphoproliferative disorders. *Hum. Pathol.* 2007, 38:1293-1304.

[145] Hadinoto V, Shapiro M, Greenough TC, Sullivan JL, Luzuriaga K,Thorley-Lawson DA: On the dynamics of acute EBV infection and the pathogenesis of infectious mononucleosis. *Blood* 2008, 111:1420-1427.

[146] Khanna R, Slade RW, Poulsen L, Moss DJ, Burrows SR, Nicholls J,Burrows JM: Evolutionary dynamics of genetic variation in Epstein-Barr virus isolates of diverse geographical origins: evidence for immune pressure-independent genetic drift. *J. Virol.* 1997, 71:8340-8346.

[147] Thorley-Lawson DA,Gross A: Persistence of the Epstein-Barr virus and the origins of associated lymphomas. *N. Engl. J. Med.* 2004, 350:1328-1337.

[148] Shaknovich R, Basso K, Bhagat G, Mansukhani M, Hatzivassiliou G, Murty VV, Buettner M, Niedobitek G, Alobeid B,Cattoretti G: Identification of rare Epstein-Barr virus infected memory B cells and plasma cells in non-monomorphic post-transplant lymphoproliferative disorders and the signature of viral signaling. *Haematologica* 2006, 91:1313-1320.

[149] Cai X, Schafer A, Lu S, Bilello JP, Desrosiers RC, Edwards R, Raab-Traub N,Cullen BR: Epstein-Barr virus microRNAs are evolutionarily conserved and differentially expressed. *PLoS Pathog.* 2006, 2:e23.

[150] Levitskaya J, Coram M, Levitsky V, Imreh S, Steigerwald-Mullen PM, Klein G, Kurilla MG,Masucci MG: Inhibition of antigen processing by the internal repeat region of the Epstein-Barr virus nuclear antigen-1. *Nature* 1995, 375:685-688.

[151] Kusano S,Raab-Traub N: An Epstein-Barr virus protein interacts with Notch. *J. Virol.* 2001, 75:384-395.

[152] Middeldorp JM, Brink AA, van den Brule AJ,Meijer CJ: Pathogenic roles for Epstein-Barr virus (EBV) gene products in EBV-associated proliferative disorders. *Crit. Rev. Oncol. Hematol.* 2003, 45:1-36.

[153] Graham JP, Moore CR,Bishop GA: Roles of the TRAF2/3 binding site in differential B cell signaling by CD40 and its viral oncogenic mimic, LMP1. *J. Immunol.* 2009, 183:2966-2973.

[154] Boehm D, Gewurz BE, Kieff E,Cahir-McFarland E: Epstein-Barr latent membrane protein 1 transformation site 2 activates NF-kappaB in the absence of NF-kappaB essential modifier residues 133-224 or 373-419. Proc Natl Acad Sci U S A 2010, 107:18103-18108.

[155] Blackburn EH, Greider CW,Szostak JW: Telomeres and telomerase: the path from maize, Tetrahymena and yeast to human cancer and aging. *Nat. Med.* 2006, 12:1133-1138.

[156] Giunco S, Dolcetti R, Keppel S, Celeghin A, Indraccolo S, Dal Col J, Mastorci K,De Rossi A: hTERT inhibition triggers Epstein-Barr virus lytic cycle and apoptosis in immortalized and transformed B cells: a basis for new therapies. *Clin. Cancer Res.* 2013, 19:2036-2047.

[157] Kondo S, Seo SY, Yoshizaki T, Wakisaka N, Furukawa M, Joab I, Jang KL,Pagano JS: EBV latent membrane protein 1 up-regulates hypoxia-inducible factor 1alpha through

Siah1-mediated down-regulation of prolyl hydroxylases 1 and 3 in nasopharyngeal epithelial cells. *Cancer Res.* 2006, 66:9870-9877.

[158] Uchida J, Yasui T, Takaoka-Shichijo Y, Muraoka M, Kulwichit W, Raab-Traub N,Kikutani H: Mimicry of CD40 signals by Epstein-Barr virus LMP1 in B lymphocyte responses. *Science* 1999, 286:300-303.

[159] Casola S, Otipoby KL, Alimzhanov M, Humme S, Uyttersprot N, Kutok JL, Carroll MC,Rajewsky K: B cell receptor signal strength determines B cell fate. *Nat. Immunol.* 2004, 5:317-327.

[160] Samanta M, Iwakiri D,Takada K: Epstein-Barr virus-encoded small RNA induces IL-10 through RIG-I-mediated IRF-3 signaling. *Oncogene* 2008, 27:4150-4160.

[161] Takada K: Role of Epstein-Barr virus in Burkitt's lymphoma. *Curr. Top Microbiol. Immunol.* 2001, 258:141-151.

[162] Iwakiri D, Zhou L, Samanta M, Matsumoto M, Ebihara T, Seya T, Imai S, Fujieda M, Kawa K,Takada K: Epstein-Barr virus (EBV)-encoded small RNA is released from EBV-infected cells and activates signaling from Toll-like receptor 3. *Journal of Experimental Medicine* 2009, 206:2091-2099.

[163] Barth S, Meister G,Grasser FA: EBV-encoded miRNAs. *Biochim. Biophys. Acta* 2011, 1809:631-640.

[164] Qiu J, Cosmopoulos K, Pegtel M, Hopmans E, Murray P, Middeldorp J, Shapiro M,Thorley-Lawson DA: A novel persistence associated EBV miRNA expression profile is disrupted in neoplasia. *PLoS Pathog.* 2011, 7:e1002193.

[165] Zomer A, Vendrig T, Hopmans ES, van Eijndhoven M, Middeldorp JM,Pegtel DM: Exosomes: Fit to deliver small RNA. *Commun. Integr. Biol.* 2010, 3:447-450.

[166] Ross N, Gandhi MK,Nourse JP: The Epstein-Barr virus microRNA BART11-5p targets the early B-cell transcription factor EBF1. *Am. J. Blood Res.* 2013, 3:210-224.

[167] Marquitz AR, Mathur A, Nam CS,Raab-Traub N: The Epstein-Barr Virus BART microRNAs target the pro-apoptotic protein Bim. *Virology* 2011, 412:392-400.

[168] Fischer E, Delibrias C,Kazatchkine MD: Expression of CR2 (the C3dg/EBV receptor, CD21) on normal human peripheral blood T lymphocytes. *J. Immunol.* 1991, 146:865-869.

[169] Tabiasco J, Vercellone A, Meggetto F, Hudrisier D, Brousset P,Fournie JJ: Acquisition of viral receptor by NK cells through immunological synapse. *J. Immunol.* 2003, 170:5993-5998.

[170] George LC, Rowe M,Fox CP: Epstein-barr virus and the pathogenesis of T and NK lymphoma: a mystery unsolved. *Curr. Hematol. Malig. Rep.* 2012, 7:276-284.

[171] De Paepe P,De Wolf-Peeters C: Diffuse large B-cell lymphoma: a heterogeneous group of non-Hodgkin lymphomas comprising several distinct clinicopathological entities. *Leukemia* 2007, 21:37-43.

[172] Alizadeh AA, Eisen MB, Davis RE, Ma C, Lossos IS, Rosenwald A, Boldrick JC, Sabet H, Tran T, Yu X, Powell JI, Yang L, Marti GE, Moore T, Hudson J, Jr., Lu L, Lewis DB, Tibshirani R, Sherlock G, Chan WC, Greiner TC, Weisenburger DD, Armitage JO, Warnke R, Levy R, Wilson W, Grever MR, Byrd JC, Botstein D, Brown PO,Staudt LM: Distinct types of diffuse large B-cell lymphoma identified by gene expression profiling. *Nature* 2000, 403:503-511.

[173] Savage KJ, Monti S, Kutok JL, Cattoretti G, Neuberg D, De Leval L, Kurtin P, Dal Cin P, Ladd C, Feuerhake F, Aguiar RC, Li S, Salles G, Berger F, Jing W, Pinkus GS,

Habermann T, Dalla-Favera R, Harris NL, Aster JC, Golub TR,Shipp MA: The molecular signature of mediastinal large B-cell lymphoma differs from that of other diffuse large B-cell lymphomas and shares features with classical Hodgkin lymphoma. *Blood* 2003, 102:3871-3879.

[174] Rosenwald A, Wright G, Chan WC, Connors JM, Campo E, Fisher RI, Gascoyne RD, Muller-Hermelink HK, Smeland EB, Giltnane JM, Hurt EM, Zhao H, Averett L, Yang L, Wilson WH, Jaffe ES, Simon R, Klausner RD, Powell J, Duffey PL, Longo DL, Greiner TC, Weisenburger DD, Sanger WG, Dave BJ, Lynch JC, Vose J, Armitage JO, Montserrat E, Lopez-Guillermo A, Grogan TM, Miller TP, LeBlanc M, Ott G, Kvaloy S, Delabie J, Holte H, Krajci P, Stokke T, Staudt LM,Lymphoma/Leukemia Molecular Profiling P: The use of molecular profiling to predict survival after chemotherapy for diffuse large-B-cell lymphoma. *N. Engl. J. Med.* 2002, 346:1937-1947.

[175] Kreisel F, Kulkarni S, Kerns RT, Hassan A, Deshmukh H, Nagarajan R, Frater JL,Cashen A: High resolution array comparative genomic hybridization identifies copy number alterations in diffuse large B-cell lymphoma that predict response to immuno-chemotherapy. *Cancer Genet.* 2011, 204:129-137.

[176] Baldwin AS: Control of oncogenesis and cancer therapy resistance by the transcription factor NF-kappaB. *J. Clin. Invest.* 2001, 107:241-246.

[177] Yoon SO, Jeon YK, Paik JH, Kim WY, Kim YA, Kim JE,Kim CW: MYC translocation and an increased copy number predict poor prognosis in adult diffuse large B-cell lymphoma (DLBCL), especially in germinal centre-like B cell (GCB) type. *Histopathology* 2008, 53:205-217.

[178] Morin RD, Johnson NA, Severson TM, Mungall AJ, An J, Goya R, Paul JE, Boyle M, Woolcock BW, Kuchenbauer F, Yap D, Humphries RK, Griffith OL, Shah S, Zhu H, Kimbara M, Shashkin P, Charlot JF, Tcherpakov M, Corbett R, Tam A, Varhol R, Smailus D, Moksa M, Zhao Y, Delaney A, Qian H, Birol I, Schein J, Moore R, Holt R, Horsman DE, Connors JM, Jones S, Aparicio S, Hirst M, Gascoyne RD,Marra MA: Somatic mutations altering EZH2 (Tyr641) in follicular and diffuse large B-cell lymphomas of germinal-center origin. *Nat. Genet.* 2010, 42:181-185.

[179] Pasqualucci L, Compagno M, Houldsworth J, Monti S, Grunn A, Nandula SV, Aster JC, Murty VV, Shipp MA,Dalla-Favera R: Inactivation of the PRDM1/BLIMP1 gene in diffuse large B cell lymphoma. *Journal of Experimental Medicine* 2006, 203:311-317.

[180] Iqbal J, Greiner TC, Patel K, Dave BJ, Smith L, Ji J, Wright G, Sanger WG, Pickering DL, Jain S, Horsman DE, Shen Y, Fu K, Weisenburger DD, Hans CP, Campo E, Gascoyne RD, Rosenwald A, Jaffe ES, Delabie J, Rimsza L, Ott G, Muller-Hermelink HK, Connors JM, Vose JM, McKeithan T, Staudt LM, Chan WC,Leukemia/Lymphoma Molecular Profiling P: Distinctive patterns of BCL6 molecular alterations and their functional consequences in different subgroups of diffuse large B-cell lymphoma. *Leukemia* 2007, 21:2332-2343.

[181] Compagno M, Lim WK, Grunn A, Nandula SV, Brahmachary M, Shen Q, Bertoni F, Ponzoni M, Scandurra M, Califano A, Bhagat G, Chadburn A, Dalla-Favera R,Pasqualucci L: Mutations of multiple genes cause deregulation of NF-kappaB in diffuse large B-cell lymphoma. *Nature* 2009, 459:717-721.

[182] Davis RE, Brown KD, Siebenlist U,Staudt LM: Constitutive nuclear factor kappaB activity is required for survival of activated B cell-like diffuse large B cell lymphoma cells. *Journal of Experimental Medicine* 2001, 194:1861-1874.

[183] Pasqualucci L, Trifonov V, Fabbri G, Ma J, Rossi D, Chiarenza A, Wells VA, Grunn A, Messina M, Elliot O, Chan J, Bhagat G, Chadburn A, Gaidano G, Mullighan CG, Rabadan R,Dalla-Favera R: Analysis of the coding genome of diffuse large B-cell lymphoma. *Nat. Genet.* 2011, 43:830-837.

[184] Morin RD, Mendez-Lago M, Mungall AJ, Goya R, Mungall KL, Corbett RD, Johnson NA, Severson TM, Chiu R, Field M, Jackman S, Krzywinski M, Scott DW, Trinh DL, Tamura-Wells J, Li S, Firme MR, Rogic S, Griffith M, Chan S, Yakovenko O, Meyer IM, Zhao EY, Smailus D, Moksa M, Chittaranjan S, Rimsza L, Brooks-Wilson A, Spinelli JJ, Ben-Neriah S, Meissner B, Woolcock B, Boyle M, McDonald H, Tam A, Zhao Y, Delaney A, Zeng T, Tse K, Butterfield Y, Birol I, Holt R, Schein J, Horsman DE, Moore R, Jones SJ, Connors JM, Hirst M, Gascoyne RD,Marra MA: Frequent mutation of histone-modifying genes in non-Hodgkin lymphoma. *Nature* 2011, 476:298-303.

[185] Pasqualucci L: The genetic basis of diffuse large B-cell lymphoma. *Curr. Opin. Hematol.* 2013, 20:336-344.

[186] Pasqualucci L, Dominguez-Sola D, Chiarenza A, Fabbri G, Grunn A, Trifonov V, Kasper LH, Lerach S, Tang H, Ma J, Rossi D, Chadburn A, Murty VV, Mullighan CG, Gaidano G, Rabadan R, Brindle PK,Dalla-Favera R: Inactivating mutations of acetyltransferase genes in B-cell lymphoma. *Nature* 2011, 471:189-195.

[187] Shilatifard A: The COMPASS family of histone H3K4 methylases: mechanisms of regulation in development and disease pathogenesis. *Annu. Rev. Biochem.* 2012, 81:65-95.

[188] Kanda H, Nguyen A, Chen L, Okano H,Hariharan IK: The Drosophila ortholog of MLL3 and MLL4, trithorax related, functions as a negative regulator of tissue growth. *Mol. Cell Biol.* 2013, 33:1702-1710.

[189] Cerchietti LC, Hatzi K, Caldas-Lopes E, Yang SN, Figueroa ME, Morin RD, Hirst M, Mendez L, Shaknovich R, Cole PA, Bhalla K, Gascoyne RD, Marra M, Chiosis G,Melnick A: BCL6 repression of EP300 in human diffuse large B cell lymphoma cells provides a basis for rational combinatorial therapy. *J. Clin. Invest.* 2010,

[190] Knutson SK, Wigle TJ, Warholic NM, Sneeringer CJ, Allain CJ, Klaus CR, Sacks JD, Raimondi A, Majer CR, Song J, Scott MP, Jin L, Smith JJ, Olhava EJ, Chesworth R, Moyer MP, Richon VM, Copeland RA, Keilhack H, Pollock RM,Kuntz KW: A selective inhibitor of EZH2 blocks H3K27 methylation and kills mutant lymphoma cells. *Nat. Chem. Biol.* 2012, 8:890-896.

[191] Jiang Y, Soong TD, Wang L, Melnick AM,Elemento O: Genome-wide detection of genes targeted by non-Ig somatic hypermutation in lymphoma. *PLoS One* 2012, 7:e40332.

[192] Bross L, Fukita Y, McBlane F, Demolliere C, Rajewsky K,Jacobs H: DNA double-strand breaks in immunoglobulin genes undergoing somatic hypermutation. *Immunity* 2000, 13:589-597.

[193] He L, Thomson JM, Hemann MT, Hernando-Monge E, Mu D, Goodson S, Powers S, Cordon-Cardo C, Lowe SW, Hannon GJ,Hammond SM: A microRNA polycistron as a potential human oncogene. *Nature* 2005, 435:828-833.

[194] Calin GA, Dumitru CD, Shimizu M, Bichi R, Zupo S, Noch E, Aldler H, Rattan S, Keating M, Rai K, Rassenti L, Kipps T, Negrini M, Bullrich F,Croce CM: Frequent deletions and down-regulation of micro- RNA genes miR15 and miR16 at 13q14 in chronic lymphocytic leukemia. *Proc. Natl. Acad. Sci. U S A* 2002, 99:15524-15529.

[195] Roehle A, Hoefig KP, Repsilber D, Thorns C, Ziepert M, Wesche KO, Thiere M, Loeffler M, Klapper W, Pfreundschuh M, Matolcsy A, Bernd HW, Reiniger L, Merz H,Feller AC: MicroRNA signatures characterize diffuse large B-cell lymphomas and follicular lymphomas. *Br. J. Haematol.* 2008, 142:732-744.

[196] Malumbres R, Sarosiek KA, Cubedo E, Ruiz JW, Jiang X, Gascoyne RD, Tibshirani R,Lossos IS: Differentiation stage-specific expression of microRNAs in B lymphocytes and diffuse large B-cell lymphomas. *Blood* 2009, 113:3754-3764.

[197] Caramuta S, Lee L, Ozata DM, Akcakaya P, Georgii-Hemming P, Xie H, Amini RM, Lawrie CH, Enblad G, Larsson C, Berglund M,Lui WO: Role of microRNAs and microRNA machinery in the pathogenesis of diffuse large B-cell lymphoma. *Blood Cancer J* 2013, 3:e152.

[198] Moingeon P, Chang HC, Wallner BP, Stebbins C, Frey AZ,Reinherz EL: CD2-mediated adhesion facilitates T lymphocyte antigen recognition function. *Nature* 1989, 339:312-314.

[199] Steidl C, Shah SP, Woolcock BW, Rui L, Kawahara M, Farinha P, Johnson NA, Zhao Y, Telenius A, Neriah SB, McPherson A, Meissner B, Okoye UC, Diepstra A, van den Berg A, Sun M, Leung G, Jones SJ, Connors JM, Huntsman DG, Savage KJ, Rimsza LM, Horsman DE, Staudt LM, Steidl U, Marra MA,Gascoyne RD: MHC class II transactivator CIITA is a recurrent gene fusion partner in lymphoid cancers. *Nature* 2011, 471:377-381.

[200] Green MR, Monti S, Rodig SJ, Juszczynski P, Currie T, O'Donnell E, Chapuy B, Takeyama K, Neuberg D, Golub TR, Kutok JL,Shipp MA: Integrative analysis reveals selective 9p24.1 amplification, increased PD-1 ligand expression, and further induction via JAK2 in nodular sclerosing Hodgkin lymphoma and primary mediastinal large B-cell lymphoma. *Blood* 2010, 116:3268-3277.

[201] Bea S, Zettl A, Wright G, Salaverria I, Jehn P, Moreno V, Burek C, Ott G, Puig X, Yang L, Lopez-Guillermo A, Chan WC, Greiner TC, Weisenburger DD, Armitage JO, Gascoyne RD, Connors JM, Grogan TM, Braziel R, Fisher RI, Smeland EB, Kvaloy S, Holte H, Delabie J, Simon R, Powell J, Wilson WH, Jaffe ES, Montserrat E, Muller-Hermelink HK, Staudt LM, Campo E, Rosenwald A,Lymphoma/Leukemia Molecular Profiling P: Diffuse large B-cell lymphoma subgroups have distinct genetic profiles that influence tumor biology and improve gene-expression-based survival prediction. *Blood* 2005, 106:3183-3190.

[202] Gross S,Walden P: Immunosuppressive mechanisms in human tumors: why we still cannot cure cancer. *Immunol. Lett.* 2008, 116:7-14.

[203] Whiteside TL: The tumor microenvironment and its role in promoting tumor growth. *Oncogene* 2008, 27:5904-5912.

[204] Kuze T, Nakamura N, Hashimoto Y, Sasaki Y,Abe M: The characteristics of Epstein-Barr virus (EBV)-positive diffuse large B-cell lymphoma: comparison between EBV(+) and EBV(-) cases in Japanese population. *Jpn. J. Cancer Res.* 2000, 91:1233-1240.

[205] Park S, Lee J, Ko YH, Han A, Jun HJ, Lee SC, Hwang IG, Park YH, Ahn JS, Jung CW, Kim K, Ahn YC, Kang WK, Park K,Kim WS: The impact of Epstein-Barr virus status on clinical outcome in diffuse large B-cell lymphoma. *Blood* 2007, 110:972-978.

[206] Oyama T, Yamamoto K, Asano N, Oshiro A, Suzuki R, Kagami Y, Morishima Y, Takeuchi K, Izumo T, Mori S, Ohshima K, Suzumiya J, Nakamura N, Abe M, Ichimura K, Sato Y, Yoshino T, Naoe T, Shimoyama Y, Kamiya Y, Kinoshita T,Nakamura S: Age-related EBV-associated B-cell lymphoproliferative disorders constitute a distinct clinicopathologic group: a study of 96 patients. *Clin. Cancer Res.* 2007, 13:5124-5132.

[207] Morales D, Beltran B, De Mendoza FH, Riva L, Yabar A, Quinones P, Butera JN,Castillo J: Epstein-Barr virus as a prognostic factor in de novo nodal diffuse large B-cell lymphoma. *Leuk. Lymphoma* 2010, 51:66-72.

[208] Gibson SE,Hsi ED: Epstein-Barr virus-positive B-cell lymphoma of the elderly at a United States tertiary medical center: an uncommon aggressive lymphoma with a nongerminal center B-cell phenotype. *Hum. Pathol.* 2009, 40:653-661.

[209] Caceres W, Cruz-Amy M,Diaz-Melendez V: AIDS-related malignancies: revisited. *P. R. Health Sci. J.* 2010, 29:70-75.

[210] Epeldegui M, Vendrame E,Martinez-Maza O: HIV-associated immune dysfunction and viral infection: role in the pathogenesis of AIDS-related lymphoma. *Immunol. Res.* 2010, 48:72-83.

[211] Collaboration of Observational HIVERESG, Bohlius J, Schmidlin K, Costagliola D, Fatkenheuer G, May M, Caro-Murillo AM, Mocroft A, Bonnet F, Clifford G, Karafoulidou A, Miro JM, Lundgren J, Chene G,Egger M: Incidence and risk factors of HIV-related non-Hodgkin's lymphoma in the era of combination antiretroviral therapy: a European multicohort study. *Antivir. Ther.* 2009, 14:1065-1074.

[212] Petrara MR, Freguja R, Gianesin K, Zanchetta M,Rossi AD: Epstein-Barr virus-driven lymphomagenesis in the context of human immunodeficiency virus type 1 infection. *Front Microbiol.* 2013, 4:311.

[213] Engels EA, Pfeiffer RM, Landgren O,Moore RD: Immunologic and virologic predictors of AIDS-related non-hodgkin lymphoma in the highly active antiretroviral therapy era. *J. Acquir. Immune Defic. Syndr* .2010, 54:78-84.

[214] Nagy N, Adori M, Rasul A, Heuts F, Salamon D, Ujvari D, Madapura HS, Leveau B, Klein G,Klein E: Soluble factors produced by activated CD4+ T cells modulate EBV latency. *Proc. Natl. Acad. Sci. U S A* 2012, 109:1512-1517.

[215] Powles T, Robinson D, Stebbing J, Shamash J, Nelson M, Gazzard B, Mandelia S, Moller H,Bower M: Highly active antiretroviral therapy and the incidence of non-AIDS-defining cancers in people with HIV infection. *J. Clin. Oncol.* 2009, 27:884-890.

[216] Franceschi S, Lise M, Clifford GM, Rickenbach M, Levi F, Maspoli M, Bouchardy C, Dehler S, Jundt G, Ess S, Bordoni A, Konzelmann I, Frick H, Dal Maso L, Elzi L, Furrer H, Calmy A, Cavassini M, Ledergerber B, Keiser O,Swiss HIVCS: Changing patterns of cancer incidence in the early- and late-HAART periods: the Swiss HIV Cohort Study. *Br. J. Cancer* 2010, 103:416-422.

[217] Castillo JJ, Beltran BE, Miranda RN, Paydas S, Winer ES,Butera JN: Epstein-barr virus-positive diffuse large B-cell lymphoma of the elderly: what we know so far. *Oncologist* 2011, 16:87-96.

[218] Carbone A: AIDS-related non-Hodgkin's lymphomas: from pathology and molecular pathogenesis to treatment. *Hum. Pathol.* 2002, 33:392-404.

[219] Ibrahim HA, Menasce LP, Pomplun S, Burke M, Bower M,Naresh KN: Epstein-Barr virus (EBV) genotypes among human immunodeficiency virus (HIV)-related B-cell lymphomas and B-cell post-transplant lymphoproliferative disorders (B-PTLD)--late-onset lymphomas, especially in the HIV setting, are associated with type-B-EBV. *Eur. J. Haematol.* 2010, 85:227-230.

[220] Conteduca V, Sansonno D, Lauletta G, Russi S, Ingravallo G,Dammacco F: H. pylori infection and gastric cancer: state of the art (review). *Int. J. Oncol.* 2013, 42:5-18.

[221] Schnittman SM, Lane HC, Higgins SE, Folks T,Fauci AS: Direct polyclonal activation of human B lymphocytes by the acquired immune deficiency syndrome virus. *Science* 1986, 233:1084-1086.

[222] Lazzi S, Bellan C, De Falco G, Cinti C, Ferrari F, Nyongo A, Claudio PP, Tosi GM, Vatti R, Gloghini A, Carbone A, Giordano A, Leoncini L,Tosi P: Expression of RB2/p130 tumor-suppressor gene in AIDS-related non-Hodgkin's lymphomas: implications for disease pathogenesis. *Hum. Pathol.* 2002, 33:723-731.

[223] Liapis K, Clear A, Owen A, Coutinho R, Greaves P, Lee AM, Montoto S, Calaminici M,Gribben JG: The microenvironment of AIDS-related diffuse large B-cell lymphoma provides insight into the pathophysiology and indicates possible therapeutic strategies. *Blood* 2013, 122:424-433.

[224] Carbone A,Gloghini A: The microenvironment of AIDS-related diffuse large B-cell lymphoma provides insight into the pathophysiology and indicates possible therapeutic strategies. *Blood* 2013, 122:459-460.

[225] Feng WH, Cohen JI, Fischer S, Li L, Sneller M, Goldbach-Mansky R, Raab-Traub N, Delecluse HJ,Kenney SC: Reactivation of latent Epstein-Barr virus by methotrexate: a potential contributor to methotrexate-associated lymphomas. *J. Natl. Cancer Inst.* 2004, 96:1691-1702.

[226] Park SH, Kim CG, Kim JY,Choe JY: Spontaneous regression of EBV-associated diffuse lymphoproliferative disease in a patient with rheumatoid arthritis after discontinuation of etanercept treatment. *Rheumatol. Int.* 2008, 28:475-477.

[227] Hasserjian RP, Chen S, Perkins SL, de Leval L, Kinney MC, Barry TS, Said J, Lim MS, Finn WG, Medeiros LJ, Harris NL,O'Malley DP: Immunomodulator agent-related lymphoproliferative disorders. *Mod. Pathol.* 2009, 22:1532-1540.

[228] Hoshida Y, Xu JX, Fujita S, Nakamichi I, Ikeda J, Tomita Y, Nakatsuka S, Tamaru J, Iizuka A, Takeuchi T,Aozasa K: Lymphoproliferative disorders in rheumatoid arthritis: clinicopathological analysis of 76 cases in relation to methotrexate medication. *J. Rheumatol.* 2007, 34:322-331.

[229] Filipovich AH, Mathur A, Kamat D,Shapiro RS: Primary immunodeficiencies: genetic risk factors for lymphoma. *Cancer Res.* 1992, 52:5465s-5467s.

[230] Leechawengwongs E,Shearer WT: Lymphoma complicating primary immunodeficiency syndromes. *Curr. Opin. Hematol.* 2012, 19:305-312.

[231] Shapiro RS: Malignancies in the setting of primary immunodeficiency: Implications for hematologists/oncologists. *Am. J. Hematol.* 2011, 86:48-55.

[232] Oyama T, Ichimura K, Suzuki R, Suzumiya J, Ohshima K, Yatabe Y, Yokoi T, Kojima M, Kamiya Y, Taji H, Kagami Y, Ogura M, Saito H, Morishima Y,Nakamura S: Senile

EBV+ B-cell lymphoproliferative disorders: a clinicopathologic study of 22 patients. *Am. J. Surg. Pathol.* 2003, 27:16-26.

[233] Fagnoni FF, Vescovini R, Mazzola M, Bologna G, Nigro E, Lavagetto G, Franceschi C, Passeri M, Sansoni P: Expansion of cytotoxic CD8+ CD28- T cells in healthy ageing people, including centenarians. *Immunology* 1996, 88:501-507.

[234] Ouyang Q, Wagner WM, Walter S, Muller CA, Wikby A, Aubert G, Klatt T, Stevanovic S, Dodi T, Pawelec G: An age-related increase in the number of CD8+ T cells carrying receptors for an immunodominant Epstein-Barr virus (EBV) epitope is counteracted by a decreased frequency of their antigen-specific responsiveness. *Mech. Ageing Dev.* 2003, 124:477-485.

[235] Adam P, Bonzheim I, Fend F, Quintanilla-Martinez L: Epstein-Barr virus-positive diffuse large B-cell lymphomas of the elderly. *Adv. Anat. Pathol.* 2011, 18:349-355.

[236] Dojcinov SD, Venkataraman G, Pittaluga S, Wlodarska I, Schrager JA, Raffeld M, Hills RK, Jaffe ES: Age-related EBV-associated lymphoproliferative disorders in the Western population: a spectrum of reactive lymphoid hyperplasia and lymphoma. *Blood* 2011, 117:4726-4735.

[237] Asano N, Yamamoto K, Tamaru J, Oyama T, Ishida F, Ohshima K, Yoshino T, Nakamura N, Mori S, Yoshie O, Shimoyama Y, Morishima Y, Kinoshita T, Nakamura S: Age-related Epstein-Barr virus (EBV)-associated B-cell lymphoproliferative disorders: comparison with EBV-positive classic Hodgkin lymphoma in elderly patients. *Blood* 2009, 113:2629-2636.

[238] Kojima M, Sugiura I, Itoh H, Shimizu K, Murayama K, Motoori T, Shimano S, Masawa N, Nakamura S: Histological varieties of Epstein-Barr virus-related lymph node lesion resembling autoimmune disease-like clinicopathological findings in middle-aged and elderly patients: a study of six cases. *Pathol. Res. Pract.* 2006, 202:609-615.

[239] Hakim FT, Gress RE: Immunosenescence: deficits in adaptive immunity in the elderly. *Tissue Antigens* 2007, 70:179-189.

[240] Ghia P, Prato G, Stella S, Scielzo C, Geuna M, Caligaris-Cappio F: Age-dependent accumulation of monoclonal CD4+CD8+ double positive T lymphocytes in the peripheral blood of the elderly. *Br. J. Haematol.* 2007, 139:780-790.

[241] Montes-Moreno S, Odqvist L, Diaz-Perez JA, Lopez AB, de Villambrosia SG, Mazorra F, Castillo ME, Lopez M, Pajares R, Garcia JF, Mollejo M, Camacho FI, Ruiz-Marcellan C, Adrados M, Ortiz N, Franco R, Ortiz-Hidalgo C, Suarez-Gauthier A, Young KH, Piris MA: EBV-positive diffuse large B-cell lymphoma of the elderly is an aggressive post-germinal center B-cell neoplasm characterized by prominent nuclear factor-kB activation. *Mod. Pathol.* 2012, 25:968-982.

[242] Nguyen-Van D, Keane C, Han E, Jones K, Nourse JP, Vari F, Ross N, Crooks P, Ramuz O, Green M, Griffith L, Trappe R, Grigg A, Mollee P, Gandhi MK: Epstein-Barr virus-positive diffuse large B-cell lymphoma of the elderly expresses EBNA3A with conserved CD8 T-cell epitopes. *Am. J. Blood Res.* 2011, 1:146-159.

[243] Dolcetti R, Dal Col J, Martorelli D, Carbone A, Klein E: Interplay among viral antigens, cellular pathways and tumor microenvironment in the pathogenesis of EBV-driven lymphomas. *Semin. Cancer Biol.* 2013, 23:441-456.

[244] Kwee I, Capello D, Rinaldi A, Rancoita PM, Bhagat G, Greiner TC, Spina M, Gloghini A, Chan WC, Paulli M, Zucca E, Tirelli U, Carbone A, Gaidano G, Bertoni F: Genomic

aberrations affecting the outcome of immunodeficiency-related diffuse large B-cell lymphoma. *Leuk Lymphoma* 2012, 53:71-76.

[245] Johannessen I, Perera SM, Gallagher A, Hopwood PA, Thomas JA,Crawford DH: Expansion in scid mice of Epstein-Barr virus-associated post-transplantation lymphoproliferative disease biopsy material. *J. Gen. Virol.* 2002, 83:173-178.

[246] Johannessen I, Bieleski L, Urquhart G, Watson SL, Wingate P, Haque T,Crawford DH: Epstein-Barr virus, B cell lymphoproliferative disease, and SCID mice: modeling T cell immunotherapy in vivo. *J. Med. Virol.* 2011, 83:1585-1596.

[247] Zhang B, Kracker S, Yasuda T, Casola S, Vanneman M, Homig-Holzel C, Wang Z, Derudder E, Li S, Chakraborty T, Cotter SE, Koyama S, Currie T, Freeman GJ, Kutok JL, Rodig SJ, Dranoff G,Rajewsky K: Immune surveillance and therapy of lymphomas driven by Epstein-Barr virus protein LMP1 in a mouse model. *Cell* 2012, 148:739-751.

[248] Bernasconi M, Ueda S, Krukowski P, Bornhauser BC, Ladell K, Dorner M, Sigrist JA, Campidelli C, Aslandogmus R, Alessi D, Berger C, Pileri SA, Speck RF,Nadal D: Early gene expression changes by Epstein-Barr virus infection of B-cells indicate CDKs and survivin as therapeutic targets for post-transplant lymphoproliferative diseases. *Int. J. Cancer* 2013, 133:2341-2350.

[249] Dai Y, Tang Y, He F, Zhang Y, Cheng A, Gan R,Wu Y: Screening and functional analysis of differentially expressed genes in EBV-transformed lymphoblasts. *Virol. J.* 2012, 9:77.

[250] Timms JM, Bell A, Flavell JR, Murray PG, Rickinson AB, Traverse-Glehen A, Berger F,Delecluse HJ: Target cells of Epstein-Barr-virus (EBV)-positive post-transplant lymphoproliferative disease: similarities to EBV-positive Hodgkin's lymphoma. *Lancet* 2003, 361:217-223.

[251] Gires O, Kohlhuber F, Kilger E, Baumann M, Kieser A, Kaiser C, Zeidler R, Scheffer B, Ueffing M,Hammerschmidt W: Latent membrane protein 1 of Epstein-Barr virus interacts with JAK3 and activates STAT proteins. *EMBO J.* 1999, 18:3064-3073.

[252] Shair KH, Bendt KM, Edwards RH, Bedford EC, Nielsen JN,Raab-Traub N: EBV latent membrane protein 1 activates Akt, NFkappaB, and Stat3 in B cell lymphomas. *PLoS Pathog.* 2007, 3:e166.

[253] Vakiani E, Basso K, Klein U, Mansukhani MM, Narayan G, Smith PM, Murty VV, Dalla-Favera R, Pasqualucci L,Bhagat G: Genetic and phenotypic analysis of B-cell post-transplant lymphoproliferative disorders provides insights into disease biology. *Hematol. Oncol.* 2008, 26:199-211.

[254] Montone KT, Hodinka RL, Salhany KE, Lavi E, Rostami A,Tomaszewski JE: Identification of Epstein-Barr virus lytic activity in post-transplantation lymphoproliferative disease. *Mod. Pathol.* 1996, 9:621-630.

[255] Draborg AH, Duus K,Houen G: Epstein-Barr virus and systemic lupus erythematosus. *Clin. Dev. Immunol.* 2012, 2012:370516.

[256] Hong GK, Kumar P, Wang L, Damania B, Gulley ML, Delecluse HJ, Polverini PJ,Kenney SC: Epstein-Barr virus lytic infection is required for efficient production of the angiogenesis factor vascular endothelial growth factor in lymphoblastoid cell lines. *J. Virol.* 2005, 79:13984-13992.

[257] Ma SD, Hegde S, Young KH, Sullivan R, Rajesh D, Zhou Y, Jankowska-Gan E, Burlingham WJ, Sun X, Gulley ML, Tang W, Gumperz JE,Kenney SC: A new model

of Epstein-Barr virus infection reveals an important role for early lytic viral protein expression in the development of lymphomas. *J. Virol.* 2011, 85:165-177.

[258] Hong GK, Gulley ML, Feng WH, Delecluse HJ, Holley-Guthrie E,Kenney SC: Epstein-Barr virus lytic infection contributes to lymphoproliferative disease in a SCID mouse model. *J. Virol.* 2005, 79:13993-14003.

[259] Nelson BP, Nalesnik MA, Bahler DW, Locker J, Fung JJ,Swerdlow SH: Epstein-Barr virus-negative post-transplant lymphoproliferative disorders: a distinct entity? *Am. J. Surg. Pathol.* 2000, 24:375-385.

[260] Shimizu N, Tanabe-Tochikura A, Kuroiwa Y,Takada K: Isolation of Epstein-Barr virus (EBV)-negative cell clones from the EBV-positive Burkitt's lymphoma (BL) line Akata: malignant phenotypes of BL cells are dependent on EBV. *J. Virol.* 1994, 68:6069-6073.

[261] Jox A, Rohen C, Belge G, Bartnitzke S, Pawlita M, Diehl V, Bullerdiek J,Wolf J: Integration of Epstein-Barr virus in Burkitt's lymphoma cells leads to a region of enhanced chromosome instability. *Ann. Oncol.* 1997, 8 Suppl 2:131-135.

[262] Theate I, Michaux L, Squifflet JP, Martin A,Raphael M: Human herpesvirus 8 and Epstein-Barr virus-related monotypic large B-cell lymphoproliferative disorder coexisting with mixed variant of Castleman's disease in a lymph node of a renal transplant recipient. *Clin. Transplant.* 2003, 17:451-454.

[263] Kapelushnik J, Ariad S, Benharroch D, Landau D, Moser A, Delsol G,Brousset P: Post renal transplantation human herpesvirus 8-associated lymphoproliferative disorder and Kaposi's sarcoma. *Br. J. Haematol.* 2001, 113:425-428.

[264] Zallio F, Primon V, Tamiazzo S, Pini M, Baraldi A, Corsetti MT, Gotta F, Bertasello C, Salvi F, Rocchetti A,Levis A: Epstein-Barr virus reactivation in allogeneic stem cell transplantation is highly related to cytomegalovirus reactivation. *Clin. Transplant.* 2013, 27:E491-497.

[265] Craig FE, Johnson LR, Harvey SA, Nalesnik MA, Luo JH, Bhattacharya SD,Swerdlow SH: Gene expression profiling of Epstein-Barr virus-positive and -negative monomorphic B-cell posttransplant lymphoproliferative disorders. *Diagn. Mol. Pathol.* 2007, 16:158-168.

[266] Morscio J, Dierickx D, Ferreiro JF, Herreman A, Van Loo P, Bittoun E, Verhoef G, Matthys P, Cools J, Wlodarska I, De Wolf-Peeters C, Sagaert X,Tousseyn T: Gene expression profiling reveals clear differences between EBV-positive and EBV-negative posttransplant lymphoproliferative disorders. *Am. J. Transplant.* 2013, 13:1305-1316.

[267] Strong MJ, Xu G, Coco J, Baribault C, Vinay DS, Lacey MR, Strong AL, Lehman TA, Seddon MB, Lin Z, Concha M, Baddoo M, Ferris M, Swan KF, Sullivan DE, Burow ME, Taylor CM,Flemington EK: Differences in gastric carcinoma microenvironment stratify according to EBV infection intensity: implications for possible immune adjuvant therapy. *PLoS Pathog.* 2013, 9:e1003341.

[268] Vogt L, Schmitz N, Kurrer MO, Bauer M, Hinton HI, Behnke S, Gatto D, Sebbel P, Beerli RR, Sonderegger I, Kopf M, Saudan P,Bachmann MF: VSIG4, a B7 family-related protein, is a negative regulator of T cell activation. *J. Clin. Invest.* 2006, 116:2817-2826.

[269] Green MR, Rodig S, Juszczynski P, Ouyang J, Sinha P, O'Donnell E, Neuberg D,Shipp MA: Constitutive AP-1 activity and EBV infection induce PD-L1 in Hodgkin

lymphomas and posttransplant lymphoproliferative disorders: implications for targeted therapy. *Clin. Cancer Res.* 2012, 18:1611-1618.

[270] Cesarman E, Chadburn A, Liu YF, Migliazza A, Dalla-Favera R,Knowles DM: BCL-6 gene mutations in posttransplantation lymphoproliferative disorders predict response to therapy and clinical outcome. *Blood* 1998, 92:2294-2302.

[271] Poirel HA, Bernheim A, Schneider A, Meddeb M, Choquet S, Leblond V, Charlotte F, Davi F, Canioni D, Macintyre E, Mamzer-Bruneel MF, Hirsch I, Hermine O, Martin A, Cornillet-Lefebvre P, Patey M, Toupance O, Kemeny JL, Deteix P,Raphael M: Characteristic pattern of chromosomal imbalances in posttransplantation lymphoproliferative disorders: correlation with histopathological subcategories and EBV status. *Transplantation* 2005, 80:176-184.

[272] Djokic M, Le Beau MM, Swinnen LJ, Smith SM, Rubin CM, Anastasi J,Carlson KM: Post-transplant lymphoproliferative disorder subtypes correlate with different recurring chromosomal abnormalities. *Genes Chromosomes Cancer* 2006, 45:313-318.

[273] Cerri M, Capello D, Muti G, Rambaldi A, Paulli M, Gloghini A, Berra E, Deambrogi C, Rossi D, Franceschetti S, Conconi A, Morra E, Pasqualucci L, Carbone A,Gaidano G: Aberrant somatic hypermutation in post-transplant lymphoproliferative disorders. *Br. J. Haematol.* 2004, 127:362-364.

[274] Abed N, Casper JT, Camitta BM, Margolis D, Trost B, Orentas R,Chang CC: Evaluation of histogenesis of B-lymphocytes in pediatric EBV-related post-transplant lymphoproliferative disorders. *Bone Marrow Transplant.* 2004, 33:321-327.

[275] Hans CP, Weisenburger DD, Greiner TC, Gascoyne RD, Delabie J, Ott G, Muller-Hermelink HK, Campo E, Braziel RM, Jaffe ES, Pan Z, Farinha P, Smith LM, Falini B, Banham AH, Rosenwald A, Staudt LM, Connors JM, Armitage JO,Chan WC: Confirmation of the molecular classification of diffuse large B-cell lymphoma by immunohistochemistry using a tissue microarray. *Blood* 2004, 103:275-282.

[276] Choi WW, Weisenburger DD, Greiner TC, Piris MA, Banham AH, Delabie J, Braziel RM, Geng H, Iqbal J, Lenz G, Vose JM, Hans CP, Fu K, Smith LM, Li M, Liu Z, Gascoyne RD, Rosenwald A, Ott G, Rimsza LM, Campo E, Jaffe ES, Jaye DL, Staudt LM,Chan WC: A new immunostain algorithm classifies diffuse large B-cell lymphoma into molecular subtypes with high accuracy. *Clin. Cancer Res.* 2009, 15:5494-5502.

[277] Brauninger A, Spieker T, Mottok A, Baur AS, Kuppers R,Hansmann ML: Epstein-Barr virus (EBV)-positive lymphoproliferations in post-transplant patients show immunoglobulin V gene mutation patterns suggesting interference of EBV with normal B cell differentiation processes. *Eur. J. Immunol.* 2003, 33:1593-1602.

[278] Kinch A, Baecklund E, Backlin C, Ekman T, Molin D, Tufveson G, Fernberg P, Sundstrom C, Pauksens K,Enblad G: A population-based study of 135 lymphomas after solid organ transplantation: The role of Epstein-Barr virus, hepatitis C and diffuse large B-cell lymphoma subtype in clinical presentation and survival. *Acta Oncol.* 2013,

[279] Capello D, Cerri M, Muti G, Berra E, Oreste P, Deambrogi C, Rossi D, Dotti G, Conconi A, Vigano M, Magrini U, Ippoliti G, Morra E, Gloghini A, Rambaldi A, Paulli M, Carbone A,Gaidano G: Molecular histogenesis of posttransplantation lymphoproliferative disorders. *Blood* 2003, 102:3775-3785.

[280] Locker J,Nalesnik M: Molecular genetic analysis of lymphoid tumors arising after organ transplantation. *Am. J. Pathol.* 1989, 135:977-987.

[281] de Wind N, Dekker M, van Rossum A, van der Valk M,te Riele H: Mouse models for hereditary nonpolyposis colorectal cancer. *Cancer Res.* 1998, 58:248-255.

[282] Saeterdal I, Bjorheim J, Lislerud K, Gjertsen MK, Bukholm IK, Olsen OC, Nesland JM, Eriksen JA, Moller M, Lindblom A,Gaudernack G: Frameshift-mutation-derived peptides as tumor-specific antigens in inherited and spontaneous colorectal cancer. *Proc. Natl. Acad. Sci. U S A* 2001, 98:13255-13260.

[283] Duval A, Raphael M, Brennetot C, Poirel H, Buhard O, Aubry A, Martin A, Krimi A, Leblond V, Gabarre J, Davi F, Charlotte F, Berger F, Gaidano G, Capello D, Canioni D, Bordessoule D, Feuillard J, Gaulard P, Delfau MH, Ferlicot S, Eclache V, Prevot S, Guettier C, Lefevre PC, Adotti F,Hamelin R: The mutator pathway is a feature of immunodeficiency-related lymphomas. *Proc. Natl. Acad. Sci. U S A* 2004, 101:5002-5007.

[284] Rinaldi A, Kwee I, Poretti G, Mensah A, Pruneri G, Capello D, Rossi D, Zucca E, Ponzoni M, Catapano C, Tibiletti MG, Paulli M, Gaidano G,Bertoni F: Comparative genome-wide profiling of post-transplant lymphoproliferative disorders and diffuse large B-cell lymphomas. *Br. J. Haematol.* 2006, 134:27-36.

[285] Rinaldi A, Capello D, Scandurra M, Greiner TC, Chan WC, Bhagat G, Rossi D, Morra E, Paulli M, Rambaldi A, Rancoita PM, Inghirami G, Ponzoni M, Moreno SM, Piris MA, Mian M, Chigrinova E, Zucca E, Favera RD, Gaidano G, Kwee I,Bertoni F: Single nucleotide polymorphism-arrays provide new insights in the pathogenesis of post-transplant diffuse large B-cell lymphoma. *Br. J. Haematol.* 2010, 149:569-577.

[286] Booman M, Douwes J, Glas AM, Riemersma SA, Jordanova ES, Kok K, Rosenwald A, de Jong D, Schuuring E,Kluin PM: Mechanisms and effects of loss of human leukocyte antigen class II expression in immune-privileged site-associated B-cell lymphoma. *Clin. Cancer Res.* 2006, 12:2698-2705.

[287] Luo WJ, Takakuwa T, Ham MF, Wada N, Liu A, Fujita S, Sakane-Ishikawa E,Aozasa K: Epstein-Barr virus is integrated between REL and BCL-11A in American Burkitt lymphoma cell line (NAB-2). *Lab. Invest.* 2004, 84:1193-1199.

[288] Blanco S, Sanz-Garcia M, Santos CR,Lazo PA: Modulation of interleukin-1 transcriptional response by the interaction between VRK2 and the JIP1 scaffold protein. PLoS One 2008, 3:e1660.

[289] Reshef R, Luskin MR, Kamoun M, Vardhanabhuti S, Tomaszewski JE, Stadtmauer EA, Porter DL, Heitjan DF,Tsai de E: Association of HLA polymorphisms with post-transplant lymphoproliferative disorder in solid-organ transplant recipients. *Am. J. Transplant.* 2011, 11:817-825.

[290] Pourfarziani V, Einollahi B, Taheri S, Nemati E, Nafar M,Kalantar E: Associations of Human Leukocyte Antigen (HLA) haplotypes with risk of developing lymphoproliferative disorders after renal transplantation. *Ann. Transplant.* 2007, 12:16-22.

[291] Lee TC, Savoldo B, Barshes NR, Rooney CM, Heslop HE, Gee AP, Caldwell Y, Scott JD,Goss JA: Use of cytokine polymorphisms and Epstein-Barr virus viral load to predict development of post-transplant lymphoproliferative disorder in paediatric liver transplant recipients. *Clin. Transplant.* 2006, 20:389-393.

[292] Udalova IA, Richardson A, Denys A, Smith C, Ackerman H, Foxwell B,Kwiatkowski D: Functional consequences of a polymorphism affecting NF-kappaB p50-p50 binding to the TNF promoter region. *Mol. Cell. Biol.* 2000, 20:9113-9119.

[293] Balkwill F: Tumor necrosis factor or tumor promoting factor? *Cytokine Growth Factor Rev.* 2002, 13:135-141.

[294] Kasztelewicz B, Jankowska I, Pawlowska J, Teisseyre J,Dzierzanowska-Fangrat K: The impact of cytokine gene polymorphisms on Epstein-Barr virus infection outcome in pediatric liver transplant recipients. *J. Clin. Virol.* 2012, 55:226-232.

[295] Zuercher E, Butticaz C, Wyniger J, Martinez R, Battegay M, Boffi El Amari E, Dang T, Egger JF, Fehr J, Mueller-Garamvogyi E, Parini A, Schaefer SC, Schoeni-Affolter F, Thurnheer C, Tinguely M, Telenti A, Rothenberger S,Swiss HIVCS: Genetic diversity of EBV-encoded LMP1 in the Swiss HIV Cohort Study and implication for NF-Kappab activation. *PLoS One* 2012, 7:e32168.

[296] Kasztelewicz B, Jankowska I, Pawlowska J, Teisseyre J,Dzierzanowska-Fangrat K: Epstein-Barr virus gene expression and latent membrane protein 1 gene polymorphism in pediatric liver transplant recipients. *J. Med. Virol.* 2011, 83:2182-2190.

[297] Jones K, Nourse JP, Morrison L, Nguyen-Van D, Moss DJ, Burrows SR,Gandhi MK: Expansion of EBNA1-specific effector T cells in posttransplantation lymphoproliferative disorders. *Blood* 2010, 116:2245-2252.

[298] Rossi D, Gaidano G, Gloghini A, Deambrogi C, Franceschetti S, Berra E, Cerri M, Vendramin C, Conconi A, Viglio A, Muti G, Oreste P, Morra E, Paulli M, Capello D,Carbone A: Frequent aberrant promoter hypermethylation of O6-methylguanine-DNA methyltransferase and death-associated protein kinase genes in immunodeficiency-related lymphomas. *Br. J. Haematol.* 2003, 123:475-478.

[299] Gerson SL: MGMT: its role in cancer aetiology and cancer therapeutics. *Nat. Rev. Cancer* 2004, 4:296-307.

[300] Leonard S, Wei W, Anderton J, Vockerodt M, Rowe M, Murray PG,Woodman CB: Epigenetic and transcriptional changes which follow Epstein-Barr virus infection of germinal center B cells and their relevance to the pathogenesis of Hodgkin's lymphoma. *J. Virol.* 2011, 85:9568-9577.

[301] Greaves P, Clear A, Coutinho R, Wilson A, Matthews J, Owen A, Shanyinde M, Lister TA, Calaminici M,Gribben JG: Expression of FOXP3, CD68, and CD20 at diagnosis in the microenvironment of classical Hodgkin lymphoma is predictive of outcome. *J. Clin. Oncol.* 2013, 31:256-262.

[302] Koch K, Hoster E, Unterhalt M, Ott G, Rosenwald A, Hansmann ML, Engelhard M, Hiddemann W,Klapper W: The composition of the microenvironment in follicular lymphoma is associated with the stage of the disease. *Hum. Pathol.* 2012, 43:2274-2281.

[303] Richendollar BG, Tsao RE, Elson P, Jin T, Steinle R, Pohlman B,Hsi ED: Predictors of outcome in post-transplant lymphoproliferative disorder: an evaluation of tumor infiltrating lymphocytes in the context of clinical factors. *Leuk. Lymphoma* 2009, 50:2005-2012.

[304] Verdonk RC, Haagsma EB, Jonker MR, Bok LI, Zandvoort JH, Kleibeuker JH, Faber KN,Dijkstra G: Effects of different immunosuppressive regimens on regulatory T-cells in noninflamed colon of liver transplant recipients. *Inflamm. Bowel. Dis.* 2007, 13:703-709.

[305] Dukers DF, Meij P, Vervoort MB, Vos W, Scheper RJ, Meijer CJ, Bloemena E,Middeldorp JM: Direct immunosuppressive effects of EBV-encoded latent membrane protein 1. *J. Immunol.* 2000, 165:663-670.

[306] Zimmermann H, Reinke P, Neuhaus R, Lehmkuhl H, Oertel S, Atta J, Planker M, Gartner B, Lenze D, Anagnostopoulos I, Riess H,Trappe RU: Burkitt post-transplantation lymphoma in adult solid organ transplant recipients: sequential immunochemotherapy with rituximab (R) followed by cyclophosphamide, doxorubicin, vincristine, and prednisone (CHOP) or R-CHOP is safe and effective in an analysis of 8 patients. *Cancer* 2012, 118:4715-4724.

[307] Picarsic J, Jaffe R, Mazariegos G, Webber SA, Ellis D, Green MD,Reyes-Mugica M: Post-transplant Burkitt lymphoma is a more aggressive and distinct form of post-transplant lymphoproliferative disorder. *Cancer* 2011, 117:4540-4550.

[308] Thorley-Lawson DA,Allday MJ: The curious case of the tumour virus: 50 years of Burkitt's lymphoma. *Nat. Rev. Microbiol.* 2008, 6:913-924.

[309] Zindy F, Eischen CM, Randle DH, Kamijo T, Cleveland JL, Sherr CJ,Roussel MF: Myc signaling via the ARF tumor suppressor regulates p53-dependent apoptosis and immortalization. *Genes Dev.* 1998, 12:2424-2433.

[310] Nagy N, Klein G,Klein E: To the genesis of Burkitt lymphoma: regulation of apoptosis by EBNA-1 and SAP may determine the fate of Ig-myc translocation carrying B lymphocytes. *Semin. Cancer Biol.* 2009, 19:407-410.

[311] Yamamoto N, Takizawa T, Iwanaga Y, Shimizu N,Yamamoto N: Malignant transformation of B lymphoma cell line BJAB by Epstein-Barr virus-encoded small RNAs. *FEBS Lett* 2000, 484:153-158.

[312] Klapproth K, Sander S, Marinkovic D, Baumann B,Wirth T: The IKK2/NF-{kappa}B pathway suppresses MYC-induced lymphomagenesis. *Blood* 2009, 114:2448-2458.

[313] Klapproth K,Wirth T: Advances in the understanding of MYC-induced lymphomagenesis. *Br. J. Haematol.* 2010, 149:484-497.

[314] Borenstein J, Pezzella F,Gatter KC: Plasmablastic lymphomas may occur as post-transplant lymphoproliferative disorders. *Histopathology* 2007, 51:774-777.

[315] Valera A, Balague O, Colomo L, Martinez A, Delabie J, Taddesse-Heath L, Jaffe ES,Campo E: IG/MYC rearrangements are the main cytogenetic alteration in plasmablastic lymphomas. *Am. J. Surg. Pathol.* 2010, 34:1686-1694.

[316] Knowles DM: Immunodeficiency-associated lymphoproliferative disorders. *Mod. Pathol.* 1999, 12:200-217.

[317] Gheorghe G, Albano EA, Porter CC, McGavran L, Wei Q, Meltesen L, Danielson SM,Liang X: Posttransplant Hodgkin lymphoma preceded by polymorphic posttransplant lymphoproliferative disorder: report of a pediatric case and review of the literature. *J. Pediatr. Hematol. Oncol.* 2007, 29:112-116.

[318] Dharnidharka VR, Douglas VK, Hunger SP,Fennell RS: Hodgkin's lymphoma after post-transplant lymphoproliferative disease in a renal transplant recipient. *Pediatr. Transplant.* 2004, 8:87-90.

[319] Jaffe ES, Nicolae A,Pittaluga S: Peripheral T-cell and NK-cell lymphomas in the WHO classification: pearls and pitfalls. *Mod. Pathol.* 2013, 26 Suppl 1:S71-87.

[320] Takahara M, Kis LL, Nagy N, Liu A, Harabuchi Y, Klein G,Klein E: Concomitant increase of LMP1 and CD25 (IL-2-receptor alpha) expression induced by IL-10 in the EBV-positive NK lines SNK6 and KAI3. *Int. J. Cancer* 2006, 119:2775-2783.

[321] Ng SB, Selvarajan V, Huang G, Zhou J, Feldman AL, Law M, Kwong YL, Shimizu N, Kagami Y, Aozasa K, Salto-Tellez M,Chng WJ: Activated oncogenic pathways and

therapeutic targets in extranodal nasal-type NK/T cell lymphoma revealed by gene expression profiling. *J. Pathol.* 2011, 223:496-510.

[322] Magro CM, Weinerman DJ, Porcu PL, Morrison CD: Post-transplant EBV-negative anaplastic large-cell lymphoma with dual rearrangement: a propos of two cases and review of the literature. *J. Cutan. Pathol.* 2007, 34 Suppl 1:1-8.

Reviewed by: Prof. Dr. Em. Christiane De Wolf-Peeters: KU Leuven, Department of Imaging and Pathology, Translational Cell and Tissue Research; University Hospitals KU Leuven, Department of Pathology, Leuven, Belgium

Biographical Sketch

Julie Morscio, MsC, is currently affiliated with the KU Leuven, Department of Imaging and Pathology, Leuven, Belgium. Research and Professional Experience: Master in Biomedical Sciences at the KU Leuven. During her studies she explored different research fields (Parkinson's Disease, adenoviral vectors and clinical immunology) during three internships in different University labs. During her master thesis in the lab of Prof. Dr. Thomas Tousseyn she got involved in a research project aiming to unravel the pathogenetic mechanisms of lymphomas arising in chronically immunosuppressed patients performing histopathological studies and gene expression analyses on human tumor samples. She continued this research starting a PhD in 2012. Her project focusses on the clinicopathological and molecular characterization of aggressive lymphomas with emphasis on the role of the Epstein-Barr virus in lymphomagenesis. She is also involved in a project aiming at the establishment of a patient-derived human lymphoma xenograft mouse models. She has published 5 papers over the last 3 years.

Thomas Tousseyn, MD, is currently affiliated with the KU Leuven, Department of Imaging and Pathology and the UZ Leuven, Department of Pathology, Leuven, Belgium. Research and Professional Experience: Medical doctor and hematopathologist, responsible for diagnostic Hematopathology and Neurodegenerative disorders at the Pathology Department of the UZ Leuven. His current research project focuses on translational research of lymphoid neoplasms, more specifically on the understanding of the molecular pathogenesis of lymphomas and the identification of prognostic biomarkers in lymphoma. Professional Appointments: Adjunct Clinical Head at Department of Pathology, UZ Leuven, Associate Professor in Faculty of Medicine, KU Leuven. He was honored with ICRETT fellowship from International Union Against Cancer (2010), Young Investigator's Award from the International Society of Neuropathology (2006), Fellowship Belgian American Educational Foundation: D. Collen Grant (2006), Aspirant-Fonds voor Wetenschappelijk Onderzoek (2003), and several research grants, including the last one "Study of the role of tyrosine phosphatases in the pathogenesis of acute lymphatic leukemia". He has published 34 papers over the last 3 years.

In: Epstein-Barr Virus (EBV)
Editor: Jan Styczynski

ISBN: 978-1-63117-476-6
© 2014 Nova Science Publishers, Inc.

Chapter V

EBV-Related Post-Transplant Lymphoproliferative Disorders (PTLD): Background, Diagnosis and Treatment

Ghaith Abu-Zeinah[1],* and Mustafa Al-Kawaaz[2]
[1]Department of Internal Medicine, New York Presbyterian Hospital/
Weill Cornell Medical Center, New York, NY, US
[2]Department of Pathology, New York Presbyterian Hospital/
Weill Cornell Medical Center, New York, NY, US

Abstract

Post-transplant lymphoproliferative disease (PTLD) is the uncontrolled proliferation of plasmacytic or lymphoid cells in the immunosuppressed, transplant patient. Although exceptions do exist, PTLD is largely due to latent Epstein-Barr virus (EBV). The expressed oncogenic viral proteins interfere with cell cycle regulation of the host's lymphoid cells, commonly B cells. This leads to the abnormal cellular proliferation in the absence of immune surveillance. Serial measurement of EBV viral load post-transplant is currently the chosen method for early detection of the disease and identifying those at risk. It is also useful for monitoring disease progression and response to treatment. However, pathology is essential to make the diagnosis and classify PTLD based on the histologic subtypes. Immunohistochemistry, flow cytometry, and other modalities are utilized to classify the subtype and predict prognosis and response to therapy. Identifying cellular markers, including CD20 expression can help guide therapy. The CD-20 monoclonal antibody rituximab has shown efficacy as monotherapy in B-cell PTLD. However it is often combined with chemotherapeutic regimens such as CHOP to yield better response rates and cover a broader category of PTLDs. The first step in treatment, however, is reduction in immunosuppression. A major and innovative new approach to treatment is that of adoptive immunotherapy. This involves transfer of EBV-specific cytotoxic T-cells (EBV-CTLs) and it had shown remarkable efficacy and safety outcomes. While initially autologous CTLs were used, currently, partially HLA-matched

---

* Address for correspondence. E-mail: gfa2001@nyp.org.

EBV-CTLs are preferred as a more cost-effective and practical alternative. Current research in the field of PTLD is investigating the use of targeted therapy in treatment. Due to the epidemiology of this disease, however, large clinical trials are lacking.

Keywords: EBV, PTLD, diagnosis, treatment, viral load, rituximab, chemotherapy, adoptive immunotherapy

1. Introduction

The herpesvirus family name was derived from the Greek word "herpein", which means "to creep". The term describes the ability of the virus to make its way into host cells and establish a life-long latent state while evading the immune system. The Epstein-Barr virus (EBV), a member of this family, demonstrates this feature within the B-lymphocytic cells.

The cytotoxic immune response is normally unable to detect and destroy latently infected B-cells. However, a primary EBV infection or a reactivation can trigger the immune response against the replicating EBV within its host. It normally serves to limit viremia and prevent both disseminated disease and EBV-induced lymphoproliferation. This response is lacking in post-transplant patients who are immunosuppressed.

A primary EBV infection in such patients, or even a reactivation, can lead to a lethal infectious mononucleosis syndrome with high mortality rates. On the other hand, latent EBV can trigger oncogenic pathways within the B-cell host. This promotes dysregulated B cell proliferation and resistance to apoptosis that ultimately progresses to a lymphoproliferative disease. The various types of lymphomas/lymphoproliferations in the setting of transplant is collectively referred to as post-transplant lymphoproliferative disease (PTLD).

1a) PTLD and Its Clinical Presentation

PTLD is the uncontrolled proliferation of plasmacytic or lymphoid cells in the hematopoietic or solid organ transplant patient, and is often life-threatening. The different subtypes lie among a continuum of disease classified by the WHO in 2008, which will be addressed in the pathology section of diagnosis *(see section 2c)*.

Clinically, PTLD has a highly variable presentation. In the transplant patient, graft rejection, infection and PTLD should always be considered with potentially any new, concerning symptoms and signs. The time frame from transplant to presentation can be helpful in making the distinction, as PTLD is more common within the first few months after transplant.

Generally, PTLD can present as a viral syndrome of infectious mononucleosis (fever, malaise, lymphadenopathy, hepatosplenomegaly) or potentially as other types of lymphomas would. More specific clinical findings can be related to the type of PTLD and the involved organ. The commonly involved organs include the skin, gastrointestinal tract, lungs, liver, and the allograft itself. In general however, PTLD presents with a constellation of non-specific signs and symptoms that usually include those illustrated in Table 1 below [1,2,3].

Table 1. Symptoms and signs that can be seen in PTLD

Symptoms	Signs
Fever, chills, night sweats	Tonsillar enlargement
Malaise	Lymphadenopathy
Weight loss	Hepatosplenomegaly
Swollen glands	Subcutaneous nodules
Abdominal pain/Nausea/Vomiting/Diarrhea	
Other organ specific symptoms (e.g., lethargy, altered mental status, seizures in CNS disease)	Other organ specific signs (acute abdomen from bowel perforation in GI disease or focal neurologic deficits from mass lesions in CNS disease)

1b) Epidemiology and Risk Factors

EBV currently remains the predominant cause of PTLD in both the adult and pediatric population. EBV related PTLD (EBV-PTLD) more often presents early after transplant, with the highest rates typically within the first year. After a solid organ transplant (SOT), the median time to primary EBV infection is 6 weeks. Reactivation, on the other hand, is more commonly seen at 2- to 3-months. However, PTLD can occur any time up to 10 years after a transplant. While EBV still remains the major cause, a significant proportion of late PTLD (21–38%) may be EBV-negative and non-B cell. These tend to present more than five years after transplant and carry a worse prognosis [1, 2, 3].

While both a primary EBV infection and a reactivation can trigger PTLD, the primary infection is much more likely to do so and is considered a major risk factor in transplant patients. Almost 90-95 % of adults worldwide have already been exposed to and are seropositive for EBV [3]. Therefore, a primary infection in the adult transplant population is much less likely than in the pediatric population, and so they have a lower risk of developing EBV-PTLD.

Besides EBV sero-status and age (of which younger age is an independent positive predictor of PTLD risk), the incidence of PTLD is also dependent on the transplanted organ. For example, the rates are highest after small intestinal transplant (up to 32%) and lowest among renal transplant recipients (1–2%) [1, 2, 4].

Mortality rates were extremely high prior to the development of current therapeutic protocols and the rituximab era. With therapy, rates have been significantly reduced, but remain highly variable and unpredictable due to the diverse nature of PTLDs and the diverse demographics of the affected population.

1c) The Virology of EBV in PTLD

The EBV virion is a linear double-stranded DNA molecule at the core within a nucleocapsid that is surrounded by an icosahedral viral envelope. Entry into host B-cell is initiated by the binding of the major envelope glycoprotein, the gp350, to the CD21 molecule on the B cell surface. The MHC II cofactor further facilitates the viral penetration and entry into the target B cell [3, 5]. What is characteristic in the establishment of latency is the fact that the linear EBV genome transforms into a circular episome. This episome associates with cellular chromosomes during mitosis to maintain viral lineage. The episome otherwise only allows the expression of 10 out of the 100 genes encoded in the viral DNA on average [3, 6]. By limiting gene expression, less EBV antigens are exposed to the T cell surveillance and EBV succeeds in establishing latency.

The EBV nuclear antigen (EBNA) 1 protein is one of the few transcribed proteins in latent EBV and serves to maintain the viral episome in the host cell. EBNA 2 on the other hand plays a key role in the proliferation and malignant transformation of EBV-infected B cells. It does so by upregulating both viral proteins (latent membrane proteins (LMP) 1 and 2) and B cell proteins. LMP1 acts as an oncogene, results in the nuclear factor κB (NFκB) pathway activation and further activation of B cell proteins that increase B-cell proliferation and/or enhances B cell resistance to apoptosis (eg. by interfering with Bcl2 or c-Myc pathways) [7]. Additionally, non-translated EBV encoded RNA (EBER) has also shown a role in oncogenesis and resistance to apoptosis [8]. By triggering oncogenic pathways, EBV can potentially lead to lymphoproliferative disorders (LDs) in both the immune-competent and immune-compromised hosts. However, it is relatively more common and aggressive in the immunocompromised.

An important question that researchers attempted to answer decades ago, was whether EBV would trigger LDs while in its latent form versus its active replicative form. In a study by Katz et al. back in 1989, DNA was extracted from biopsy samples of immunocompromised patients with lymphoproliferative diseases. All samples showed evidence that EBV episomal DNA was present, a finding consistent with latent EBV. Meanwhile, only 40% of samples had linear EBV DNA, which served as evidence for the active, replicating form of the virus [9].

In 1994, Rea et al. designed a study in attempt to answer this question in patients with EBV-related B cell PTLD [10]. They found the EBV-PTLD B cells to exhibit varying patterns of latent viral gene expression, as opposed to the replicative. Each pattern was characterized by a different combination of latency genes being expressed. The pattern observed was related to the form of B-cell PTLD (eg. monomorphic vs polymorphic). On the other hand, the study group found molecular evidence of replicative cycle in 5 out of 9 of the cases. Only 3 of those had late viral proteins to indicate the production of complete virions. In conclusion, findings suggested that active viral replication is occasionally present but not necessarily a driving force for PTLD development, especially given that only few had complete production of virions.

While more recent results point to an important role for lytic EBV infection in the development of B cell lymphomas in immunocompetent hosts [11], the role of lytic infection in EBV-induced PTLD remains unclear. Therefore, as far as we know, EBV-PTLD is driven by latent EBV. Understanding the concept of EBV latency in PTLD progression provides insight into the current and potential future therapeutic modalities for treatment. This will be re-addressed as treatment options are discussed (*see section 4*).

2. Diagnosis

The clinical presentation by itself is neither sensitive nor specific (section 1a) in diagnosing PTLD. To support our clinical suspicion, a number of important tests can be done. Viral load measurement is one useful screening tool, with good sensitivity. Combining the clinical findings with the results of viral load testing and imaging, serves to increase our pre-test probability of making the diagnosis by pathology. The histologic examination of a specimen is absolutely necessary to make the diagnosis when PTLD is clinically suspected. The diagnosis of EBV+ PTLD requires the demonstration of EBV DNA, RNA, or protein in the biopsy tissue. This section will address the use of viral load testing and findings on pathology in PTLD.

2a) Viral Load Monitoring

The memory B cells hosting latent EBV are thought to be immortalized. Their number, almost 1 to 50 B cells per million, remains stable over the years [3, 12]. In an immune-competent host, this number remains in equilibrium. While viral latency mechanisms prevent the number from diminishing (immortalization), a functioning immune response normally prevents the numbers from rising (cytotoxic response against viral reactivation and lymphoproliferation).

This equilibrium is disturbed in the immunocompromised host. In the absence of T cell surveillance, these EBV-B cells are free to proliferate, whether at a normal rate or abnormally as in LDs. Thus, an EBV seropositive transplant patient, devoid of functional T cell immunity, is expected to have a higher number of EBV-infected memory B cells in the peripheral blood than that in the immunocompetent individual [13].

In immunosuppressed or transplant patients, a primary EBV infection, a re-activation and PTLD are all associated with higher numbers of EBV-B cells in the peripheral blood. This is where the interpretation of viral load and the work of Riddler et al in 1994 become worth mentioning [13]. The study group took samples from 23 transplant patients, 12 of which developed PTLD. While excluding the PTLD cohort, the EBV seropositive recipients had a higher number of EBV genomes per peripheral blood lymphocytes (PBL) compared to immunocompetent controls. This supports our discussion earlier that immunosuppression by itself leads to higher viral loads. However, the increase was no more than 10-fold higher than the 0.1-5 EBV genomes/10^6 PBL seen in the control group.

The 10-fold limit is what differentiated this cohort from the patients with active EBV infection and those with PTLD. Recipients who were seronegative and developed a primary EBV infection had uncontrolled viremia with levels of EBV-infected PBLs up to 400 times the level in controls (in this case the control is a cohort of immunocompetent individuals with acute infectious mononucleosis (IM) with an estimated load of 1.0 to 50 EBV genomes/10^6 PBL [14]).

For our main cohort, the transplant patients who developed PTLD, a significantly higher number of EBV-infected PBLs was noted. The majority of individuals in the group had viral load levels more than or equal to 300,000 EBV genomes per 10^5 PBL. Therefore, quantifying the rise in viral load can help differentiate PTLD from the other clinical scenarios associated with an elevated load.

Subsequent to this study, several groups have sought interest in evaluating the utility of EBV viral load in detection of PTLD. The term 'viral load' can mean different things in each of these studies. Therefore, one must be aware of what the numbers really mean in relation to the sample being tested (whole blood, cellular component (PBLs) or plasma). For instance, understanding the difference between EBV DNA levels in whole blood as opposed to those within PBLs can prove very helpful for diagnostic purposes.

An elevated viral load from a whole blood sample can indicate one of two things. One is an increase in number of circulating lymphocytes containing latent EBV. Another is an increase in EBV levels in serum, likely due to actively replicating virions that lyse their way out of the host lymphocytes. Splitting whole blood into serum and cellular component helps us differentiate the etiology of elevated viral load.

This was studied by Stevens et al. in a prospective analysis [15]. EBV DNA load in whole blood samples (cellular + serum) from lung transplant (LTx) patients with and without PTLD was measured. As high as 78% of samples from the PTLD patients had DNA levels above the cutoff value of their quantitative competitive PCR (qc-PCR). Simultaneously, only 3.4% of whole blood samples from non-PTLD LTx patients had EBV DNA load above the cutoff value. Parallel samples of serum all had EBV DNA below cutoff values, indicating that the cellular compartment is main source of EBV DNA in this scenario.

This had shed further light on the question brought up earlier (*section 1c*) on whether EBV is latent or active in PTLD development. The absence of significant elevation in serum EBV load suggests lack of lytic viral replication. In this situation EBV was mostly confined within the cellular compartment, suggesting that PTLD develops in the setting of latent EBV expression. The significance of knowing this will become apparent when treatment strategies are discussed (*see section 3*).

Further evidence by Stevens et al. suggests that EBV viral load monitoring is a useful screening tool for early detection of PTLD. In their study, EBV viral load was markedly elevated in PTLD even prior to diagnosis. Thus, the level should be closely monitored in such a population, especially since the doubling time of EBV + cells can be as short as 56 hours [15]. Following the rate at which the load increases during serial measurements might be another approach to screening [15-17].

Other studies, such as Wagner et al. and collegues [18], also found significantly higher EBV viral load in PTLD patients than other cohorts. However, their findings in relation to the tested blood samples were somewhat contradictory to those Stevens et al. They found better specificity for diagnosing PTLD using plasma samples as opposed to peripheral blood monocytes (PBMCs). When plasma was analyzed, a value of greater than 1,000 EBV genomes per100 μl plasma had both a sensitivity and specificity of 100% for diagnosing PTLD. On the other hand, a value of greater than 5,000 EBV genomes per microgram DNA of peripheral blood monocytes (PBMC) was 100% sensitive but only 89% specific.

This is an example of the many differences in studies that make standardization of EBV viral load detection for the diagnosis of PTLD extremely difficult. Many studies, in addition to the ones mentioned, reported different threshold values with varying sensitivities (ranging from 60–100%) and specificities (71–100%) [16, 19-21]. Several PCR techniques, various segments of amplified EBV DNA, different blood components and different specimens from transplant patients all accounts for such variability [22]. Very few studies targeted EBV RNA, but results were inconsistent [22].

Stevens et al. went a step further and attempted to standardize diagnostic testing for PTLD with EBV viral load [22]. Despite his proposal, as of yet there seems to be no standard protocol and cutoff values that institutions worldwide or nationwide can adopt. The few things we can agree on at this point are the following:

1) EBV DNA load in whole blood is significantly higher in the majority of PTLD patients than those without PTLD
2) Whole blood or cell-associated EBV loads are always higher than those found in plasma, and in fact loads can be significantly high in the cellular compartment and remain undetectable in plasma [15-16, 22-25]. This would theoretically make plasma viral load a test of lower sensitivity and poorer negative predictive value

Different transplant centers vary in regards to their definition of high-risk patients and their methods of viral load measurements. This makes a controlled comparison to identify the ideal test a difficult task. While real time quantitative PCR assays is now commonly regarded as the detection method of choice, the choice of sample is still a matter of debate and remains institution dependent. In attempt to identify the superior test, Tsai et al. performed a two-arm prospective trial on EBV PCR in the diagnosis and monitoring of PTLD [26].

The findings support our earlier argument that plasma would not be the screening test of choice given its lower sensitivity and negative predictive value (77% and 86% respectively), but can be utilized as a confirmatory test given a superior specificity and positive predictive value (100% for both). On the other hand, whole blood for EBV PCR should be used for screening given a superior sensitivity and NPV (92% and 93% respectively) [26]. This suggests that plasma could be used for confirmatory testing after a positive result on the whole blood sample. However, the diagnosis of PTLD ultimately requires pathology, so it is unclear whether the result of the plasma testing would alter clinical decision to biopsy.

2b) Other Markers and Imaging

Another marker to combine with viral load was initially suggested by Smets et al. [27]. In their article published in 2002, they described measuring anti-EBV T lymphocytes (EBV-TL) in correlation with EBV viral load in PTLD patients. Based on their results, high viral load in combination with low EBV-TL count (<2/mm^3) were parameters that can be combined to achieve a higher positive predictive index (no patient had PTLD whenever the count was >2 /mm^3, achieving a positive predictive index of 100% in this study). Simultaneously, they concluded that rapid EBV-TL increase, combined with decreasing viral load, would be a marker of healing from PTLD. Others looked at the absolute CD4 and CD8 T cell counts as well as the EBV-specific CD4 and CD8 T cell responses in relation to EBV load. Low absolute CD4 count was thought to be a risk factor and possible predictor of PTLD [28].

Imaging techniques including ultrasound, endoscopy, CT, FDG-PET scanning, and MRI are used to help diagnosing, staging and evaluating response to treatment in PTLD. Each of the techniques has a wide spectrum of imaging features of which a few are more specific and allow early detection of possible disease. To go through such features is beyond the scope of this chapter [16, 29-32].

2c) Pathology

i. Histologic Morphology and Immunophenotyping of PTLD Categories

PTLD is a group of different abnormal lymphoid proliferations, manifested as lymphoid hyperplasia and neoplasms. This disease is classified into several categories with different prognostic outcomes. The diagnosis and categorization of PTLD is made after examining the morphology, immunophenotyping, clonality and the presence of EBV [33, 34].

The WHO classification includes the following types of PTLD: Early lesion, Polymorphic PTLD, Monomorphic PTLD and classical Hodgkin lymphoma-type PTLD.

Early lesions can be subdivided into plasmacytic hyperplasia and infectious mononucleosis-like PTLD. Plasmacytic hyperplasia shows plasma cells and lymphocytes with preserved architecture. Infectious mononucleosis-like PTLD is mostly characterized by T-cells and plasma cells with associated lymphoid hyperplasia. These lesions have polyclonal B-cells and the majority is EBV positive. Nelson et al reviewed 15 cases of early PTLD. They correlated clinical history, morphology, clonal status and the presence of EBV with staining intensity of an antibody pS6, which is an effector target of rapamycin. They concluded that their early PTLD cases were mostly compromised of plasmacytic hyperplasia, developed mostly in tonsils and adenoids, had an increased intensity of pS6 staining and a good prognosis with modification of immunosuppression [34, 35].

Polymorphic PTLD is characterized by architectural effacement along with complete maturation with presence of B-cells at different stages (Immunoblasts, Lymphocytes and Plasma cells). These lesions can show light chain restriction. The presence of EBV is a helpful clue to favor the diagnosis of Polymorphic PTLD over allograft rejection.

Monomorphic PTLD is subdivided into B-cell (Diffuse large B-cell lymphoma, Plasma cell myeloma, Plasmacytoma-like lesions, Burkitt lymphoma and indolent small B-cell lymphomas) and T-cell neoplasms (peripheral T-cell lymphoma, and hepatosplenic T-cell lymphoma). In regards to morphology, both B-cell lymphoma and T-cell lymphomas usually demonstrate architectural effacement. B-cell lymphomas must satisfy the conventional criteria for the lymphoma subtypes. They cells are predominately monoclonal. T-cell lymphomas show features similar to conventional T/NK-cell lymphoma. B-cell lymphomas in PTLD usually express CD19, CD20 and CD79a, whereas T-cell lymphomas express CD4/CD8, CD30 and ALK. Jonson et al looked at 30 B-cell monomorphic PTLD cases. They used the following panels: EBER, CD20, CD3/bcl-6, CD10, MUM-1/IRF4, CD138, and bcl-2. Their results demonstrated wide variety of histologic and genetic spectrum in B-cell monomorphic PTLD. They also revealed an association between EBV presence and non-germinal center phenotype which implies that EBV-PTLD shares some features with lymphomas manifesting in immunocompetent patients [34, 36].

Classical Hodgkin lymphoma (CHL)-type PTLD demonstrates architectural effacement and resembles CHL morphologically. Fulfillment of CHL criteria is also required for the diagnosis. These lesions usually express CD15 and CD30; however CD15 negativity does not rule out the diagnosis of CHL-PTLD. EBV is present in the majority of the cases.

Pitman et al studied 5 cases of CHL like PTLD. The study included a characterization of immunophenotype, the presence of EBV, clonal status, and clinical outcome. They concluded that several significant differences exist in terms of immunophenotypic characterization, molecular genetics and clinical course. These differences suggest a critical distinction between HL-PTLD and HL-like PTLD in regards to the clinical course and outcome [34, 37].

ii. Cytogenetic Analysis

The cytogenetic characterization of PTLD is somewhat challenging due to the presence of multiple heterogeneous subtypes. Vakiani et. al conducted cytogenetic characterization on 28 PTLD cases (1 mononucleosis like, 17 monomorphic PTLD, 9 polymorphic and 1 Hodgkin's lymphoma PTLD). After the karyotype was identified, they were linked to some other important variants (presence of EBV and clinical course). The following chromosomal abnormalities were identified: chromosomal breaks at (1q11-21, 14q32, 16p13, 11q23-24 and 8q24), gains of chromosomes (7, X, 2 and 12) and loss of chromosome 22. Their results showed that the presence of a cytogenetic abnormality did not correlate with presence of EBV, phenotype or clinical prognosis [38]. Dijokic et al assessed 36 cases of PTLD. They examined their karyotype and the correlation to laboratory findings, histopathology and clinical outcome. These cases had 2 early-lesion PTLD, 13 polymorphic PTLD, 18 B-cell monomorphic PTLD and 3 T-cell monomorphic PTLD. Their results showed cytogenetic abnormalities in 72% of B-cell monomorphic lesions, 100% of T-cell monomorphic lesions, 15% of polymorphic lesions and non in early lesions. Monomorphic PTLD cases had the following abnormalities: trisomy 9, trisomy 11, rearrangement of 8q24.1 (MYC), 3q27 and 14q32. It was also noted that MYC rearrangement and T-cell PTLD with cytogenetic abnormality was associated with poor prognosis. Trisomy 9 and trisomy 11 associated PTLD, early after transplant, correlates with good prognosis [39]. Delecluse et al reported two cases of fatal EBV related PTLD in heart transplant patients. Both cases were monomorphic and had multiple chromosomal abnormalities. MYC rearrangement was among those genetic abnormalities [40]. Some other cytogenetic abnormalities are associated with poor prognosis. However; more studies are needed to characterize the different chromosomal abnormalities and their association with clinical outcome in the setting of PTLD.

3. Treatment and Prevention

Monitoring EBV viral load in patients at high risk for PTLD is essential in order to pre-emptively treat for and prevent progression of disease. When the EBV viral load reaches critical levels in the immunosuppressed recipients and PTLD is confirmed, it is imperative to reduce or completely withdraw immunosuppression. Therefore, the first step, before any therapy is administered, is to reduce the dose of the calcineurin inhibitors and anti-lymphocytic therapy and assess the patient's clinical response and changes in viral load.

PTLD not responsive to reduction in immunosuppressive therapy requires urgent treatment. Given the previously high mortality from PTLD and the relatively small number of cases, phase III clinical trials are lacking in this field. However, a number of different monotherapies and combination regimens have been investigated in pilot studies and phase II clinical trials.

Currently rituximab is considered first line therapy in B-cell PTLD with CD20-positive expression. Chemotherapy, whether with CHOP or other regimens, is occasionally combined with rituximab therapy especially when rituximab monotherapy yields poor clinical response. Alternatively, adoptive immunotherapy, achieved by transferring EBV-specific cytotoxic T lymphocyte cell lines (EBV-CTLs) to the patient, has shown remarkable results in terms of safety and efficacy in achieving remission. There remain no standardized guidelines for therapy as multiple therapeutic combinations have been used to treat the different subtypes of this disease and response rates have varied [41-44].

The use of antiviral therapy, such as the commonly prescribed ganciclovir, remains controversial. It's efficacy is limited when treating latent EBV within host B-cells. This is due to both a lack of thymidine kinase within the infected B cell and a lack of active viral replication. However, it is thought to play a role in prevention, especially when combined with arginine butyrate, an activator of thymidine kinase.

3a) Antiviral Therapy

At this point in our discussion we have established our understanding of PTLD as the active proliferation of latently infected EBV-lymphocytes. I emphasize the description of EBV as being "latent". The virology of EBV was briefly discussed (*section 1c*), describing how latent viral expression can lead to dysregulated B cell proliferation through Bcl2 pathway disruption. The virus need not be actively proliferating.

Antivirals such as ganciclovir and acyclovir are nucleoside analogs that have a strong affinity to viral polymerase enzyme and can be somewhat effective in treatment of EBV during active DNA replication. DNA replication is limited during latency. Also, the expression of the thymidine kinase enzyme that activates the antiviral drugs is lacking in EBV-infected B cells. For these reasons, antiviral treatment has mostly shown to be ineffective in the treatment of PTLD [45].

Although it's utility has not been established, antiviral therapy for PTLD prophylaxis was explored by many investigators through retrospective studies [45, 46]. Certain benefits of prophylactic antiviral therapy were observed in specific transplant populations. For instance, Funch et al. found that prophylactic anti-viral use was associated with up to 83% reduction in the risk of PTLD in renal transplant patients when ganciclovir was used [46]. Ganciclovir was found to be superior to acyclovir.

Accordingly, Mentzer et al. proposed a strategy to utilize ganciclovir for the treatment of EBV-PTLD. The strategy entails pharmacologically inducing the thymidine kinase in EBV-infected B cells. To do so, arginine butyrate is given prior to ganciclovir therapy. The initial pilot study included six patients with chemo-resistant EBV- PTLD or EBV-lymphoma. The proposed combination therapy produced complete clinical responses in four of six patients, with a partial response occurring in a fifth patient. Pathologic examination in two of three patients demonstrated complete necrosis of the EBV lymphoma, with no residual disease.

Positive results in terms of clinical response were also noted in the phase I/II study by the group. Their phase II trial of 'arginine butyrate and ganciclovir/valganciclovir in EBV(+) lymphoid malignancies' was initiated in 2009 but later terminated [47-49].This combination therapy currently remains under ongoing debate.

An interesting alternative strategy has been suggested to create a scenario where antiviral therapy could be effective. Cohen et al. suggested inducing lytic EBV infection in PTLD tumor cells by targeting specific viral genes [50]. More research is needed to determine how to optimize the efficacy of antiviral treatment in PTLD.

3b) Rituximab Immunotherapy and/or Chemotherapy

Pathologic determination of the PTLD subtype and CD20 expression is important to guide whether anti-B-cell monoclonal antibody therapy would have an anticipated benefit in achieving remission from PTLD. As noted in several single center studies, anti-B-cell monoclonal antibody therapy with rituximab seemed to be effective in achieving remission [51-53]. Observed complications were a partly CD20-negative relapse of PTLD and a hypogammaglobulinemia [52]. With otherwise fewer complications and lower morbidity profile than chemotherapy, rituximab was considered first line therapy and that chemotherapy should be reserved for resistant cases only [53].

Choquet et al. designed the first prospective trial (phase II) to evaluate the efficacy and safety of rituximab therapy for B-PTLD after SOT. Forty-six patients with untreated B-PTLD, not responding to tapering of immunosuppression, were included. With rituximab therapy, the overall survival rate at 1 year was 67%. This provided further evidence to the efficacy of this regimen [54]. It was proposed that combining rituximab with other treatments may yield better survival outcomes. Subsequently, a retrospective study evaluated PTLD patients receiving rituximab and/or chemotherapy for overall response rate (ORR), time to treatment failure (TTF) and overall survival (OS). The rituximab group had a lower ORR and OS (68% and 31 months, respectively) than the chemotherapy group (74% and 42 months), but no patient died from rituximab toxicity. Toxicity of chemotherapy was marked, and so again, the recommendation was to reserve chemotherapy for patients who fail rituximab, have EBV-negative tumors or need a rapid response [55].

Orjuela et al., who have previously demonstrated a >80% complete response (CR) rate with cyclophosphamide/prednisone (Cy/Pred) chemotherapy alone, investigated the combination of Cy/Pred with rituximab as treatment for PTLD patients (post SOT) in a pilot study. Among the six patients, the overall response rate was 100% (five CRs and one PR). There were no grade III or IV toxicities and no infectious complications related to the combination therapy [56].

Secondary to the promising findings, Trappe et al. conducted a prospective, international multi-center phase 2 trial published in the Lancet Oncology in 2012 [43]. The study evaluated whether the use of rituximab followed by CHOP chemotherapy would improve the outcome of patients with PTLD. The patient population was SOT adult patients with CD20-positive PTLD that failed to respond to immunosuppression reduction. They received rituximab monotherapy, immediately followed by CHOP if progression of disease was observed. 70 patients were eligible to receive treatment. PTLD was of late type in 76%, mostly monomorphic (96%). Not surprisingly, given most of the PTLD was of the late type, only 44% were histologically EBV associated. In patients who completed the planned combination therapy, response rates were promising with 90% achieving complete or partial response (95% CI 79-96) - 68% had CR (95% CI 55-78). Unfortunately, as the toxicity of chemotherapy was emphasized earlier, the study observed 11% mortality that was considered

CHOP-associated. Overall, however, the results supported the use of sequential immunochemotherapy with rituximab and CHOP in PTLD [43].

Trials combining rituximab with different chemotherapeutic regimens for PTLD are ongoing. A phase II clinical trial sponsored by the Massachusettes General Hospital is determining whether the addition of bortezomib to rituximab can increase the rate of complete remissions and cures of PTLD after SOT or HSCT [57]. Bortezomib is the first therapeutic proteasome inhibitor, and has shown significant activity against lymphoma cells caused by EBV [58]. It is currently FDA approved here in the US to treat multiple myeloma and Mantle Cell Lymphoma.

In the setting of hematopoietic stem cell transplant (HSCT), chemotherapy did not seem to contribute to improved survival of patients who developed PTLD [42]. Rather, the preemptive use of rituximab and EBV-cytotoxic T lymphocytes (CTL) significantly reduced the risk of death due to EBV-PTLD in HSCT recipients with survival rates of 89.7% and 94.1%, respectively. The rates were reported in a paper by Styczynski et al. that analyzed outcomes of several studies in the field of PTLD after HSCT [42].

3c. Adoptive Immunotherapy

As mentioned in the introduction, the first step in PTLD management is always reduction in immunosuppression. The purpose is to allow the host's innate cytotoxic T-cell response to overcome the lymphoproliferative burden. However, in the majority of situations this is not sufficient. Specifically, EBV seronegative recipients do not have an immunologic memory against EBV epitopes and lack EBV-specific CTLs (EBV-CTLs).

A turning point in PTLD therapy was when the concept of adoptive immunotherapy was applied in the treatment of PTLD. Adoptive immunotherapy refers to transfer of immune-derived cells (in this case cytotoxic T cells (CTLs)) to a host for the purpose of cancer treatment. In the 1990s, Khanna et al. developed a protocol for activating autologous EBV-specific CTL lines *in vitro* from patients who acquired EBV-PTLD. The adoptive transfer of the activated EBV-CTLs into a single patient with active PTLD was coincident with a very significant regression of the PTLD [59]. The therapeutic potential of adoptive immunotherapy was demonstrated in multiple studies and clinical trials that followed.

The utility of pre-emptive therapy with autologous EBV-specific CTLs for PTLD prevention was tested by Comoli et al. The study group targeted patients that had elevated EBV viral load and were considered at risk of developing PTLD. From the 7 who received infusions of EBV-specific CTLs, 5 had a 1.5- to 3-log decrease in EBV DNA. They concluded that a pre-emptive treatment approach guided by EBV viral load may be safely used as prophylaxis against EBV-PTLD [60]. Other studies had similar success pre-emptively treating patients at risk [61].

Despite its efficacy, treatment with autologous CTLs is labor intensive and expensive. The use of partially human leukocyte antigen (HLA)-matched EBV-specific CTL grown ex vivo was considered a less expensive potential alternative. In 2001, Haque et al. had reported complete regression of EBV-PTLD using partially (HLA)-matched EBV-CTLs in an 18-month old child who had a small bowel transplant. There was no subsequent evidence of infusion-related toxicity or graft-versus-host disease [62]. Accordingly, Haque et al proceeded with a phase I/II trial where patients with progressive PTLD, unresponsive to conventional treatment, were given infusions of the partly HLA-matched EBV-CTLs. The cell lines were taken from a frozen bank of CTLs derived from healthy blood donors. Three of the five patients who received therapy had complete remission and two had no clinical response [63]. Treatment was deemed effective and the group commenced with a phase II multicenter trial including 33 PTLD patients who failed conventional therapy.

In 2007, the results of the trial were published. The response rate (complete or partial) was 64% at 5 weeks and 52% at 6 months. That, and the absence of adverse effects, yielded a safe, effective and rapid therapy for PTLD, while bypassing the need to grow autologous CTLs [64]. Third party partially HLA-matched EBV-specific CTLs have also been successfully used to treat PTLD in cord blood transplant (CBT) patients [65].

The use of partly HLA-matched CTLs has proven less time consuming and costly than generation of autologous CTLs. Efforts are currently directed at establishing protocols that generates third party EBV-CTLs quickly and efficiently for use in urgent situations. One rapid isolation protocol was designed using haplo-identical donor cells [66].

The problem that remains, however, is that up until recently, EBV-lymphoblastoid cell lines (LCL) are used as a stimulating agent ex vivo to make EBV-CTLs. Although effective, the isolation protocol is still time consuming. More recent studies are examining the use of immunogenic EBV-peptide pools as the stimulating agents [67] Another recent rapid protocol involves isolation of polyclonal EBNA-1 -specific T cells. Infusion of this cell line is considered a feasible and well-tolerated therapeutic option [68].

Moreover, CTLs are now being engineered to confer resistance to common immunosuppressive therapy such as tacrolimus (FK506) [69,70]. This would allow delivery of PTLD therapy without having to withdraw immunosuppression and risk graft rejection.

The field of adoptive immunotherapy has been developing rapidly and results continue to look more promising. Other interesting potential therapies and prevention strategies are discussed in the next section.

3d. Other Therapies and the Future

The promising future of adoptive immunotherapy, and the potential for antiviral therapy were both discussed earlier. In addition to that, a number of other exciting modalities have been suggested. For prevention of PTLD, research is ongoing on developing a vaccine to prevent PTLD in transplant patients [41, 71]. Other future therapeutic interventions may include the use of mammalian target of rapamycin (mTOR) inhibitors and targeted immunotherapy with antibodies to interleukin-6, galectin-1, CDKs and survivin [41, 72, 73].

Ouyang et al. reported that primary PTLDs overexpress galectin-1 (Gal-1) [72]. Gal-1 is a carbohydrate-binding lectin that induces tolerogenic dendritic cells and triggers the selective apoptosis of T cells that would otherwise target the PTLD. In other words, the presence of Gal-1 makes the host's immune system more tolerant to the antigens expressed by the PTLD cells. Their results show that antibody-mediated Gal-1 neutralization may represent a novel immunotherapeutic strategy for PTLD and other Gal-1-expressing tumors [72]. On the other hand, targeting CDKs and survivin by specific inhibitors has also shown potential in treating EBV-LDs, especially given their over-expression in EBV-B cell PTLD [73].

Conclusion

Post-transplant lymphoproliferative disease (PTLD) is the uncontrolled proliferation of plasmacytic or lymphoid cells in the immunosuppressed, transplant patient and is largely caused by latent Epstein-Barr virus (EBV)

Serial measurement of EBV viral load post-transplant is currently the chosen method for early detection and monitoring progression and response to treatment.

Histologic examination of biopsy samples is required to make the diagnosis and determine the subtype. This would determine and guide therapy.

Large clinical trials in this field are lacking and further research is needed to standardize treatment approaches. Our knowledge is based mostly on retrospective studies, pilot studies, reported cases and phase II trials.

The first step in treatment is always reduction in immunosuppression.

Rituximab has shown safety and efficacy as monotherapy in PTLD

Chemotherapeutic regimens, such as CHOP, are often combined with rituximab to yield better response rates and cover a broader category of PTLDs.

Adoptive immunotherapy involves the transfer of EBV-specific cytotoxic T-cells (EBV-CTLs). This treatment modality has shown impressive efficacy and safety outcomes.

More recent studies have found great therapeutic potential with targeted therapy.

Glossary

Adoptive Immunotherapy

Providing a host with an adopted immunity against cancer by transferring naturally occuring or engineered T cells, mostly of cytotoxic nature, that are active against specific epitopes expressed by cancer cells.

CHOP Chemotherapy

A combination chemotherapy regimen composed of **C**yclophosphamide, **H**ydroxydaunorubicin (also called doxorubicin), **O**ncovin (also called vincristine), and **P**rednisone, and is considered a standard of treatment for certain lymphomas including Hodgkin's lymphoma.

Epstein-Barr Virus (EBV)

It is a virus from the family of herpes virus and one of the most common viruses in humans. The EBV virion is a linear double-stranded DNA molecule at the core within a nucleocapsid that is surrounded by an icosahedral viral envelope.

Ganciclovir

A nucleoside analog that has a strong affinity to viral polymerase enzyme and acts as an antiviral by terminating the viral DNA replication process. It requires thymidine kinase for activation.

Post-Transplant Lymphoproliferative Disease (PTLD)

The uncontrolled proliferation of plasmacytic or lymphoid cells in the hematopoietic or solid organ transplant patient

Targeted Therapy

A form of therapy applied in cancer treatment that involves the use of medications that are specific to a target molecule only present within rapidly dividing cancer cells as opposed other host cells.

Thymidine Kinase

An enzyme that can be found in most living cells and has a key role in DNA synthesis and cell division. It is required for the action of a number of antiviral agents, including ganciclovir.

References

[1] Allen U, Preiksaitis J. Epstein–Barr virus and post-transplant lymphoproliferative disorder in solid organ transplant recipients. *Am J Transplant* 2009; 9(Suppl 4): S87–S96.

[2] Green M, Michaels MG. Epstein–Barr Virus Infection and post-transplant lymphoproliferative disorder. *Am J Transplant* 2013; 13: 41-54.

[3] Cohen JI. Epstein–Barr virus infection. *N Engl J Med* 2000; 343:481–492.

[4] Green M, Webber S. Post-transplantation lymphoproliferative disorders. *Pediatr Clin North Amer 2003*; 50: 1471–1491.

[5] Li Q, Spriggs MK, Kovats S, Turk SM, Comeau MR, Nepom B, Hutt-Fletcher LM. Epstein-Barr virus uses HLA class II as a cofactor for infection of B lymphocytes. *J Virol* 1997;71:4657-4662.

[6] Harris A, Young BD, Griffin BE. Random association of Epstein-Barr virus genomes with host cell metaphase chromosomes in Burkitt's lymphoma-derived cell lines. *J Virol* 1985;56:328–332.

[7] Wang D, Liebowitz D, Kieff E. An EBV membrane protein expressed in immortalized lymphocytes transforms established rodent cells. *Cell* 1985;43:831-840.

[8] Komano J, Maruo S, Kurozumi K, Oda T, Takada K. Oncogenic role of Epstein-Barr virus-encoded RNAs in Burkitt's lymphoma cell line Akata. *J Virol* 1999;73:9827-9831.

[9] Katz BZ, Raab-Traub N, Miller G. Latent and replicating forms of Epstein-Barr virus DNA in lymphomas and lymphoproliferative diseases. *J Infect Dis* 1989;160:589–598.

[10] Rea D, Fourcade C, Leblond V, Rowe M, Joab I, Edelman L, Bitker MO, Gandjbakhch I, Suberbielle C, Farcet JP, et al. Patterns of Epstein-Barr virus latent and replicative gene expression in Epstein-Barr virus B cell lymphoproliferative disorders after organ transplantation. *Transplantation* 1994;58:317–324.

[11] Ma S D, Hegde S, Young KH, Sullivan R, Rajesh D, Zhou Y, Jankowska-Gan E, Burlingham WJ, Sun X, Gulley ML, Tang W, Gumperz JE, Kenney SC. A new model of Epstein–Barr virus infection reveals an important role for early lytic viral protein expression in the development of lymphomas. *J Virol* 2011;85:165–177.

[12] Babcock GJ, Decker LL, Volk M, Thorley-Lawson DA. EBV persistence in memory B cells *in vivo. Immunity* 1998;9:395-404.

[13] Riddler SA, Breinig MC, McKnight JLC. Increased levels of circulating Epstein-Barr virus (EBV)-infected lymphocytes and decreased EBV nuclear antigen antibody responses are associated with the development of post-transplant lymphoproliferative disease in solid-organ transplant recipients. *Blood* 1994; 84: 972-984.

[14] Rocchi G, deFelici A, Ragona G, Heinz A. Quantitative evaluation of Epstein-Barr virus infected mononuclear peripheral blood leukocytes in infectious mononucleosis. *N Engl J Med* 1977;296:132-134.

[15] Stevens SJC, Verschuuren EAM, Pronk I, Van Der Bij W, Harmsen MC, The TH, Meijer CJLM, Van Den Brule AJC, Middeldorp JM. Frequent monitoring of Epstein-Barr virus DNA load in unfractionated whole blood is essential for early detection of post-transplant lymphoproliferative disease in high-risk patients. *Blood* 2001; 97:1165-1171.

[16] Bakker NA, Van Imhoff GW, Verschuuren EAM, Van Son WJ. Presentation and early detection of post-transplant lymphoproliferative disorder after solid organ transplantation. *Transplant International* 2007;20: 207-218.

[17] Holman CJ, Karger AB, Mullan BD, Brundage RC, Balfour HH. Quantitative Epstein-Barr virus shedding and its correlation with the risk of post-transplant lymphoproliferative disorder. *Clinical Transplantation* 2012;26:741-747.

[18] Wagner HJ, Wessel M, Jabs W, Smets F, Fischer L, Offner G, Bucsky P. Patients at risk for development of post-transplant lymphoproliferative disorder: Plasma versus peripheral blood mononuclear cells as material for quantification of Epstein-Barr viral load by using real-time quantitative polymerase chain reaction. *Transplantation* 2001;72:1012-1019.

[19] Limaye AP, Huang ML, Atienza EE, Ferrenberg JM, Corey L. Detection of Epstein–Barr virus DNA in sera from transplant recipients with lymphoproliferative disorders. *J Clin Microbiol,* 1999; 37: 1113-1116.

[20] Rowe DT, Webber S, Schauer EM, Reyes J, Green M. Epstein–Barr virus load monitoring: its role in the prevention and management of post-transplant lymphoproliferative disease. *Transpl Infect Dis* 2001; 3: 79-87.

[21] Tsai DE, Nearey M, Hardy CL, Tomaszewski JE, Kotloff RM, Grossman RA, Olthoff KM, Stadtmauer EA, Porter DL, Schuster SJ, Luger SM, Hodinka RL. Use of EBV

PCR for the diagnosis and monitoring of post-transplant lymphoproliferative disorder in adult solid organ transplant patients. *Am J Transplant* 2002; 2: 946-954.

[22] Stevens SJ, Verschuuren EA, Verkuijlen SA, Van Den Brule AJ, Meijer CJ, Middeldorp JM. Role of Epstein-Barr virus DNA load monitoring in prevention and early detection of post-transplant lymphoproliferative disease. *Leuk Lymphoma* 2002; 43:831-840.

[23] Rowe DT, Webber S, Schauer EM, Reyes J, Green M. Epstein–Barr virus load monitoring: its role in the prevention and management of post-transplant lymphoproliferative disease. *Transplant Infect Dis* 2001; 3:79–87.

[24] Rose C, Green M, Webber S, Ellis D, Reyes J, Rowe D. Pediatric solid-organ transplant recipients carry chronic loads of Epstein–Barr virus exclusively in the immunoglobulin D-negative B-cell compartment. *J Clin Microbiol* 2001; 39:1407–1415.

[25] Meerbach A, Gruhn B, Egerer R, Reischl U, Zintl F, Wutzler P. Semiquantitative PCR analysis of Epstein–Barr virus DNA in clinical samples of patients with EBV-associated diseases. *J Med Virol* 2001;65:348–357.

[26] Tsai DE, Douglas L, Andreadis C, Vogl DT, Arnoldi S, Kotloff R, Svoboda J, Bloom RD, Olthoff KM, Brozena SC, Schuster SJ, Stadtmauer EA, Robertson ES, Wasik MA, Ahya VN. EBV PCR in the diagnosis and monitoring of post-transplant lymphoproliferative disorder: Results of a two-arm prospective trial. *Am J Transplantation* 2008;8:1016-1024.

[27] Smets F, Latinne D, Bazin H, Reding R, Otte JB, Buts JP, Sokal EM. Ratio between Epstein-Barr viral load and anti-Epstein-Barr virus specific T-cell response as a predictive marker of post-transplant lymphoproliferative disease. *Transplantation* 2002;73:1603-1610.

[28] Sebelin-Wulf K, Nguyen TD, Oertel S, Papp-Vary M, Trappe RU, Schulzki A, Pezzutto A, Riess H, Subklewe M. Quantitative analysis of EBV-specific CD4/CD8 T cell numbers, absolute CD4/CD8 T cell numbers and EBV load in solid organ transplant recipients with PLTD. *Transplant Immunology* 2007;17: 203-210.

[29] Marom EM, McAdams HP, Butnor KJ, Coleman RE. Positron emission tomography with fluoro-2-deoxy-d-glucose (FDG-PET) in the staging of post transplant lymphoproliferative disorder in lung transplant recipients. J Thorac Imaging 2004; 19: 74-78.

[30] O'Conner AR, Franc BL. FDG PET imaging in the evaluation of post-transplant lymphoproliferative disorder following renal transplantation. Nucl Med Commun 2005; 26: 1107-1111.

[31] Bakker NA, Pruim J, De Graaf W, Van Son WJ, Van der Jagt EJ, Van Imhoff GW. PTLD visualization by FDG-PET: improved detection of extranodal localizations. *Am J Transplant* 2006; 6: 19841985.

[32] Russ PD, Way DE, Pretorius DH, Manco-Johnson ML, Weil R III. Post-transplant lymphoma. Sonographic characteristics of renal allograft involvement. *J Ultrasound Med* 1987; 6: 453-456.

[33] Nalesnik MA. The diverse pathology of post-transplant lymphoproliferative disorders: The importance of a standardized approach. *Transplant Infect Dis* 2001;3:88-96.

[34] Swerdlow, Steven H. *WHO Classification of Tumours of Haematopoietic and Lymphoid Tissues*. Lyon, France: International Agency for Research on Cancer, 2008.

[35] Nelson BP, Wolniak KL, Evens A, Chenn A, Maddalozzo J, Proytcheva M. Early post-transplant lymphoproliferative disease. *Am J Clin Pathol* 2012;138:568-578.

[36] Johnson LR, Nalesnik MA, Swerdlow SH. Impact of Epstein-Barr virus in monomorphic B-cell post-transplant lymphoproliferative disorders: A histogenetic study. *Am J Surg Pathol* 2006;30:1604-1612.

[37] Pitman SD, Huang Q, Zuppan CW, Rowsell EH, Cao JD, Berdeja JG, Weiss LM, Wang J. Hodgkin lymphoma-like post-transplant lymphoproliferative disorder (HL-like PTLD) simulates monomorphic B-cell PTLD both clinically and pathologically. *Am J Surg Pathol* 2006;30:470-476.

[38] Vakiani E, Nandula SV, Subramaniyam S, Keller CE, Alobeid B, Murty VV, Bhagat G. Cytogenetic analysis of B-cell post-transplant lymphoproliferations validates the World Health Organization classification and suggests inclusion of florid follicular hyperplasia as a precursor lesion. *Hum Pathol* 2007;38:315-325.

[39] Djokic M, Le Beau MM, Swinnen LJ, Smith SM, Rubin CM, Anastasi J, Carlson KM. Post-transplant lymphoproliferative disorder subtypes correlate with different recurring chromosomal abnormalities. Genes Chromosomes Cancer 2006;45:313-318.

[40] Delecluse HJ, Rouault JP, Ffrench M, Dureau G, Magaud JP, Berger F. Post-transplant lymphoproliferative disorders with genetic abnormalities commonly found in malignant tumours. *Br J Haematol* 1995;89:90-97.

[41] Murukesan V, Mukherjee S. Managing post-transplant lymphoproliferative disorders in solid-organ transplant recipients: A review of immunosuppressant regimens. *Drugs* 2012;72:1631-1643.

[42] Styczynski J, Einsele H, Gil L, Ljungman P. Outcome of treatment of Epstein-Barr virus-related post-transplant lymphoproliferative disorder in hematopoietic stem cell recipients: A comprehensive review of reported cases. *Transplant Infect Dis* 2009;11:383-392.

[43] Trappe R, Oertel S, Leblond V, Mollee P, Sender M, Reinke P, Neuhaus R, Lehmkuhl H, Horst HA, Salles G, Morschhauser F, Jaccard A, Lamy T, Leithäuser M, Zimmermann H, Anagnostopoulos I, Raphael M, Riess H, Choquet S; German PTLD Study Group; European PTLD Network. Sequential treatment with rituximab followed by CHOP chemotherapy in adult B-cell post-transplant lymphoproliferative disorder (PTLD): The prospective international multicentre phase 2 PTLD-1 trial. *Lancet Oncol* 2012;13:196-206.

[44] Comoli P, Maccario R, Locatelli F, Valente U, Basso S, Garaventa A, Tomà P, Botti G, Melioli G, Baldanti F, Nocera A, Perfumo F, Ginevri F. Treatment of EBV-related post-renal transplant lymphoproliferative disease with a tailored regimen including EBV-specific T cells. *Am J Transplant* 2005;5: 1415-1422.

[45] Frey NV, Tsai DE. The management of post-transplant lymphoproliferative disorder. *Med Oncol* 2007;24: 125-136.

[46] Funch DP, Walker AM, Schneider G, Ziyadeh NJ, Pescovitz MD. Ganciclovir and acyclovir reduce the risk of post-transplant lymphoproliferative disorder in renal transplant recipients. *Am J Transplant* 2005;5: 2894-2900.

[47] Mentzer SJ, Perrine SP, Faller DV. Epstein-Barr virus post-transplant lymphoproliferative disease and virus-specific therapy: Pharmacological re-activation of viral target genes with arginine butyrate. *Transplant Infect Dis* 2001;3:177-185.

[48] Perrine SP, Hermine O, Small T, Suarez F, O'Reilly R, Boulad F, Fingeroth J, Askin M, Levy A, Mentzer SJ, Di Nicola M, Gianni AM, Klein C, Horwitz S, Faller DV. A phase 1/2 trial of arginine butyrate and ganciclovir in patients with Epstein-Barr virus-associated lymphoid malignancies. *Blood* 2007;109:2571-2578.

[49] HemaQuest Pharmaceuticals Inc. US national institute of Health, clinicaltrials.gov. *Study of arginine butyrate and ganciclovir/valganciclovir in EBV(+) lymphoid malignancies* (NCT00917826). 2011. Retrieved from website: http://clinicaltrials.gov/ct2/show/study/NCT00917826. Accessed Dec. 15, 2013

[50] Cohen JI, Bollard CM, Khanna R, Pittaluga S. Current understanding of the role of Epstein-Barr virus in lymphomagenesis and therapeutic approaches to EBV-associated lymphomas. *Leuk Lymph* 2008;49 (suppl. 1):27-34.

[51] Leblond V, Sutton L, Dorent R, Davi F, Bitker MO, Gabarre J, Charlotte F, Ghoussoub JJ, Fourcade C, Fischer A, et al. Lymphoproliferative disorders after organ transplantation: A report of 24 cases observed in a single center. *J Clin Oncol* 1995;13: 961-968.

[52] Verschuuren EAM, Stevens SJC, Van Imhoff GW, Middeldorp JM, De Boer C, Koeter G, The TH, Van Der Bij W. Treatment of post-transplant lymphoproliferative disease with rituximab: The remission, the relapse, and the complication. *Transplantation* 2002;73:100-104.

[53] Ganne V, Siddiqi N, Kamaplath B, Chang CC, Cohen EP, Bresnahan BA, Hariharan S. Humanized anti-CD20 monoclonal antibody (Rituximab) treatment for post-transplant lymphoproliferative disorder. *Clin Transplant* 2003;17: 417-422.

[54] Choquet S, Leblond V, Herbrecht R, Socié G, Stoppa AM, Vandenberghe P, Fischer A, Morschhauser F, Salles G, Feremans W, Vilmer E, Peraldi MN, Lang P, Lebranchu Y, Oksenhendler E, Garnier JL, Lamy T, Jaccard A, Ferrant A, Offner F, Hermine O, Moreau A, Fafi-Kremer S, Morand P, Chatenoud L, Berriot-Varoqueaux N, Bergougnoux L, Milpied N. Efficacy and safety of rituximab in B-cell post-transplantation lymphoproliferative disorders: results of a prospective multicenter phase 2 study. *Blood* 2006;107:3053–3057.

[55] Elstrom RL, Andreadis C, Aqui NA, Ahya VN, Bloom RD, Brozena SC, Olthoff KM, Schuster SJ, Nasta SD, Stadtmauer EA, Tsai DE. Treatment of PTLD with rituximab or chemotherapy. *Am J Transplant* 2006; 6:569-576.

[56] Orjuela M, Gross TG, Cheung YK, Alobeid B, Morris E, Cairo MS. A pilot study of chemoimmunotherapy (cyclophosphamide, prednisone, and rituximab) in patients with post-transplant lymphoproliferative disorder following solid organ transplantation. *Clin Cancer Res* 2003; 9:3945s-3952s.

[57] Jeremy A. US national institute of Health, clinicaltrials.gov. Bortezomib Plus Rituximab for EBV+ PTLD (NCT01058239). 2013. Retrieved from website: http://clinicaltrials.gov/show/NCT01058239. Accessed Dec. 15, 2013

[58] Zou P, Kawada J, Pesnicak L, Cohen JI. Bortezomib induces apoptosis of Epstein-Barr virus (EBV)-transformed B cells and prolongs survival of mice inoculated with EBV-transformed B cells. *J Virol* 2007;81:10029–10036.

[59] Khanna R, Bell S, Sherritt M, Galbraith A, Burrows SR, Rafter L, Clarke B, Slaughter R, Falk MC, Douglass J, Williams T, Elliott SL, Moss DJ. Activation and adoptive transfer of Epstein-Barr virus-specific cytotoxic T cells in solid organ transplant

patients with post-transplant lymphoproliferative disease. *Proc Natl Acad Sci* U S A 1999;96:10391-10396.

[60] Comoli P, Labirio M, Basso S, Baldanti F, Grossi P, Furione M, Viganò M, Fiocchi R, Rossi G, Ginevri F, Gridelli B, Moretta A, Montagna D, Locatelli F, Gerna G, Maccario R. Infusion of autologous Epstein-Barr virus (EBV)-specific cytotoxic T cells for prevention of EBV-related lymphoproliferative disorder in solid organ transplant recipients with evidence of active virus replication. *Blood* 2002; 99:2592-2598.

[61] Savoldo B, Goss JA, Hammer MM, Zhang L, Lopez T, Gee AP, Lin YF, Quiros-Tejeira RE, Reinke P, Schubert S, Gottschalk S, Finegold MJ, Brenner MK, Rooney CM, Heslop HE. Treatment of solid organ transplant recipients with autologous Epstein Barr virus-specific cytotoxic T lymphocytes (CTLs). *Blood* 2006;108:2942-2949.

[62] Haque T, Taylor C, Wilkie GM, Murad P, Amlot PL, Beath S, McKiernan PJ, Crawford DH. Complete regression of post-transplant lymphoproliferative disease using partially HLA-matched Epstein Barr virus-specific cytotoxic T cells. *Transplantation* 2001;72:1399-1402.

[63] Haque T, Wilkie GM, Taylor C, Amlot PL, Murad P, Iley A, Dombagoda D, Britton KM, Swerdlow AJ, Crawford DH. Treatment of Epstein-Barr-virus-positive post-transplantation lymphoproliferative disease with partly HLA-matched allogeneic cytotoxic T cells. *Lancet* 2002;360:436-442.

[64] Haque T, Wilkie GM, Jones MM, Higgins CD, Urquhart G, Wingate P, Burns D, McAulay K, Turner M, Bellamy C, Amlot PL, Kelly D, MacGilchrist A, Gandhi MK, Swerdlow AJ, Crawford DH. Allogeneic cytotoxic T-cell therapy for EBV-positive post-transplantation lymphoproliferative disease: Results of a phase 2 multicenter clinical trial. *Blood* 2007;110:1123-1131.

[65] Barker JN, Doubrovina E, Sauter C, Jaroscak JJ, Perales MA, Doubrovin M, Prockop SE, Koehne G, O'Reilly RJ. Treatment of EBV-associated post-transplantation lymphoma after cord blood transplantation using third-party EBV-specific cytotoxic T lymphocytes. *Blood* 2010;116: 5045-5049.

[66] Uhlin M, Okas M, Gertow J, Uzunel M, Brismar TB, Mattsson J. A novel haplo-identical adoptive CTL therapy as a treatment for EBV-associated lymphoma after stem cell transplantation. *Cancer Immunol Immunother* 2010;59:473-477.

[67] Wang Y, Aissi-Rothe L, Virion JM, De Carvalho Bittencourt M, Ulas N, Audonnet S, Salmon A, Clement L, Venard V, Jeulin H, Stoltz JF, Decot V, Bensoussan D. Combination of Epstein-Barr virus nuclear antigen 1, 3 and lytic antigen BZLF1 peptide pools allows fast and efficient stimulation of Epstein-Barr virus-specific T cells for adoptive immunotherapy. *Cytotherapy* 2014;16:122-134.

[68] Icheva V, Kayser S, Wolff D, et al. Adoptive transfer of Epstein-Barr virus (EBV) nuclear antigen 1-specific T cells as treatment for EBV reactivation and lymphoproliferative disorders after allogeneic stem-cell transplantation. *J Clin Oncol* 2013;31: 39-48.

[69] De Angelis B, Dotti G, Quintarelli C, Huye LE, Zhang L, Zhang M, Pane F, Heslop HE, Brenner MK, Rooney CM, Savoldo B. Generation of Epstein-Barr virus-specific cytotoxic T lymphocytes resistant to the immunosuppressive drug tacrolimus (FK506). *Blood* 2009;114:4784-4791.

[70] Brewin J, Mancao C, Straathof K, Karlsson H, Samarasinghe S, Amrolia PJ, Pule M. Generation of EBV-specific cytotoxic T cells that are resistant to calcineurin inhibitors

for the treatment of post-transplantation lymphoproliferative disease. *Blood* 2009;114:4792-4803.
[71] Omiya R, Buteau C, Kobayashi H, Paya CV, Celis E. Inhibition of EBV-induced lymphoproliferation by CD4+ T cells specific for an MHC class II promiscuous epitope. *J Immunol* 2002;169:2172-2179.
[72] Ouyang J, Juszczynski P, Rodig SJ, Green MR, O'Donnell E, Currie T, Armant M, Takeyama K, Monti S, Rabinovich GA, Ritz J, Kutok JL, Shipp MA. Viral induction and targeted inhibition of galectin-1 in EBV + post-transplant lymphoproliferative disorders. *Blood* 2011;117: 4315-4322.
[73] Bernasconi M, Ueda S, Krukowski P, Bornhauser BC, Ladell K, Dorner M, Sigrist JA, Campidelli C, Aslandogmus R, Alessi D, Berger C, Pileri SA, Speck RF, Nadal D. Early gene expression changes by Epstein-Barr virus infection of B-cells indicate CDKs and survivin as therapeutic targets for post-transplant lymphoproliferative diseases. *Int J Cancer* 2013;133:2341-2350.

Biographical Sketch

Ghaith Abu-Zeinah, MD, is currently affiliated with New York Presbyterian Hospital / Weill Cornell. Department of Medicine. Education: He obtained his degree at Weill Cornell Medical College in Qatar, Doha, Qatar. He is on residency at Department of Internal Medicine at New York Presbyterian Hospital / Weill Cornell, New York, NY, USA. He has published 5 publications over last 3 years.

Mustafa Al-Kawaaz, MD, is currently affiliated with New York Presbyterian Hospital / Weill Cornell. Department of Medicine. Education: He obtained his degree at Weill Cornell Medical College in Qatar, Doha, Qatar. He is on residency at Department of Pathology at New York Presbyterian Hospital / Weill Cornell, New York, NY, USA.

In: Epstein-Barr Virus (EBV)
Editor: Jan Styczynski

ISBN: 978-1-63117-476-6
© 2014 Nova Science Publishers, Inc.

Chapter VI

Differences between EBV-Associated Post-Transplant Lymphoproliferative Disorders after Hematopoietic Stem Cell Transplantation and Solid Organ Transplantation

*Jan Styczynski**
Department of Pediatric Hematology and Oncology,
Collegium Medicum, Nicolaus Copernicus University, Bydgoszcz, Poland

Abstract

This chapter presents similarities and differences in the biology, course and therapy of post-transplant lymphoproliferative disorders (PTLD) after hematopoietic stem cell transplantation (HSCT) and solid organ transplantation (SOT). This review is focused on a comparison of key features of EBV-associated PTLD between HSCT and SOT recipients, with respect to the epidemiology and risk factors for EBV-PTLD in these distinct populations. In addition, current concepts and practices in the diagnosis, management and prevention of EBV-PTLD in HSCT and SOT settings are highlighted. PTLD after HSCT occurs in about 3% of patients, with differences between various types of transplantation. The following risk factors for PTLD development after HSCT are recognized: unrelated or HLA-mismatched transplant, cord blood transplant, in vitro or in vivo T-cell depletion, the use of thymoglobulin or anti-CD3 antibodies, serological EBV incompatibility between donor and recipient, and splenectomy. PTLD after SOT occurs more frequently than after HSCT. Risk factors for PTLD in SOT recipients should be differentiated between early and late PTLD. Risk factors for early PTLD include: primary EBV infection, young recipient age, type of organ transplanted, multiple organ transplantation, CMV mismatch or CMV disease, OKT3 and polyclonal anti-lymphocyte antibodies, and high intensity of immunosuppressive therapy. Risk factors for late PTLD

---

[*] Address for correspondence: Department of Pediatric Hematology and Oncology; Collegium Medicum, Nicolaus Copernicus University; ul. Curie-Sklodowskiej 9; 85-094 Bydgoszcz, Poland. E-mail: jstyczynski@cm.umk.pl

include: duration of immunosuppression; type of organ transplanted, and older recipient age. The following first-line treatment of PTLD is recommended: (i) anti-proliferative therapy with anti-CD20 therapy (rituximab); (ii) reduction of immunosuppression (RI); (iii) immunotherapy with either in vitro generated EBV-specific cytotoxic T-cells, or an infusion of donor lymphocytes (DLI) in order to restore T-cell reactivity. All other therapies, sometimes historically conventionalized, such as chemotherapy, surgery, or the use of antiviral agents, interferon or intravenous immunoglobulins (IVIG), are of low value and are thus used rarely nowadays. The use of rituximab for EBV-related PTLD is a therapy of choice after HSCT. Recent data show that RI when applied in combination with rituximab significantly improves the outcome of HSCT patients. Reduction or withdrawal of immunosuppression remains the gold standard for first-line PTLD therapy after SOT, while rituximab is regarded as a second-line therapy in this setting. Another issue addressed in this chapter is the relapse of PTLD, which is extremely rare after HSCT, and not uncommon in SOT recipients. Definitions related to therapy response and PTLD relapse are being proposed in this chapter. It has also been suggested that patients with a history of previous treatment for PTLD, undergoing second transplantation, should receive prophylactic rituximab after stem cell infusion.

Keywords: Epstein-Barr virus; post-transplant lymphoproliferative disorder; hematopoietic stem cell transplantation; solid organ transplantation; rituximab; reduction of immunosuppression; PTLD relapse

Abbreviations

ATG	Anti-thymocyte globulin
CD	Cluster of differentiation
CHOP	Cyclophosphamide-Adriamycin-Vincristin-Prednisone
CMV	Cytomegalovirus
CNS	Central nervous system
CR	Complete remission
CT	Computed tomography
CTL	Cytotoxic T-cell
DLI	Donor Lymphocytes Infusion
DNA	Deoxyribonucleic acid
EBER	Epstein-Barr Virus-encoded RNA
EBNA	Epstein-Barr Virus nuclear antigen
EBV	Epstein-Barr Virus nuclear antigen
ECIL	European Conference on Infections in Leukemia
GVHD	Graft-versus-host-disease
HD-MTX	High-dose methotrexate
HHV	Human Herpes Virus
HL	Hodgkin Lymphoma
HLA	Human Leukocyte Antigen
HSC	Hematopoietic stem cell
HSCT	Hematopoietic stem cell transplantation
IFN	Interferon
IM	Infectious mononucleosis

IT	Intrathecal
IVIG	Intravenous immunglobulin
MRD	Matched Related Donor
MTX	Methotrexate
MUD	Matched Unrelated Donor
NAT	Nucleic acid testing
NHL	Non-Hodgkin lymphoma
NK-cell	Natural killer cell
PCR	Polymerase chain reaction
PET	Positron emission tomography
PTLD	Post-transplant lymphoproliferative disorder
RI	Reduction of immunosuppression
SOT	Solid organ transplantation
WHO	World Health Organization

Introduction

Post-transplant lymphoproliferative disorder (PTLD) following hematopoietic stem cell transplantation (HSCT) or solid organ transplantation (SOT) is a life-threatening form of post-transplant malignancy [1]. Its occurrence is often associated with the Epstein-Barr virus (EBV) and profound immunosuppressive therapy [2]. PTLD might have a variable presentation [3].

EBV infection may be associated with a heterogeneous group of diseases, including non-neoplastic and neoplastic diseases, such as infectious mononucleosis (IM), various types of lymphomas, or nasopharyngeal carcinoma. Primary EBV infection or reactivation usually induces an asymptomatic infection or IM in immunocompetent people. If the balance between EBV-infected cells and the immune system is disrupted, EBV may result in a wide spectrum of diseases, ranging from fever to lymphoproliferative diseases in immunocompromised people. In recipients of allogeneic HSCT, the spectrum of diseases includes asymptomatic EBV DNA-emia, fever, PTLD, and end-organ diseases (pneumonia, encephalitis/myelitis, and hepatitis).

Solid organ transplantation is an accepted therapy for a wide range of conditions associated with end-stage diseases of the heart, kidney, lung, liver, as well as intestine and pancreas. The success of an organ transplantation surgery is dependent upon the use of immunosuppressive agents to prevent or treat rejection of the allograft [2]. However, successful management of rejection comes at the cost of increased susceptibility to infections in the post-transplant period. This is particularly true of herpes viruses in general, and EBV in particular. Because EBV is exceptionally prevalent in the general population, the possibility of developing an infection and disease due to this virus is a frequent cause of concern for recipients of organ transplantation [2].

EBV is closely involved in the pathogenesis of PTLD. It is an oncogenic DNA-virus belonging to the γ-herpesvirus family. EBV is acquired by the vast majority of the population: 90%-95% of adult individuals worldwide are seropositive. In a healthy individual, there exists a very tight balance between EBV-infected B-cells and anti-EBV immunity, manifested primarily by EBV-specific, CD8-positive cytotoxic T-lymphocytes (EBV-CTL).

Manifestations of EBV-Related Diseases

EBV infection after transplantation can manifest in a number of various diseases (Table 1) [4]. While the application of a classification scheme for EBV-related diseases is useful, it is important to note that EBV presents as a continuous spectrum of illnesses, and benign manifestations can evolve to more serious syndromes within individual patients. Furthermore, non-PTLD viral syndromes are not always benign, and fatal viral sepsis may occur in the absence of mass lesions [2]. Pediatric transplant patients have a higher risk for PTLD than adults because many pediatric patients had not yet been exposed to EBV at the time of transplantation and develop a primary EBV infection, a condition strongly associated with PTLD development. Several very rare manifestations of EBV infection have been reported, including brain tumor as an unusual presentation of PTLD [5], EBV-associated enteritis with ulcers characterized by numerous plasma cells and lymphoepithelial-like lesions after stem cell transplantation [6], and post-transplant EBV-associated smooth muscle tumors [7]. EBV-positive T-cell PTLDs are very rare occurrences and are associated with a very poor prognosis. EBV encephalitis diagnosed by EBV-specific PCR and antibody testing in the cerebrospinal fluid in an immunocompromised patient who presented with psychiatric symptoms and cognitive dysfunction in the absence of any neurological impairments or infectious signs has also been reported [8]. EBV-associated PTLD accompanied by EBV-associated pneumonia after transplant is rare. Cytology of bronchoalveolar lavage (BAL) fluid and a lung biopsy may help establish the diagnosis. Those patients with PTLD accompanied by EBV-associated pneumonia who developed hyperpyrexia and dyspnea progressed rapidly, and eventually all died within 2 weeks of the onset of PTLD [9].

Table 1. Manifestations of EBV-related diseases after transplantation

- Asymptomatic infection
- Infectious mononucleosis
    - Typical
    - Fulminant, severe
- EBV hepatitis
- Lymphocytic interstitial pneumonitis
- Meningoencephalitis
- Post-transplant lymphoproliferative disease (PTLD)
    - Early lesions
    - Polymorphic PTLD
    - Monomorphic PTLD

Biology and Pathogenesis of EBV-PTLD after HSCT and SOT

Biology of EBV-PTLD after HSCT and SOT

Transplantation of solid organs and hematopoietic stem cells is accompanied by a profound disturbance of immune function mediated by immunosuppressive drugs or delayed immune reconstitution. Impaired T-cell control of EBV-infected B cells leads to PTLD in up to 11% of patients after HSCT and 20% after SOT [2,10,11].

Pathogenesis is the key to understand potential therapy and prevention measures for both HSCT and SOT recipients. Following HSCT, EBV-infected B cells in PTLD are almost always of donor origin, because host-latent EBV infection is eradicated by myeloablative conditioning regimens [12]. Following SOT, though PTLD cells are of recipient origin, the source of EBV can be from the donor, the recipient or a primary infection via natural oral transmission (Table 2).

Table 2. Key features of EBV-PTLD in HSCT and SOT settings

	HSCT	SOT
Primary source of EBV	Donor	Recipient
Site of infection	Donor B cell	Recipient B cell
Responsible effector cell	Donor CD8+ T cell	Recipient CD8+ T cell
Peak incidence	60 days after HSCT Rare >6 months	First year after SOT Late cases can occur
Incidence range	1-11%	1-20%
Key risk factors	T cell depletion Anti-lymphocyte antibodies Stimulation of B cell proliferation	Recipient EBV negative Anti-lymphocyte antibodies Age Organ transplanted
Range of infection	Asymptomatic infection Infectious mononucleosis EBV hepatitis Lymphocytic interstitial pneumonitis Meningoencephalitis PTLD	Asymptomatic infection Nonspecific viral syndrome Infectious mononucleosis EBV hepatitis EBV enteritis PTLD EBV+ spindle cell tumors

Histological changes observed in PTLD are similar to lymphomas occurring in non-transplant patients, with the vast majority being B-cell lymphomas, although T-cell and Hodgkin's lymphomas, or even plasma-cell disease-resembling myelomas, may occur sporadically. Up to 30% of PTLDs following SOT will be EBV-negative and/or non-B-cell, whereas an EBV-negative or non-B-cell disease following HSCT is exceedingly rare [4].

The World Health Organization (WHO) has provided standardized criteria for the pathologic evaluation of lesions associated with EBV in transplant recipients [2,13,14]. However, histological grades of multiple lesions obtained simultaneously from the same patient may vary, potentially limiting the accuracy of pathologic assessment [15]. Histological characterization of PTLD is the same in the HSCT and SOT settings, and is used in accordance with the WHO classification of PTLD, where PTLDs are divided into four groups: early lesions (plasmacytic hyperplasia or infectious mononucleosis-like PTLD), polymorphic PTLD, monomorphic PTLD (B- and T/NK-cell types, with further classification into subtypes), and classical Hodgkin lymphoma-type PTLD. After SOT, the onset of viral syndrome, infectious mononucleosis and polymorphic PTLD occurs primarily within the first year, whereas monomorphic PTLD and lymphoma tend to occur later [2]. Monomorphic or lymphomatous PTLD resembles non-Hodgkin lymphoma; it is more aggressive, occurs later after transplantation, and is rarely responsive to a reduction of immunosuppression [5,16].

The pathogenesis of PTLDs is a result of EBV-induced transformation of B cells in the setting of anti-EBV cellular immunity being impaired due to iatrogenic immunosuppression. Both CD8+ and CD4+ T regulatory cells are required for cellular immunity. Graft-versus-host disease (GVHD) prevention strategies that indiscriminately remove T cells from the graft inadvertently increase the risk of PTLD [17]. Thus, risk factors for PTLD after HSCT include the use of a T-cell-depleted allograft and the application of anti-thymocyte globulin (ATG) or anti-CD3 monoclonal antibody as part of the GVHD prevention strategy [18]. Interestingly, agents that deplete both B cells and T cells, such as the anti-CD52 monoclonal antibody, alemtuzumab, do not appear to increase the risk of PTLD [19].

Incidence of PTLD after HSCT

In the HSCT setting, the type of transplant is an important risk factor for PTLD development. PTLD following autologous HSCT is rare [4]. In comparison to autologous HSCT, recipients of allogeneic HSCT are at an increased risk for developing PTLD, which presents clinically as aggressive and frequently fatal lymphomas [20,21]. Its incidence is low (about 1%) following HSCT from matched related donors (MRD), probably due to an early reconstitution of EBV-CTL activity (which may be as early as 30 days post-transplant) [4,21,22]. PTLD is more common to unrelated donor HSCT [4,21], as EBV-CTL recovery is delayed in the case of unrelated donor use, compared with MRD use [22]. However, human leukocyte antigen (HLA) disparity, which is more common in unrelated donor HSCT, may also induce chronic B-cell stimulation and proliferation, which could predispose a patient to develop PTLD.

In a recent extensive multicenter study, the overall EBV-PTLD frequency after HSCT in the participating centers was 3.22 % (144/4466), and ranged from 1.16% in matched family donor (MFD), 2.86% in mismatched family donor (MMFD), 3.97% in matched unrelated donor (MUD), and 11.24% in mismatched unrelated donor (MMUD) recipients. Overall, the frequency of PTLD after alternative donor (MMFD or unrelated donor) allo-HSCT was 4.75% and the PTLD frequency after cord blood transplantation (CBT) was 4.06%. PTLDs were diagnosed at a median of 2 months after HSCT (range 0.5-53). An early onset of PTLD occurred in 109 patients (75.7%). Eight patients (6%) developed PTLD in the first month, whereas 16 patients (11.1%) were diagnosed later than 6 months after HSCT [11].

Incidence of PTLD after SOT

PTLD after SOT usually occurs within the first 36 months after transplant with a frequency that varies according to the type of solid organ graft as well as the type, intensity, and duration of immunosuppressive therapy used [19,23]. PTLD is relatively uncommon in kidney transplants, but can be seen in up to 15-20% of lung transplants which involve transplantation of greater amounts of lymphoid tissue [19]. Thus, another major risk factor for the development of PTLD is EBV-seronegative status of the host who receives an organ from an EBV+ donor [24]. EBV infection is frequently acquired in adolescence; therefore, seronegative pediatric transplant recipients are at a particular risk for PTLD. As regards the cell of origin, B-cell PTLDs present early with 80-90% of cases occurring in the first year and mostly in the first 6 months, whereas PTLDs of T/NK-cell origin are more likely to develop late after transplantation [11,25,26].

Strategies such as monitoring PCR viral load have been developed in order to detect EBV reactivation prior to the development of lymphoma [27,28]. The incidence of EBV reactivation monitored in this fashion can be as high as 15% but, unfortunately, not all PTLDs are heralded by a rise in the viral load [27,29]. Nonetheless, pre-emptive treatment strategies are becoming increasingly common in the era of reduced-intensity conditioning HSCT, given its greater reliance on immunosuppression relative to conventional myeloablative HSCT procedures [19].

The incidence of PTLD after SOT varies according to the age of the patient and the type of the transplanted organ. The type of solid organ allograft has also been identified as a risk factor, with low-risk patients (including kidney, heart and liver transplant recipients) having about 1-5% risk, compared with high-risk patients (namely lung, small bowel and multiple organ transplant recipients) having a 5-15% risk for developing PTLD [30]. The risk is the lowest following renal transplantation, moderate after heart transplantation, and the highest after lung, small intestine and multivisceral transplantation, reaching 31% patients [31,32].

Differences relative to transplanted organs arise primarily due to the varying level of immunosuppression. The higher incidence of PTLD following lung and small intestine transplantation can be attributed to aggressive immunosuppression and to the presence of preexisting lymphoid tissue in these organs, which is then transferred to the recipient, increasing the probability of EBV infection [33]. The frequency of PTLD after SOT is higher in childhood, regardless of the transplanted organ: the incidence is 2 to 3-fold, compared to adults. Pediatric patients are often EBV-seronegative, and PTLD after SOT is usually induced by a primary EBV infection [31,33]. The organ-specific cumulative 1-year incidence rates for children and adults are: for kidney transplant 1.3% vs <0.2%; for heart transplant 1.6% vs 0.3%; for liver 2.1% vs 0.25%; for lungs 4% vs 1%. The corresponding cumulative 5-year incidence rates for children and adults are: for kidney transplant 2.4% vs <0.6%; for heart transplant 5.7% vs 0.7%; for liver 4.7% vs 1.1%; for lungs 16% vs 1.5%. The overall incidence is 2.4%-5.8% after combined heart and lung transplantation, and may be as high as 20% after small bowel transplantation [2,31,32].

As regards the age of donor and recipient, their EBV serostatus and recipient EBV naivety implying younger age constitute the strongest risk factors for PTLD following SOT [4,21]. Exposure to EBV begins early in life, with approximately 50% of children in developed countries becoming seropositive by 5 years of age [34]. Children have an increased risk for developing PTLD after organ transplantation because they are more often EBV-naive than adults before a transplantation surgery. Over 90% of pediatric PTLD cases are of B-cell origin, CD20 positive, and most are associated with EBV infection [35].

Risk Factors for PTLD in HSCT

Risk factors related to the HSCT setting can be divided into the following categories: donor-related factors (unrelated or mismatched donor, unrelated cord blood, older recipient age, older donor age); the preparative regimen (Total Body Irradiation, T-cell depletion, and especially the use of anti-T-cell monoclonal antibodies); immunosuppression (the use of ATG, ALG or anti-CD3 monoclonal antibodies) and a combination of the above-mentioned key factors [4].

PTLD in the post-HSCT setting originates predominantly from donor B cells and typically occurs within the first 6 months after transplant, before reconstitution of the EBV-specific CTL (cytotoxic T lymphocytes) response [36]. The range of risk factors includes the degree of mismatch between donor and recipient, manipulation of the graft to deplete T cells and the degree of immunosuppression used to prevent the graft-versus-host disease (GVHD) [37]. A high incidence of PTLD in both pediatric and adult patients after transplantation following reduced intensity conditioning (RIC) regimens using ATG or alemtuzumab has also been reported [38,39]. This likely reflects both the delayed recovery of EBV-specific immunity after such transplants and the persistence of recipient-derived B cells.

Zallio et al showed that the main factors significantly associated with a high risk for PTLD after HSCT were as follows: (i) unrelated vs. sibling donor (26% vs. 7%), (ii) T-cell depletion (29% vs. 6%), (iii) graft-versus-host disease (GVHD; 30% vs. 7%), and (iv) cytomegalovirus (CMV) reactivation (29% vs. 4%) [40]. Multivariate analysis showed that CMV reactivation was the only independent variable associated with EBV reactivation. The authors concluded that: (i) a single infusion of rituximab is able to prevent the risk of progression into EBV-related PTLD; and (ii) CMV reactivation is strongly associated with EBV reactivation; therefore, an intensive EBV monitoring strategy could be advisable in case of CMV reactivation [40].

The impact of immunosuppression on PTLD occurrence is important. In general, the risk is correlated with the intensity of immunosuppression, particularly T-cell-specific immunosuppression, and cumulative exposure. Anti-T-cell antibodies are the most potent suppressants of EBV-CTL activity, followed by T-cell activation inhibitors, such as cyclosporin and tacrolimus. Patients treated with corticosteroids, anti-metabolites (i.e., azathioprine, mycophenolate mofetil or methotrexate), or the mTOR inhibitors (rapamycin) have a relatively lower risk for PTLD [2,41].

Following HSCT, T-cell depletion (TCD) is the strongest risk factor for PTLD [4,21]. TCD methods that remove T-cells in a selective manner confer a higher risk for PTLD than methods that completely deplete lymphocytes from the stem cell graft, which include the use of alemtuzumab, elutriation or positive CD34 cell selection [4]. Pan-lymphocyte depletion methods decrease the number of EBV-infected B cells and T cells, which may delay B-cell proliferation until the EBV-CTL function recovers [4,42,43]. In HSCT, the recipient's age and EBV status are not recognized as risk factors for PTLD, although the risk increases with donor age and it has been speculated that this is due to a lower number of EBV-CTLs as age increases [4].

In general, any factor that stimulates B-cell proliferation and/or decreases or delays T-cell immunity will increase the risk for PTLD. It has to be underlined that improved measures of detection and management of EBV infections has led to a reduction in PTLD rates over time, regardless of graft type [2].

Risk Factors for PTLD in SOT

Risk factors for PTLD in SOT recipients should be differentiated between early and late PTLD. Risk factors for early PTLD include: primary EBV infection (EBV-seropositive patients are not devoid of risk, especially in the case of intestine transplantation); young recipient age; type of organ transplanted; CMV mismatch or CMV disease; OKT3 and polyclonal anti-lymphocyte antibodies. Risk factors for late PTLD include: duration of immunosuppression; type of organ transplanted, and older recipient age [44]. There exists contradictory and controversial evidence for the role of the following risk factors for primary disease: tacrolimus in pediatric recipients; HLA matching; certain cytokine gene polymorphisms; preexisting chronic immune stimulation; hepatitis C infection; viral strain virulence (EBV-1 vs. EBV-2 and LMP1 deletion mutants) [44]. Risk factors include the exposure to a calcineurin inhibitor, but there has been no increased risk in patients treated with anti-T-lymphocyte antibodies [45].

The severe impairment of T-cell function in SOT recipients as a result of the required immunosuppressive post-transplantation regimen also places these patients at a risk for the development of PTLD, although in this setting the majority of cases are of recipient origin [36]. The strongest risk factors are the degree of immunosuppression and the development of primary infection after transplant. Higher incidence rates are therefore seen in lung and small bowel transplants, as well as in EBV-seronegative pediatric patients receiving a transplant from an EBV-seropositive donor [46].

The prevalence of EBV-related PTLD in SOT recipients depends on several factors, such as the type of organ transplanted, the EBV immunological status of the donor and the recipient, and the type and intensity of immunosuppressive drugs [47]. The overall risk for PTLD in recipients is between 1% and 2%, but the type of transplanted organ is an important risk factor. Recipients without previous infection with EBV (i.e., IgG negative) are at the greatest risk for PTLD [5,47]. CD4+ cell count at day +30 is a predictive factor for EBV DNA-emia and may help identify patients requiring closer monitoring. Although only 3% of patients progressed to PTLD and all were successfully managed, EBV reactivation was associated with higher treatment-related mortality, mainly because of subsequent infections [20]. Cumulative occurrence can be as high as 12-20% by 7-12 years after liver transplantation [2].

Spectrum of EBV-Associated Diseases in Recipients of Allogeneic HSCT

EBV infection can be either primary (new infection occurring in an immunologically naive patient) or secondary, the latter being due to either the reactivation of latent EBV in the transplant recipient under the pressure of immune suppression or a reinfection with a new EBV strain [2]. In general, primary infection is associated with a more clinically significant disease while secondary infection tends to be mild or even asymptomatic [2,48].

Fever and lymphadenopathy are the most common symptoms and signs, and are usually associated with a rapidly progressive multiorgan failure and death if not treated in PTLD [49]. A growing body of data suggests that PTLD is only the tip of the iceberg of post-transplantation EBV-associated diseases [49]. The incidence of PTLD varies among allo-HSCT recipients depending on the number of risk factors. However, there are only scattered reports about EBV-associated diseases other than PTLD [6,8,9,49]. In the study of 263 recipients undergoing allo-HSCT who were prospectively analyzed for the incidence, clinical characteristics, and prognosis of the spectrum of EBV-associated diseases, the 3-year cumulative incidence of the total of EBV-associated diseases, PTLDs, EBV fever, and EBV end-organ diseases (pneumonia, encephalitis/myelitis, and hepatitis) were 15.6±2.5%, 9.9±2.0%, 3.3±1.3%, and 3.3±1.2% (2.2±1.0%, 1.6±0.8%, and 0.9±0.6%), respectively. Fever was the most common symptom of EBV-associated diseases. Patients with PTLD had a better response rate to rituximab-based treatments compared with those with EBV end-organ diseases, including PTLD accompanied by EBV end-organ diseases. The 3-year overall survival was 37.3±13.7%, 100.0%, and 0.0±0.0% in patients with PTLD, EBV fever, and EBV end-organ diseases, respectively[49]. The authors concluded that EBV-associated diseases other than PTLD are not rare in the recipients of allo-HSCT; the clinical manifestations of EBV end-organ diseases are similar to PTLD, and EBV end-organ diseases have had a poorer response to rituximab-based therapy compared with PTLD [49].

Variation in the severity and extent of disease is felt to be related to the degree of immunosuppression and the adequacy of the host immune response [2]. Symptomatic EBV infection and PTLD are more common after primary EBV infection: 4% of children undergoing solid organ transplantation developed PTLD, while it happened to almost all children with primary EBV infection in this population between 1 month and 5 years after transplant [50].

EBV-Negative PTLD

A growing number of cases of EBV-negative PTLD have been reported. In general, EBV-negative PTLDs are seen more frequently in adult compared to pediatric SOT recipients [2]. These cases tend to present later (>5 years after transplant) and to a large extent account for the observed bimodal pattern of timing of presentation of PTLD, with early cases being predominantly EBV-positive and late cases being increasingly EBV-negative [45,51]. Recent data from a French kidney transplant registry suggest that an increasing number of cases of EBV-negative PTLD present between 7 and 10 years after transplant, and an increased risk for PTLD is observed as long as 10 years after transplantation [51]. Data from the pediatric heart transplant registry likewise suggest that EBV-negative PTLD is increasingly being diagnosed also in children presenting late after transplant [2].

Diagnosis of PTLD after Transplantation

The diagnosis of PTLD is based on four steps: First – a physical examination, including an examination for tonsillitis, adenopathy and organomegaly. Second – imaging, including a CT of the chest and abdomen. Other possible imaging techniques include endoscopy in case of gastro-intestinal symptoms or a head CT scan. Very important information can be obtained from a PET scan, as there is an increasing wealth of experience with this method [52]. Third – a biopsy obtained from lesions for histologic confirmation, including EBER stains and molecular studies [13]. Fourth – EBV viral load tested using PCR [1]. Any suspicious lesions should undergo imaging studies and, if necessary, a biopsy and a histological evaluation.

Diagnostic workup for suspected PTLD should routinely include: a complete blood count, a differential diagnosis, platelets, serum electrolytes, calcium, BUN and creatinine, liver function tests, uric acid, lactate dehydrogenase, quantitative immunoglobulins, stools for occult bleeding, flow cytometry of lymphocytes (when possible), imaging (a chest radiograph: anteroposterior and lateral, a PET scan or a CT scan of the neck/chest/abdomen/pelvis), a core needle or excisional biopsy of the lesion and assays for the presence of EBV: EBV serology (anti-EBNA, i.e., Epstein-Barr nuclear antigens, the Viral Capsid Antigen and the Early Antigen), EBV viral load from peripheral blood, as well as EBER (EBV-encoded RNA) and CD20 histochemistry studies of pathological samples.

The diagnosis of PTLD is usually limited to lymphoid masses that are often extranodal. A particularly difficult presentation of PTLD is the very rapidly progressive disseminated disease that clinically resembles a septic shock or GVHD, which almost always results in death and is often being diagnosed at autopsy. This very fulminant disease appears to be more common following HSCT than SOT [4].

EBV DNA-Emia in Diagnosis of PTLD

There is a high correlation between EBV DNA-emia in peripheral blood and the development of an EBV disease, including PTLD. Usually, EBV DNA-emia occurs prior to the onset of clinical symptoms. The presence of high value of EBV DNA-emia seems to be highly sensitive, but not specific for PTLD, especially in patients with a prior history of EBV disease after transplantation [2,4,28]. Due to the lack of standardization of PCR measurements for EBV DNA-emia, predictive values and relationships between an increasing risk and an increasing viral load are not established. Perhaps a new WHO standard for nucleic acid testing (NAT) will allow to facilitate the analysis of such correlations.

According to the guidelines of ECIL (the European Conference on Infections in Leukemia), an early recognition of EBV viremia reactivation at a molecular level by means of real-time quantitative polymerase chain reaction (RQ-PCR) to measure EBV DNA load is recommended in post-transplant high-risk patients. Though different techniques have been used to assess EBV DNA load, there are currently no data for selecting the most optimal method; however, an analysis of EBV load in whole blood is preferred in the majority of centers. Due to technical aspects, it is not recommended to test EBV load in peripheral blood lymphocytes. Screening for EBV DNA should start at the day of HSCT, and it should last for 3 months with the frequency of at least once a week in high-risk EBV PCR-negative patients; longer monitoring is recommended in patients on treatment for GVHD, after haplo-HSCT, and in those having experienced an early EBV reactivation. In EBV DNA-positive patients with rising EBV DNA load, a more frequent sampling might be considered. The selected strategy should depend on an individual assessment of a patient. The diagnosis of EBV reactivation should be made based on quantitative data. As regards the threshold value, various data are reported and related to local experience. Mostly, 100 gEq/mL by PCR in whole blood or plasma is used. Current data does not allow to establish a threshold value calculation for EBV load for the diagnosis of PTLD (or other end-organ EBV disease) in HSCT patients. It is also not possible to correlate the peak EBV viral loads with clinical disease manifestations [1].

Management of EBV-PTLD

The following first-line treatment of PTLD is recommended: (i) anti-proliferative therapy with anti-CD20 therapy (rituximab); (ii) reduction of immunosuppressive therapy; (iii) immunotherapy with either in vitro generated EBV-specific cytotoxic T-cells, or an infusion of donor lymphocytes (DLI) in order to restore T-cell reactivity. All other therapies, sometimes historically conventionalized, such as chemotherapy, surgery, or the use of antiviral agents, interferon or intravenous immunoglobulins (IVIG) are of low value and are used rarely nowadays. Specific strategies for the management of PTLD after HSCT and SOT are presented in Table 3.

In a large retrospective study published in 1999, mortality rates reached almost 85% after the development of PTLD [21]. After the introduction of rituximab, more recent reports of mortality rates ranging from 0-60% have been issued [3,11]. Nevertheless, despite the use of rituximab and adoptive cellular therapy, overall survival rates still remain to be improved, as deaths due to sepsis, GVHD or underlying cancer recurrence are being common. Randomized studies that address the optimal management and prevention of PTLD are largely lacking.

Table 3. Specific strategies in therapy of PTLD

	HSCT	SOT
Rituximab	Promising (1st line therapy)	Promising (2nd line therapy)
Reduction of immunosuppression	Rarely effective	Frequently effective (1st line therapy)
Adoptive immunotherapy	Effective when available	Experimental and unproven
Chemotherapy	Poorly tolerated. Very poor outcomes.	Effective but potentially poorly tolerated. Promising data with use of modified protocol to limit toxicity.
Antiviral agents	Unproven	Unproven
Interferon	Limited or no experience	Unproven
IVIG	Limited or no experience	Unproven

Rituximab

The use of rituximab for EBV-related PTLD is a therapy of choice after HSCT. Out of 144 patients with EBV-PTLD after HSCT treated with rituximab, 69.4% survived. Multivariable analysis showed that a poor response of PTLD to rituximab was associated with an age ≥30 years, the involvement of extra-lymphoid tissue, acute GVHD, and a lack of reduction of immunosuppression upon PTLD diagnosis. In the prognostic model, the PTLD mortality increased with the growing number of factors: 0-1, 2 or 3 factors being associated with the mortality of 7%, 37% and 72%, respectively. Immunosuppression tapering was associated with a lower PTLD mortality (16% vs 39%) and a decrease of EBV DNA-emia in peripheral blood during therapy was predictive of better survival. Thus, over two-thirds of patients with EBV-PTLD survived after a rituximab-based treatment. Reduction of immunosuppression was associated with improved outcome, while older age, an extranodal disease, and acute GVHD predicted poor outcome [11]. Rituximab was shown to be effective also when administered intrathecally in central nervous system involvement [53]. On the other hand, the use of rituximab brings long-term (6-12 months) B-cell depletion, sometimes requiring intravenous immunoglobulin supplementation. Additionally, rituximab therapy bears high costs [4].

The use of rituximab in the SOT population is much more controversial. The efficacy and safety of the anti-CD20 antibody rituximab used as first-line treatment has been tested in CD20-positive PTLD patients after SOT unresponsive to immunosuppression reduction in 3 prospective clinical trials [54-56]. Two independently performed, multicenter, prospective phase 2 trials administered the rituximab monotherapy at a dose of 375 mg/m^2 weekly for 4 consecutive weeks. Complete remission (CR) rates were 9/17 (52%) and 12/43 (28%), respectively. However, a combined analysis of both trials demonstrated that 34/60 patients (57%) experienced disease progression within 12 months of completing the rituximab therapy, including 9/35 (26%) treatment responders [54,55]. An extended therapy with rituximab may increase the CR rate, but whether this translates into improved overall survival is unclear [57]. From published reports, it appears that >50% of patients with PTLD will respond to rituximab, but as many as 15-20% will suffer a relapse/progression [58].

Reduction of Immunosuppression

Reduction of immunosuppression is thought to be rarely successful in the HSCT setting, although some successes were reported when RI was used as a strategy for pre-emptive therapy [59,60]. Recent data show, however, that RI when applied in combination with rituximab significantly improves the outcome [11].

Reduction/withdrawal of immunosuppression (RI) remains the gold standard for first-line PTLD therapy after SOT [24]. The response to RI varies greatly, from 20% to 86% [24,61]. This is most dramatically seen in cardiothoracic transplant recipients, where complete cardiovascular collapse and subsequent death have been reported in >20% of patients [4,62]. RI is rarely successful as the sole intervention in PTLD following HSCT, because the major defect consists in delayed EBV-CTL recovery, and not suppression of EBV-CTL function. The obvious danger of RI is an increased risk of rejection or GVHD [4].

Reduction of immunosuppression is an accepted first-line therapy in most situations in SOT patients. Reduced immune suppression is the key in the management of EBV-PTLD. Recent data confirms the role of reduced immune suppression, particularly in adults. Nevertheless, in about 35-40% of cases, treatment failures are observed together with reduced immune suppression due to either tumor unresponsiveness or a significant rejection [2].

Chemotherapy in PTLD

Chemotherapy in PTLD after SOT is not usually indicated as the first-line therapy. Chemotherapy has traditionally been reserved for the refractory and/or relapsing PTLD cases [4]. It can be considered for initial use in monomorphic PTLD occurring late in the post-transplant course. Different multiple regimens have been used, such as CHOP, ACVBP, or ProMACE-CytaBOM [63-65]; however, there are no comparisons among chemotherapy regimens in clinical trials. There is an increased likelihood of infectious morbidity and mortality seen in transplant patients when compared to similar chemotherapy regimens used in a non-transplant setting. Overall response rates in the SOT setting have been determined as 65-75% including late mortality [58,66]. The newer approach is to limit the use of chemotherapy to only those patients who fail rituximab or to combine chemotherapy with the application of rituximab [67].

Current pediatric treatment protocols for CD20-positive PTLD are based on rituximab therapy with or without reduced-intensity chemotherapy regimens [15]. By contrast, the most recent studies on adults used rituximab in combination with standard-dose CHOP-based regimens [68]. Whether the rate of patients with durable remissions after rituximab monotherapy differs between children and adults is currently under investigation. In addition to reduced immunosuppression, pediatric classical Hodgkin Lymphoma (HL) PTLD is treated similarly to HL in non-transplanted patients [69]. One study in children with PTLD following SOT used a low-dose chemotherapy approach in which 75% of patients achieved remission and there were no deaths from therapy; however, the relapse rate was 18% [70].

PTLD of the central nervous system (CNS) is a rare complication of solid organ transplantation (SOT) and there is currently no consensus on an optimal therapy. Recurrent PTLD following rituximab and front-line chemotherapy represents a particularly difficult therapeutic challenge. High-dose methotrexate (HD-MTX) is an effective therapy for CNS PTLD and recurrent PTLD in which rituximab and CHOP chemotherapy have failed. A complete response of CNS PTLD was achieved with HD-MTX and intrathecal (IT) MTX. A total of 5 cycles of HD-MTX (2.5 gm/m^2/dose on day 1) were delivered over 5 months, with IT therapy given simultaneously (2 mg/dose IT × 2-3 days Q10 days beginning on day 7-10 of each HD-MTX cycle). Cycles of HD-MTX were repeated approximately every 28 days. Following the completion of systemic chemotherapy, 5 additional months of only IT chemotherapy were administered, initially with metronomic IT MTX and subsequently with IT cytarabine (15mg/dose ×3 days, administered Q21 days) [71].

Chemotherapy for PTLD after HSCT is not recommended due to poor toleration in HSCT patients who had usually been heavily pretreated with chemotherapy and/or conditioning before hematopoietic stem cell transplantation [3,11].

Cellular Therapy

Donor leukocyte infusions have been successful in treating PTLD post-HSCT; however, in order to achieve efficacy, the donor must be EBV-positive, in which case severe GVHD may occur [72,73]. Data on efficacy are very limited as DLI has usually been used in combination with other treatment modalities. Overall survival was reported as 16/39 (41.0%) patients [3]. To circumvent these complications, ex vivo-generated EBV-CTL have proved to offer a very effective prophylactic measure, pre-emptive therapy and treatment for PTLD post-HSCT [74].

Enhancement of anti-EBV cellular immunity is an attractive approach to treat PTLD. EBV-specific cytotoxic T lymphocytes (CTL) can be isolated and expanded in vitro from EBV-seropositive stem cell donors or third-party donors. CTLs used to prevent and/or treat PTLD were first applied successfully in allogeneic HSCT recipients with the stem cell donor's peripheral blood used as a source of EBV-specific CTL. Because, in most circumstances, EBV-specific CTLs have to be generated in vitro or isolated, requiring time for generation and expansion, the first choice for the treatment of EBV-PTLD is the administration of anti-CD20 monoclonal antibodies. The overall response rates to anti-EBV CTL therapy in the HSCT setting were 94.1% (127/135 patients) for the pre-emptive therapy, and 88.2% (15/17 patients) for the therapy of EBV-PTLD disease [3].

The use of EBV-CTL in SOT is complex [4]. Several groups have demonstrated the ability to generate autologous EBV-CTL for SOT patients with PTLD [75-77]. As opposed to HSCT, in SOT patients these cells do not persist; repeated infusions are required. Additionally, EBV-CTL activity did not correlate with reduced EBV levels [75-77]. T-cell lines were obtained from healthy volunteers and banked for use in treating PTLD patients, with some success [78]. Although very attractive, this approach remains prohibitive for most centers due to the high level of technology required, regulatory issues and costs [4].

Antiviral Therapy for PTLD

In spite of a relatively wide range of antiviral drugs, practically none of them can be recommended for EBV infections. This is due to the lack of activity of thymidine kinase in latent EBV virus in the phase of PTLD. EBV infection can be lytic, latent or immortalizing. PTLD lesions typically consist of EBV-immortalized B-cells, thus only a minority of cells express lytic antigens of EBV. Although acyclovir and ganciclovir can inhibit lytic EBV infection, these drugs are not useful in the latent or immortalized stadium. Moreover, there is a lack of prospective, comparative data on the latter. If this is the case, EBV viral loads can even rise with the use of antivirals. Currently, there is no antiviral drug that can be used against EBV. Theoretically, maribavir is the drug exhibiting potential activity against CMV and EBV; however, the trial with maribavir in the prophylaxis against CMV has failed [79].

The efficacy of antiviral therapy in treating PTLD is difficult to ascertain as it is almost always used in conjunction with other potentially effective treatments. A novel approach has been used recently, where viral replication is promoted with the use of arginine butyrate, which upregulates the expression of EBV thymidine kinase. Ganciclovir is also given, which causes an abortive replicative cycle and no virion production, but cell death occurs [80].

Surgical Therapy

Surgical therapy is of little benefit in PTLD after SOT and is not used in HSCT patients. Unfortunately, a disease which can be classified as resectable occurs in only a small percentage of PTLD patients [81]. The inapplicability of surgical therapy seems to be due to its effectiveness in curing mainly localized diseases [82].

Pre-Emptive Therapy

Pre-emptive therapy is defined as any agents or EBV-specific T cells given to an asymptomatic patient with EBV detected in a screening assay [1]. For pre-emptive therapy to be successful, one must have a method of reliably identifying patients who are at a high risk before they develop disease [4]. Several reports demonstrate that viral load is increased at the time of PTLD diagnosis [72,74,83]. There are no blinded, prospective studies to determine the predictive value of quantitative PCR for the development of PTLD [81]. The strongest data for EBV viral load predicting patients at a risk for PTLD is in the setting of recipients of TCD HSCT grafts [84]. The optimal timing for EBV viral load monitoring is debated, as PTLD can develop very rapidly [4,28]. As there exists a great variability between different methods and/or laboratories, the interpretation of EBV DNA-emia should be done with great caution. Threshold value calculation for EBV load for the diagnosis of PTLD in HSCT patients should be performed on the basis of local data. The predictive value of EBV DNA-emia can be greatly enhanced by combining it with measures of anti-EBV T-cell immunity [4,85,86].

Since EBV-CTL immunity recovers 1-6 months post-HSCT, it has become standard practice at many centers for patients receiving TCD, either ex vivo or in vivo, to be monitored by EBV PCR weekly for up to 6 months after transplant, with rituximab administered pre-emptively in patients with rising or persistently positive EBV viral loads [4].

Pre-emptive administration of rituximab has been shown to reduce the risk for PTLD development. The prospective study of monitoring of EBV D+/R- (Donor/Recipient) in 34 adults after kidney transplantation reported as follows: 3 out of 6 patients D+/R- discharged without monitoring developed PTLD and all lost their grafts, while all 6 patients with positive EBV-DNA-emia and the presence of clinical symptoms who were treated pre-emptively with rituximab did not develop PTLD [87].

Prevention of EBV-PTLD

Prophylaxis of EBV-DNA-emia (EBV reactivation) is defined as any agents given to an asymptomatic patient to prevent EBV reactivation in a seropositive recipient (or when the donor is seropositive).

The ECIL recommendations suggest that high-risk HSCT patients should be tested for EBV serology before allo-HSCT. If a patient is found to be seronegative, the risk for PTLD is higher. Also, HSCT donors should be tested for EBV serology before transplantation, particularly in cases of mismatched donors or when T-depletion is planned. When there is a choice, the selection of a seronegative donor might be beneficial, as EBV might be transmitted with the graft. CD34-positive selection does not prevent EBV-PTLD. The risk in HLA-identical sibling transplant recipients not receiving T-cell depletion is low, and no routine screening for EBV is recommended. For patients with hematological malignancies receiving standard chemotherapy and in autologous HSCT recipients, EBV infection is of small importance. No routine diagnostics for EBV are recommended in these groups of patients, both before and after therapy. However, additional risk factors, such as alemtuzumab treatment (and possibly the use of fludarabine, other nucleoside analogs or infliximab), might cause prolonged immunosuppression lasting for up to 6 months, causing a higher risk for EBV reactivation. The use of alemtuzumab in vivo in the non-myeloablative conditioning might have resulted in the delay in EBV-specific T-cell recovery and increased virus infections. Poor or negative data regarding EBV prophylaxis are available. The prevention of EBV reactivation in allo-HSCT recipients cannot be based on antiviral prophylaxis. Ganciclovir can reduce EBV replication, but neither ganciclovir/foscarnet nor cidofovir therapy/prophylaxis have any impact on the development of EBV-PTLD, and so antiviral agents are not recommended (Table 4). In case of high EBV load, B-cell depletion before allo-HSCT or the prophylactic use of rituximab early after allo-HSCT are optional. Immune globulin used for the prevention of EBV reactivation or disease is not recommended in patients undergoing HSCT. Routine antiviral prophylaxis for EBV is not recommended in the autologous HSCT setting and in other therapies as well. In fact, many patients are already receiving antiviral therapy when PTLD develops, and no studies support the use of antiviral prophylaxis to prevent PTLD following HSCT [1].

The utility of antiviral prophylaxis following SOT is rather controversial [4]. In the SOT setting, there is limited experience related to the prophylaxis of PTLD. Since viral replication induces B-cell lysis, the use of antivirals such as ganciclovir to prevent PTLD has been questioned [24]. Some reports indicate the opposite effect and the development of EBV-PTLD despite continuous ganciclovir or acyclovir prophylaxis [88-90]. With respect to the prophylactic use of antiviral therapy against EBV, there is a lack of concurrent controls [91,92] or any control group [93], or a failure to account for concurrent events. Prospective trial in pediatric liver transplantation setting failed to show benefit [94].

Table 4. Prevention of EBV-PTLD

	HSCT	SOT
Preemptive therapy - Reduction of IS - Rituximab - Adoptive immunotherapy	Ineffective Effective and recommended Effective and recommended if available	Appears effective and recommended Limited data Unproven
Antiviral drugs	Unproven	Unproven
Immunoprophylaxis - Active immunization - Passive immunization	Not available Unproven	Not available Unproven

Prognostic Factors in PTLD

Several variables have been identified as predictive indicators for prognosis in the management of PTLD. However, prognostic factors are not always consistent across studies. The extent to which findings can be generalized across centers is limited by the absence of a standardized approach to the pathologic diagnosis and treatment of PTLD. Factors that have been associated with poorer outcomes after SOT include: poor performance status, a multisite disease, a central nervous system disease, T- or NK-cell PTLD, spindle cell PTLD, EBV-negative PTLD, the abnormal cells leading to PTLD of recipient origin as opposed to donor-origin, a co-infection with hepatitis B or C, a monoclonal disease, the presence of mutation of proto-oncogenes or tumor suppressor genes [44]. PTLD with multisite involvement portends a worse prognosis [70,95].

Relapse of PTLD

A relapse of PTLD is extremely rare after hematopoietic stem cell transplantation (HSCT), while it is not uncommon in solid organ transplant (SOT) recipients. So far, there is only one report of a very late relapse of PTLD, which occurred 10 years after allogeneic HSCT in childhood, 9 years after cessation of immunosuppressive therapy [96], whereas reports of refractory PTLD are relatively common. In our database, there is a 5-year old boy after 2 allogeneic HSCTs, who developed polymorphic B-cell PTLD after each transplant. He was treated successfully with rituximab in both cases. Possible factors contributing to PTLD relapse in the presented case included: second HSCT, an in vivo T-cell depletion using ATG, donor HLA match of 9/10, immunosuppression, and pediatric age. On the other hand, the patient had no symptoms of GVHD, and he was serologically matched for EBV-IgG with the donor.

This case suggests that patients with a history of previous treatment for PTLD, undergoing a second transplant, should receive prophylactic rituximab after stem cell infusion (e.g., at day +5).

The following definitions related to therapy response and PTLD relapse are being proposed: Partial response – a decrease of at least 50% in initial changes, with decreases in EBV DNA-emia; Complete remission – resolution of all symptoms of PTLD, including clearance of EBV DNA-emia; Relapsed PTLD – when PTLD occurs after complete remission upon therapy for initial PTLD, with an at least 3-month interval; Refractory PTLD – when no partial response is observed after 4 weeks of therapy, or no complete remission is observed after 8 weeks of therapy.

So far, 70 cases of relapsed PTLD after SOT were reported [54,70,71,97-123], of which 50% were pediatric patients. PTLD occurred after transplantation of the heart (47%), kidney (33%), liver (17%) or lung (3%). Pathology results of initial and relapsed PTLD were: both monomorphic (52%), both polymorphic (15%), a shift from polymorphic to monomorphic (33%); no shift from monomorphic to polymorphic PTLD has been reported. Therapy of PTLD after SOT most often included rituximab or chemotherapy treatment (e.g., CHOP).

Conclusion

In conclusion, this chapter was focused on a comparison of key features of EBV-associated PTLD between HSCT and SOT recipients, with respect to the epidemiology, risk factors, management and prevention of EBV-PTLD in these settings. PTLD after HSCT occurs in about 3% of patients, with differences between various types of transplantation. PTLD after SOT occurs more often than after HSCT. The use of rituximab for EBV-related PTLD is a therapy of choice after HSCT. Recent data show that RI when applied in combination with rituximab significantly improves the outcome of HSCT patients. Reduction or withdrawal of immunosuppression remains the gold standard for first-line PTLD therapy after SOT, while rituximab is regarded as second-line therapy in this setting. Although attractive, cellular adoptive therapy is not available for most HSCT centers, and it is not available for most SOT recipients. All other therapies, sometimes historically conventionalized, such as chemotherapy, surgery, or the use of antiviral agents, interferon or IVIG, are of low value and are used rarely nowadays.

Determining the right prophylaxis or therapy for any given patient with PTLD remains a major clinical problem. Obstacles that still exist consist in the heterogeneity of disease and patient populations, as well as divergent approaches to immunosuppression and therapeutic interventions. To overcome such obstacles, collaboration among infectious disease specialists, pathologists, transplant physicians and oncologists is needed. We need to develop consensus on the definitions of PTLD and interventions that can be tested in large, prospective, multicenter trials.

Glossary

Primary EBV infection
New EBV infection occurring in an immunologically naive patient.

Secondary EBV infection
Infection occurring either due to reactivation of latent EBV in the transplant recipient under the pressure of immune suppression or reinfection with a new EBV strain.

Ultra-early onset PTLD
PTLD occurring within the first month post-transplantation [124]

Very late PTLD
PTLD occurring >10 years after transplantation

Complete remission of PTLD
Resolution of all symptoms of PTLD, including clearance of EBV-DNA-emia.

Partial response of PTLD
Decrease of at least 50% of initial changes, with decreases of EBV-DNA-emia.

Relapsed PTLD

Diagnosed when PTLD occurs after complete remission for therapy for initial PTLD, with at least 3 months interval.

Refractory PTLD

Diagnosed when no partial response is observed after 4 weeks of therapy, or no complete remission is observed after 8 weeks of therapy.

Summary Points List

- PTLD is a major complication of HSCT and SOT mostly driven by EBV infection, with different incidence related to various types of transplantation. PTLD after HSCT occurs in about 3% of patients, while PTLD after SOT occurs more often.
- Following major risk factors of PTLD development after HSCT are recognized: unrelated or HLA-mismatched transplant, T-cell depletion in vitro or in vivo, and serological EBV incompatibility between donor and recipient.
- Risk factors for PTLD in SOT recipients should be separated between early and late PTLD: risk factors for early PTLD include: primary EBV infection, young recipient age, type of organ transplanted, multiple organ transplantation, CMV mismatch or CMV disease, OKT3 and polyclonal anti-lymphocyte antibodies, and high intensity of immunosuppressive therapy; while risk factors for late PTLD include: duration of immunosuppression; type of organ transplanted and older recipient age.
- The following first line treatment of PTLD is recommended: (i) anti-proliferative therapy with anti-CD20 therapy (rituximab); (ii) reduction of immunosuppression (RI); (iii) immunotherapy with either in vitro generated EBV-specific cytotoxic T-cells, or infusion of donor lymphocytes (DLI) in order to restore T-cell reactivity. All other therapies, sometimes historically determined, such as chemotherapy, antiviral agents, surgery, interferon or intravenous immunoglobulins (IVIG) have low value and are used rarely nowadays.
- The use of rituximab for EBV-related PTLD is a therapy of choice after HSCT. Recent data show that RI when applied in combination with rituximab significantly improves the outcome of HSCT patients. Reduction or withdrawal of immunosuppression remains the gold standard for first-line PTLD therapy after SOT, while rituximab is regarded as second line therapy in this setting.
- Patients with history of previous treatment of PTLD, undergoing second transplant, should receive prophylactic rituximab after stem cell infusion.

Future Issue List

- Productive areas of investigation related to PTLD therapy should include: identifying which patients will benefit from RI; improving methods for predicting high-risk patients; developing safe and effective pre-emptive therapies, identifying those for

whom rituximab therapy is most likely to be of use; and finally, developing more effective, less toxic therapies for patients with resistant or aggressive disease.
- The incidence of symptomatic EBV disease and PTLD should decrease in the future.
- Evaluation and standardization of EBV viral load measurement is expected.
- Controlled trials of pre-emptive management modalities, including role of reduced immunosuppression with/without rituximab are necessary.
- Continued research on optimal treatment for specific categories of PTLD will include the specific regimens with/without rituximab. Future directions are focused on broadening the applicability of cellular therapies and ultimately being able to include the use of T-cells as upfront therapy with CD20 directed antibodies.
- Use of "third party" EBV CTLs in therapy of PTLD by the use of "banks" of characterized HLA-typed EBV-specific T-cell lines for third party use.
- Prevention of EBV infection in HSCT and SOT recipients would require an effective EBV vaccine.

References

[1] Styczynski J, Reusser P, Einsele H, de la Camara R, Cordonnier C, Ward KN, Ljungman P, Engelhard D: Management of HSV, VZV and EBV infections in patients with hematological malignancies and after SCT: Guidelines from the Second European Conference on Infections in Leukemia. *Bone Marrow Transplant* 2009;43:757-770.

[2] Green M, Michaels MG: Epstein-Barr virus infection and posttransplant lymphoproliferative disorder. *Am. J. Transplant* 2013;13 Suppl 3:41-54; quiz 54.

[3] Styczynski J, Einsele H, Gil L, Ljungman P: Outcome of treatment of Epstein-Barr virus-related post-transplant lymphoproliferative disorder in hematopoietic stem cell recipients: A comprehensive review of reported cases. *Transpl. Infect Dis.* 2009;11:383-392.

[4] Gross TG: Treatment for Epstein-Barr virus-associated PTLD. Herpes 2009;15:64-67.

[5] Azarpira N, Torabineghad S, Rakei M: Brain tumor as an unusual presentation of posttransplant lymphoproliferative disorder. *Exp. Clin. Transplant* 2009;7:58-61.

[6] Tashiro Y, Goto M, Takemoto Y, Sato E, Shirahama H, Utsunomiya A, Eizuru Y, Yonezawa S: Epstein-Barr virus-associated enteritis with multiple ulcers after stem cell transplantation: First histologically confirmed case. *Pathol. Int.* 2006;56:530-537.

[7] Jonigk D, Laenger F, Maegel L, Izykowski N, Rische J, Tiede C, Klein C, Maecker-Kolhoff B, Kreipe H, Hussein K: Molecular and clinicopathological analysis of Epstein-Barr virus-associated posttransplant smooth muscle tumors. *Am. J. Transplant* 2012;12:1908-1917.

[8] Behr J, Schaefer M, Littmann E, Klingebiel R, Heinz A: Psychiatric symptoms and cognitive dysfunction caused by Epstein-Barr virus-induced encephalitis. *Eur. Psychiatry* 2006;21:521-522.

[9] Liu QF, Fan ZP, Luo XD, Sun J, Zhang Y, Ding YQ: Epstein-Barr virus-associated pneumonia in patients with post-transplant lymphoproliferative disease after hematopoietic stem cell transplantation. *Transpl. Infect Dis.* 2010;12:284-291.

[10] Hussein K, Tiede C, Maecker-Kolhoff B, Kreipe H: Posttransplant lymphoproliferative disorder in pediatric patients. *Pathobiology* 2013;80:289-296.
[11] Styczynski J, Gil L, Tridello G, Ljungman P, Donnelly JP, van der Velden W, Omar H, Martino R, Halkes C, Faraci M, Theunissen K, Kalwak K, Hubacek P, Sica S, Nozzoli C, Fagioli F, Matthes S, Diaz MA, Migliavacca M, Balduzzi A, Tomaszewska A, Camara Rde L, van Biezen A, Hoek J, Iacobelli S, Einsele H, Cesaro S: Response to rituximab-based therapy and risk factor analysis in Epstein Barr virus-related lymphoproliferative disorder after hematopoietic stem cell transplant in children and adults: A study from the Infectious Diseases Working Party of the European Group for Blood and Marrow Transplantation. *Clin. Infect Dis.* 2013;57:794-802.
[12] Gratama JW, Oosterveer MA, Zwaan FE, Lepoutre J, Klein G, Ernberg I: Eradication of Epstein-Barr virus by allogeneic bone marrow transplantation: Implications for sites of viral latency. *Proc. Natl. Acad. Sci. USA* 1988;85:8693-8696.
[13] Campo E, Swerdlow SH, Harris NL, Pileri S, Stein H, Jaffe ES: The 2008 WHO classification of lymphoid neoplasms and beyond: Evolving concepts and practical applications. *Blood* 2011;117:5019-5032.
[14] Jaffe ES: The 2008 who classification of lymphomas: Implications for clinical practice and translational research. *Hematology Am. Soc. Hematol Educ. Program* 2009:523-531.
[15] Gross TG, Orjuela MA, Perkins SL, Park JR, Lynch JC, Cairo MS, Smith LM, Hayashi RJ: Low-dose chemotherapy and rituximab for posttransplant lymphoproliferative disease (PTLD): A children's oncology group report. *Am. J. Transplant* 2012;12:3069-3075.
[16] Harris NL, Ferry JA, Swerdlow SH: Posttransplant lymphoproliferative disorders: Summary of society for hematopathology workshop. *Semin. Diagn Pathol.* 1997;14:8-14.
[17] Mautner J, Bornkamm GW: The role of virus-specific CD4+ t cells in the control of Epstein-Barr virus infection. *Eur. J. Cell Biol* 2012;91:31-35.
[18] Landgren O, Gilbert ES, Rizzo JD, Socie G, Banks PM, Sobocinski KA, Horowitz MM, Jaffe ES, Kingma DW, Travis LB, Flowers ME, Martin PJ, Deeg HJ, Curtis RE: Risk factors for lymphoproliferative disorders after allogeneic hematopoietic cell transplantation. *Blood* 2009;113:4992-5001.
[19] Roschewski M, Wilson WH: EBV-associated lymphomas in adults. *Best Pract. Res. Clin. Haematol.* 2012;25:75-89.
[20] Patriarca F, Medeot M, Isola M, Battista ML, Sperotto A, Pipan C, Toffoletti E, Dozzo M, Michelutti A, Gregoraci G, Geromin A, Cerno M, Savignano C, Rinaldi C, Barbone F, Fanin R: Prognostic factors and outcome of Epstein-Barr virus dnaemia in high-risk recipients of allogeneic stem cell transplantation treated with preemptive rituximab. *Transpl. Infect Dis.* 2013;15:259-267.
[21] Curtis RE, Travis LB, Rowlings PA, Socie G, Kingma DW, Banks PM, Jaffe ES, Sale GE, Horowitz MM, Witherspoon RP, Shriner DA, Weisdorf DJ, Kolb HJ, Sullivan KM, Sobocinski KA, Gale RP, Hoover RN, Fraumeni JF, Jr., Deeg HJ: Risk of lymphoproliferative disorders after bone marrow transplantation: A multi-institutional study. *Blood* 1999;94:2208-2216.
[22] Marshall NA, Howe JG, Formica R, Krause D, Wagner JE, Berliner N, Crouch J, Pilip I, Cooper D, Blazar BR, Seropian S, Pamer EG: Rapid reconstitution of Epstein-Barr

virus-specific T lymphocytes following allogeneic stem cell transplantation. *Blood* 2000;96:2814-2821.

[23] Evens AM, Roy R, Sterrenberg D, Moll MZ, Chadburn A, Gordon LI: Post-transplantation lymphoproliferative disorders: Diagnosis, prognosis, and current approaches to therapy. *Curr. Oncol. Rep.* 2010;12:383-394.

[24] Paya CV, Fung JJ, Nalesnik MA, Kieff E, Green M, Gores G, Habermann TM, Wiesner PH, Swinnen JL, Woodle ES, Bromberg JS: Epstein-Barr virus-induced posttransplant lymphoproliferative disorders. ASTS/ASTP EBV-PTLD task force and the Mayo Clinic organized international consensus development meeting. *Transplantation* 1999;68:1517-1525.

[25] Draoua HY, Tsao L, Mancini DM, Addonizio LJ, Bhagat G, Alobeid B: T-cell post-transplantation lymphoproliferative disorders after cardiac transplantation: A single institutional experience. *Br. J. Haematol.* 2004;127:429-432.

[26] Nelson BP, Nalesnik MA, Bahler DW, Locker J, Fung JJ, Swerdlow SH: Epstein-Barr virus-negative post-transplant lymphoproliferative disorders: A distinct entity? *Am. J. Surg. Pathol.* 2000;24:375-385.

[27] Peric Z, Cahu X, Chevallier P, Brissot E, Malard F, Guillaume T, Delaunay J, Ayari S, Dubruille V, Le Gouill S, Mahe B, Gastinne T, Blin N, Saulquin B, Harousseau JL, Moreau P, Milpied N, Coste-Burel M, Imbert-Marcille BM, Mohty M: Features of Epstein-Barr virus (EBV) reactivation after reduced intensity conditioning allogeneic hematopoietic stem cell transplantation. *Leukemia* 2011;25:932-938.

[28] Gil L, Styczynski J, Komarnicki M: Strategy of pre-emptive management of Epstein-Barr virus post-transplant lymphoproliferative disorder after stem cell transplantation: Results of european transplant centers survey. *Contemp Oncol* (Pozn) 2012;16:338-340.

[29] Nourse JP, Jones K, Gandhi MK: Epstein-Barr virus-related post-transplant lymphoproliferative disorders: Pathogenetic insights for targeted therapy. *Am. J. Transplant* 2011;11:888-895.

[30] Opelz G, Dohler B: Lymphomas after solid organ transplantation: A collaborative transplant study report. *Am. J. Transplant* 2004;4:222-230.

[31] Vegso G, Hajdu M, Sebestyen A: Lymphoproliferative disorders after solid organ transplantation-classification, incidence, risk factors, early detection and treatment options. *Pathol. Oncol. Res.* 2011;17:443-454.

[32] Nassif S, Kaufman S, Vahdat S, Yazigi N, Kallakury B, Island E, Ozdemirli M: Clinicopathologic features of post-transplant lymphoproliferative disorders arising after pediatric small bowel transplant. *Pediatr. Transplant* 2013;17:765-773.

[33] Tsao L, Hsi ED: The clinicopathologic spectrum of posttransplantation lymphoproliferative disorders. *Arch. Pathol. Lab. Med.* 2007;131:1209-1218.

[34] Cohen JI: Epstein-Barr virus infection. *N. Engl. J. Med.* 2000;343:481-492.

[35] Holmes RD, Sokol RJ: Epstein-Barr virus and post-transplant lymphoproliferative disease. *Pediatr Transplant* 2002;6:456-464.

[36] Craddock J, Heslop HE: Adoptive cellular therapy with t cells specific for EBV-derived tumor antigens. *Update Cancer Ther.* 2008;3:33-41.

[37] Gottschalk S, Rooney CM, Heslop HE: Post-transplant lymphoproliferative disorders. *Annu Rev Med* 2005;56:29-44.

[38] Cohen JM, Sebire NJ, Harvey J, Gaspar HB, Cathy C, Jones A, Rao K, Cubitt D, Amrolia PJ, Davies EG, Veys P: Successful treatment of lymphoproliferative disease complicating primary immunodeficiency/immunodysregulatory disorders with reduced-intensity allogeneic stem-cell transplantation. *Blood* 2007;110:2209-2214.

[39] Brunstein CG, Weisdorf DJ, DeFor T, Barker JN, Tolar J, van Burik JA, Wagner JE: Marked increased risk of Epstein-Barr virus-related complications with the addition of antithymocyte globulin to a nonmyeloablative conditioning prior to unrelated umbilical cord blood transplantation. *Blood* 2006;108:2874-2880.

[40] Zallio F, Primon V, Tamiazzo S, Pini M, Baraldi A, Corsetti MT, Gotta F, Bertassello C, Salvi F, Rocchetti A, Levis A: Epstein-Barr virus reactivation in allogeneic stem cell transplantation is highly related to cytomegalovirus reactivation. *Clin. Transplant* 2013;27:E491-497.

[41] Caillard S, Dharnidharka V, Agodoa L, Bohen E, Abbott K: Posttransplant lymphoproliferative disorders after renal transplantation in the united states in era of modern immunosuppression. *Transplantation* 2005;80:1233-1243.

[42] Gross TG, Hinrichs SH, Winner J, Greiner TC, Kaufman SS, Sammut PH, Langnas AN: Treatment of post-transplant lymphoproliferative disease (PTLD) following solid organ transplantation with low-dose chemotherapy. *Ann. Oncol.* 1998;9:339-340.

[43] Gross TG, Hinrichs SH, Davis JR, Mitchell D, Bishop MR, Wagner JE: Depletion of EBV-infected cells in donor marrow by counterflow elutriation. *Exp. Hematol.* 1998;26:395-399.

[44] Allen UD, Preiksaitis JK: Epstein-Barr virus and posttransplant lymphoproliferative disorder in solid organ transplantation. *Am. J. Transplant* 2013;13 Suppl 4:107-120.

[45] Faull RJ, Hollett P, McDonald SP: Lymphoproliferative disease after renal transplantation in australia and new zealand. *Transplantation* 2005;80:193-197.

[46] Smith JM, Corey L, Healey PJ, Davis CL, McDonald RA: Adolescents are more likely to develop posttransplant lymphoproliferative disorder after primary Epstein-Barr virus infection than younger renal transplant recipients. *Transplantation* 2007;83:1423-1428.

[47] Lim WH, Russ GR, Coates PT: Review of Epstein-Barr virus and post-transplant lymphoproliferative disorder post-solid organ transplantation. *Nephrology* (Carlton) 2006;11:355-366.

[48] Green M, Webber S: Posttransplantation lymphoproliferative disorders. *Pediatr Clin. North Am.* 2003;50:1471-1491.

[49] Xuan L, Jiang X, Sun J, Zhang Y, Huang F, Fan Z, Guo X, Dai M, Liu C, Yu G, Zhang X, Wu M, Huang X, Liu Q: Spectrum of Epstein-Barr virus-associated diseases in recipients of allogeneic hematopoietic stem cell transplantation. *Transplantation* 2013;96:560-566.

[50] Ho M, Jaffe R, Miller G, Breinig MK, Dummer JS, Makowka L, Atchison RW, Karrer F, Nalesnik MA, Starzl TE: The frequency of Epstein-Barr virus infection and associated lymphoproliferative syndrome after transplantation and its manifestations in children. *Transplantation* 1988;45:719-727.

[51] Caillard S, Lamy FX, Quelen C, Dantal J, Lebranchu Y, Lang P, Velten M, Moulin B: Epidemiology of posttransplant lymphoproliferative disorders in adult kidney and kidney pancreas recipients: Report of the french registry and analysis of subgroups of lymphomas. *Am. J. Transplant* 2012;12:682-693.

[52] Dierickx D, Tousseyn T, Requile A, Verscuren R, Sagaert X, Morscio J, Wlodarska I, Herreman A, Kuypers D, Van Cleemput J, Nevens F, Dupont L, Uyttebroeck A, Pirenne J, De Wolf-Peeters C, Verhoef G, Brepoels L, Gheysens O: The accuracy of positron emission tomography in the detection of posttransplant lymphoproliferative disorder. *Haematologica* 2013;98:771-775.

[53] Czyzewski K, Styczynski J, Krenska A, Debski R, Zajac-Spychala O, Wachowiak J, Wysocki M: Intrathecal therapy with rituximab in central nervous system involvement of post-transplant lymphoproliferative disorder. *Leuk Lymphoma* 2013;54:503-506.

[54] Oertel SH, Verschuuren E, Reinke P, Zeidler K, Papp-Vary M, Babel N, Trappe RU, Jonas S, Hummel M, Anagnostopoulos I, Dorken B, Riess HB: Effect of anti-CD20 antibody rituximab in patients with post-transplant lymphoproliferative disorder (PTLD). *Am. J. Transplant* 2005;5:2901-2906.

[55] Choquet S, Leblond V, Herbrecht R, Socie G, Stoppa AM, Vandenberghe P, Fischer A, Morschhauser F, Salles G, Feremans W, Vilmer E, Peraldi MN, Lang P, Lebranchu Y, Oksenhendler E, Garnier JL, Lamy T, Jaccard A, Ferrant A, Offner F, Hermine O, Moreau A, Fafi-Kremer S, Morand P, Chatenoud L, Berriot-Varoqueaux N, Bergougnoux L, Milpied N: Efficacy and safety of rituximab in B-cell post-transplantation lymphoproliferative disorders: Results of a prospective multicenter Phase 2 study. *Blood* 2006;107:3053-3057.

[56] Gonzalez-Barca E, Domingo-Domenech E, Capote FJ, Gomez-Codina J, Salar A, Bailen A, Ribera JM, Lopez A, Briones J, Munoz A, Encuentra M, de Sevilla AF: Prospective phase ii trial of extended treatment with rituximab in patients with B-cell post-transplant lymphoproliferative disease. *Haematologica* 2007;92:1489-1494.

[57] Zimmermann H, Trappe RU: EBV and posttransplantation lymphoproliferative disease: What to do? *Hematology Am. Soc. Hematol. Educ. Program* 2013;2013:95-102.

[58] Lee JJ, Lam MS, Rosenberg A: Role of chemotherapy and rituximab for treatment of posttransplant lymphoproliferative disorder in solid organ transplantation. *Ann Pharmacother* 2007;41:1648-1659.

[59] Cesaro S, Murrone A, Mengoli C, Pillon M, Biasolo MA, Calore E, Tridello G, Varotto S, Alaggio R, Zanesco L, Palu G, Messina C: The real-time polymerase chain reaction-guided modulation of immunosuppression enables the pre-emptive management of Epstein-Barr virus reactivation after allogeneic haematopoietic stem cell transplantation. *Br. J. Haematol.* 2005;128:224-233.

[60] Cesaro S, Pegoraro A, Tridello G, Calore E, Pillon M, Varotto S, Abate D, Barzon L, Mengoli C, Carli M, Messina C: A prospective study on modulation of immunosuppression for Epstein-Barr virus reactivation in pediatric patients who underwent unrelated hematopoietic stem-cell transplantation. *Transplantation* 2010;89:1533-1540.

[61] Hayashi RJ, Kraus MD, Patel AL, Canter C, Cohen AH, Hmiel P, Howard T, Huddleston C, Lowell JA, Mallory G, Jr., Mendeloff E, Molleston J, Sweet S, DeBaun MR: Posttransplant lymphoproliferative disease in children: Correlation of histology to clinical behavior. *J. Pediatr Hematol. Oncol.* 2001;23:14-18.

[62] Aull MJ, Buell JF, Trofe J, First MR, Alloway RR, Hanaway MJ, Wagoner L, Gross TG, Beebe T, Woodle ES: Experience with 274 cardiac transplant recipients with posttransplant lymphoproliferative disorder: A report from the israel penn international transplant tumor registry. *Transplantation* 2004;78:1676-1682.

[63] Swinnen LJ: Durable remission after aggressive chemotherapy for post-cardiac transplant lymphoproliferation. *Leuk Lymphoma* 1997;28:89-101.

[64] Swinnen LJ, Mullen GM, Carr TJ, Costanzo MR, Fisher RI: Aggressive treatment for postcardiac transplant lymphoproliferation. *Blood* 1995;86:3333-3340.

[65] Swinnen LJ, LeBlanc M, Grogan TM, Gordon LI, Stiff PJ, Miller AM, Kasamon Y, Miller TP, Fisher RI: Prospective study of sequential reduction in immunosuppression, interferon alpha-2b, and chemotherapy for posttransplantation lymphoproliferative disorder. *Transplantation* 2008;86:215-222.

[66] Choquet S, Trappe R, Leblond V, Jager U, Davi F, Oertel S: Chop-21 for the treatment of post-transplant lymphoproliferative disorders (PTLD) following solid organ transplantation. *Haematologica* 2007;92:273-274.

[67] Knight JS, Tsodikov A, Cibrik DM, Ross CW, Kaminski MS, Blayney DW: Lymphoma after solid organ transplantation: Risk, response to therapy, and survival at a transplantation center. *J. Clin. Oncol.* 2009;27:3354-3362.

[68] Trappe R, Oertel S, Leblond V, Mollee P, Sender M, Reinke P, Neuhaus R, Lehmkuhl H, Horst HA, Salles G, Morschhauser F, Jaccard A, Lamy T, Leithauser M, Zimmermann H, Anagnostopoulos I, Raphael M, Riess H, Choquet S: Sequential treatment with rituximab followed by CHOP chemotherapy in adult B-cell post-transplant lymphoproliferative disorder (PTLD): The prospective international multicentre phase 2 PTLD-1 trial. *Lancet Oncol.* 2012;13:196-206.

[69] Dharnidharka VR, Douglas VK, Hunger SP, Fennell RS: Hodgkin's lymphoma after post-transplant lymphoproliferative disease in a renal transplant recipient. *Pediatr Transplant* 2004;8:87-90.

[70] Gross TG, Bucuvalas JC, Park JR, Greiner TC, Hinrich SH, Kaufman SS, Langnas AN, McDonald RA, Ryckman FC, Shaw BW, Sudan DL, Lynch JC: Low-dose chemotherapy for Epstein-Barr virus-positive post-transplantation lymphoproliferative disease in children after solid organ transplantation. *J. Clin. Oncol.* 2005;23:6481-6488.

[71] Twist CJ, Castillo RO: Treatment of recurrent posttransplant lymphoproliferative disorder of the central nervous system with high-dose methotrexate. *Case Rep. Transplant* 2013;2013:765230.

[72] Lucas KG, Burton RL, Zimmerman SE, Wang J, Cornetta KG, Robertson KA, Lee CH, Emanuel DJ: Semiquantitative Epstein-Barr virus (EBV) polymerase chain reaction for the determination of patients at risk for EBV-induced lymphoproliferative disease after stem cell transplantation. *Blood* 1998;91:3654-3661.

[73] Papadopoulos EB, Ladanyi M, Emanuel D, Mackinnon S, Boulad F, Carabasi MH, Castro-Malaspina H, Childs BH, Gillio AP, Small TN, et al.: Infusions of donor leukocytes to treat Epstein-Barr virus-associated lymphoproliferative disorders after allogeneic bone marrow transplantation. *N. Engl. J. Med.* 1994;330:1185-1191.

[74] Rooney CM, Smith CA, Ng CY, Loftin SK, Sixbey JW, Gan Y, Srivastava DK, Bowman LC, Krance RA, Brenner MK, Heslop HE: Infusion of cytotoxic T cells for the prevention and treatment of Epstein-Barr virus-induced lymphoma in allogeneic transplant recipients. *Blood* 1998;92:1549-1555.

[75] Bollard CM, Savoldo B, Rooney CM, Heslop HE: Adoptive T-cell therapy for EBV-associated post-transplant lymphoproliferative disease. *Acta Haematol.* 2003;110:139-148.

[76] Mathew JM, Garcia-Morales RO, Carreno M, Jin Y, Fuller L, Blomberg B, Cirocco R, Burke GW, Ciancio G, Ricordi C, Esquenazi V, Tzakis AG, Miller J: Immune responses and their regulation by donor bone marrow cells in clinical organ transplantation. *Transpl. Immunol.* 2003;11:307-321.

[77] Sherritt MA, Bharadwaj M, Burrows JM, Morrison LE, Elliott SL, Davis JE, Kear LM, Slaughter RE, Bell SC, Galbraith AJ, Khanna R, Moss DJ: Reconstitution of the latent t-lymphocyte response to Epstein-Barr virus is coincident with long-term recovery from posttransplant lymphoma after adoptive immunotherapy. *Transplantation* 2003;75:1556-1560.

[78] Savoldo B, Rooney CM, Quiros-Tejeira RE, Caldwell Y, Wagner HJ, Lee T, Finegold MJ, Dotti G, Heslop HE, Goss JA: Cellular immunity to Epstein-Barr virus in liver transplant recipients treated with rituximab for post-transplant lymphoproliferative disease. *Am. J. Transplant* 2005;5:566-572.

[79] Marty FM, Ljungman P, Papanicolaou GA, Winston DJ, Chemaly RF, Strasfeld L, Young JA, Rodriguez T, Maertens J, Schmitt M, Einsele H, Ferrant A, Lipton JH, Villano SA, Chen H, Boeckh M: Maribavir prophylaxis for prevention of cytomegalovirus disease in recipients of allogeneic stem-cell transplants: A Phase 3, double-blind, placebo-controlled, randomised trial. *Lancet Infect Dis.* 2011;11:284-292.

[80] Perrine SP, Hermine O, Small T, Suarez F, O'Reilly R, Boulad F, Fingeroth J, Askin M, Levy A, Mentzer SJ, Di Nicola M, Gianni AM, Klein C, Horwitz S, Faller DV: A phase 1/2 trial of arginine butyrate and ganciclovir in patients with Epstein-Barr virus-associated lymphoid malignancies. *Blood* 2007;109:2571-2578.

[81] Gross TG, Steinbuch M, DeFor T, Shapiro RS, McGlave P, Ramsay NK, Wagner JE, Filipovich AH: B cell lymphoproliferative disorders following hematopoietic stem cell transplantation: Risk factors, treatment and outcome. *Bone Marrow Transplant* 1999;23:251-258.

[82] Trofe J, Buell JF, Beebe TM, Hanaway MJ, First MR, Alloway RR, Gross TG, Succop P, Woodle ES: Analysis of factors that influence survival with post-transplant lymphoproliferative disorder in renal transplant recipients: The Israel Penn International Transplant Tumor Registry experience. *Am. J. Transplant* 2005;5:775-780.

[83] Rowe DT, Webber S, Schauer EM, Reyes J, Green M: Epstein-Barr virus load monitoring: Its role in the prevention and management of post-transplant lymphoproliferative disease. *Transpl. Infect Dis.* 2001;3:79-87.

[84] van Esser JW, van der Holt B, Meijer E, Niesters HG, Trenschel R, Thijsen SF, van Loon AM, Frassoni F, Bacigalupo A, Schaefer UW, Osterhaus AD, Gratama JW, Lowenberg B, Verdonck LF, Cornelissen JJ: Epstein-Barr virus (EBV) reactivation is a frequent event after allogeneic stem cell transplantation (SCT) and quantitatively predicts EBV-lymphoproliferative disease following T-cell-depleted SCT. *Blood* 2001;98:972-978.

[85] Meij P, van Esser JW, Niesters HG, van Baarle D, Miedema F, Blake N, Rickinson AB, Leiner I, Pamer E, Lowenberg B, Cornelissen JJ, Gratama JW: Impaired recovery of Epstein-Barr virus (EBV)-specific CD8+ T lymphocytes after partially T-depleted allogeneic stem cell transplantation may identify patients at very high risk for

progressive EBV reactivation and lymphoproliferative disease. *Blood* 2003;101:4290-4297.

[86] Smets F, Latinne D, Bazin H, Reding R, Otte JB, Buts JP, Sokal EM: Ratio between Epstein-Barr viral load and anti-Epstein-Barr virus specific t-cell response as a predictive marker of posttransplant lymphoproliferative disease. *Transplantation* 2002;73:1603-1610.

[87] Martin SI, Dodson B, Wheeler C, Davis J, Pesavento T, Bumgardner GL: Monitoring infection with Epstein-Barr virus among seromismatch adult renal transplant recipients. *Am. J. Transplant* 2011;11:1058-1063.

[88] Opelz G, Daniel V, Naujokat C, Fickenscher H, Dohler B: Effect of cytomegalovirus prophylaxis with immunoglobulin or with antiviral drugs on post-transplant non-hodgkin lymphoma: A multicentre retrospective analysis. *Lancet Oncol.* 2007;8:212-218.

[89] Funch DP, Walker AM, Schneider G, Ziyadeh NJ, Pescovitz MD: Ganciclovir and acyclovir reduce the risk of post-transplant lymphoproliferative disorder in renal transplant recipients. *Am. J. Transplant* 2005;5:2894-2900.

[90] Srivastava T, Zwick DL, Rothberg PG, Warady BA: Posttransplant lymphoproliferative disorder in pediatric renal transplantation. *Pediatr Nephrol.* 1999;13:748-754.

[91] Darenkov IA, Marcarelli MA, Basadonna GP, Friedman AL, Lorber KM, Howe JG, Crouch J, Bia MJ, Kliger AS, Lorber MI: Reduced incidence of Epstein-Barr virus-associated posttransplant lymphoproliferative disorder using preemptive antiviral therapy. *Transplantation* 1997;64:848-852.

[92] Malouf MA, Chhajed PN, Hopkins P, Plit M, Turner J, Glanville AR: Anti-viral prophylaxis reduces the incidence of lymphoproliferative disease in lung transplant recipients. *J. Heart Lung Transplant* 2002;21:547-554.

[93] Davis CL, Harrison KL, McVicar JP, Forg PJ, Bronner MP, Marsh CL: Antiviral prophylaxis and the Epstein Barr virus-related post-transplant lymphoproliferative disorder. *Clin. Transplant* 1995;9:53-59.

[94] Green M, Kaufmann M, Wilson J, Reyes J: Comparison of intravenous ganciclovir followed by oral acyclovir with intravenous ganciclovir alone for prevention of cytomegalovirus and Epstein-Barr virus disease after liver transplantation in children. *Clin. Infect Dis.* 1997;25:1344-1349.

[95] Leblond V, Dhedin N, Mamzer Bruneel MF, Choquet S, Hermine O, Porcher R, Nguyen Quoc S, Davi F, Charlotte F, Dorent R, Barrou B, Vernant JP, Raphael M, Levy V: Identification of prognostic factors in 61 patients with posttransplantation lymphoproliferative disorders. *J. Clin. Oncol.* 2001;19:772-778.

[96] Helgestad J, Rosthoj S, Pedersen MH, Johansen P, Iyer V, Ostergaard E, Heilmann C: Very late relapse of PTLD 10 yr after allogeneic hsct and nine yr after stopping immunosuppressive therapy. *Pediatr. Transplant* 2013.

[97] Weissmann DJ, Ferry JA, Harris NL, Louis DN, Delmonico F, Spiro I: Posttransplantation lymphoproliferative disorders in solid organ recipients are predominantly aggressive tumors of host origin. *Am. J. Clin Pathol* 1995;103:748-755.

[98] Wu TT, Swerdlow SH, Locker J, Bahler D, Randhawa P, Yunis EJ, Dickman PS, Nalesnik MA: Recurrent Epstein-Barr virus-associated lesions in organ transplant recipients. *Hum. Pathol.* 1996;27:157-164.

[99] Shapiro R, Nalesnik M, McCauley J, Fedorek S, Jordan ML, Scantlebury VP, Jain A, Vivas C, Ellis D, Lombardozzi-Lane S, Randhawa P, Johnston J, Hakala TR, Simmons RL, Fung JJ, Starzl TE: Posttransplant lymphoproliferative disorders in adult and pediatric renal transplant patients receiving tacrolimus-based immunosuppression. *Transplantation* 1999;68:1851-1854.

[100] Gross TG: Low-dose chemotherapy for children with post-transplant lymphoproliferative disease. *Recent Results Cancer Res.* 2002;159:96-103.

[101] Verschuuren EA, Stevens SJ, van Imhoff GW, Middeldorp JM, de Boer C, Koeter G, The TH, van Der Bij W: Treatment of posttransplant lymphoproliferative disease with rituximab: The remission, the relapse, and the complication. *Transplantation* 2002;73:100-104.

[102] Dotti G, Fiocchi R, Motta T, Mammana C, Gotti E, Riva S, Cornelli P, Gridelli B, Viero P, Oldani E, Ferrazzi P, Remuzzi G, Barbui T, Rambaldi A: Lymphomas occurring late after solid-organ transplantation: Influence of treatment on the clinical outcome. *Transplantation* 2002;74:1095-1102.

[103] Fridell JA, Jain A, Reyes J, Biederman R, Green M, Sindhi R, Mazariegos GV: Causes of mortality beyond 1 year after primary pediatric liver transplant under tacrolimus. *Transplantation* 2002;74:1721-1724.

[104] Bobey NA, Stewart DA, Woodman RC: Successful treatment of posttransplant lymphoproliferative disorder in a renal transplant patient by autologous peripheral blood stem cell transplantation. *Leuk Lymphoma* 2002;43:2421-2423.

[105] Wolf MT, Mildenberger E, Lennert T, Anagnostopoulos I, Zinn C, Paul K, Keitzer R, Versmold H: Pulmonary re-occurrence of post-transplant lymphoproliferative disease with hypogammaglobulinaemia. *Eur. J. Pediatr* 2003;162:180-183.

[106] Oertel SH, Papp-Vary M, Anagnostopoulos I, Hummel MW, Jonas S, Riess HB: Salvage chemotherapy for refractory or relapsed post-transplant lymphoproliferative disorder in patients after solid organ transplantation with a combination of carboplatin and etoposide. *Br. J. Haematol.* 2003;123:830-835.

[107] Al-Akash SI, Al Makadma AS, Al Omari MG: Rapid response to rituximab in a pediatric liver transplant recipient with post-transplant lymphoproliferative disease and maintenance with sirolimus monotherapy. *Pediatr Transplant* 2005;9:249-253.

[108] Bonatti H, Hoefer D, Rogatsch H, Margreiter R, Larcher C, Antretter H: Successful management of recurrent Epstein-Barr virus-associated multilocular leiomyosarcoma after cardiac transplantation. *Transplant. Proc.* 2005;37:1839-1844.

[109] Nozu K, Iijima K, Fujisawa M, Nakagawa A, Yoshikawa N, Matsuo M: Rituximab treatment for posttransplant lymphoproliferative disorder (PTLD) induces complete remission of recurrent nephrotic syndrome. *Pediatr Nephrol.* 2005;20:1660-1663.

[110] Tsai DE, Aqui NA, Tomaszewski JE, Olthoff KM, Ahya VN, Kotloff RM, Bloom RD, Brozena SC, Hodinka RL, Stadtmauer EA, Schuster SJ, Nasta SD, Porter DL, Luger SM, Klumpp TR: Serum protein electrophoresis abnormalities in adult solid organ transplant patients with post-transplant lymphoproliferative disorder. *Clin. Transplant* 2005;19:644-652.

[111] Jain AB, Marcos A, Pokharna R, Shapiro R, Fontes PA, Marsh W, Mohanka R, Fung JJ: Rituximab (chimeric anti-CD20 antibody) for posttransplant lymphoproliferative disorder after solid organ transplantation in adults: Long-term experience from a single center. *Transplantation* 2005;80:1692-1698.

[112] Flanagan KH, Brennan DC: EBV-associated recurrent hodgkin's disease after renal transplantation. *Transpl. Int.* 2006;19:338-341.

[113] Oertel S, Trappe RU, Zeidler K, Babel N, Reinke P, Hummel M, Jonas S, Papp-Vary M, Subklewe M, Dorken B, Riess H, Gartner B: Epstein-Barr viral load in whole blood of adults with posttransplant lymphoproliferative disorder after solid organ transplantation does not correlate with clinical course. *Ann. Hematol.* 2006;85:478-484.

[114] Trappe R, Riess H, Babel N, Hummel M, Lehmkuhl H, Jonas S, Anagnostopoulos I, Papp-Vary M, Reinke P, Hetzer R, Dorken B, Oertel S: Salvage chemotherapy for refractory and relapsed posttransplant lymphoproliferative disorders (PTLD) after treatment with single-agent rituximab. *Transplantation* 2007;83:912-918.

[115] Bingler MA, Feingold B, Miller SA, Quivers E, Michaels MG, Green M, Wadowsky RM, Rowe DT, Webber SA: Chronic high Epstein-Barr viral load state and risk for late-onset posttransplant lymphoproliferative disease/lymphoma in children. *Am. J. Transplant* 2008;8:442-445.

[116] Boothpur R, Brennan DC: Didactic lessons from the serum lactate dehydrogenase posttransplant: A clinical vignette. *Am. J. Transplant* 2008;8:862-865.

[117] Krishnamurthy S, Hassan A, Frater JL, Paessler ME, Kreisel FH: Pathologic and clinical features of Hodgkin lymphoma-like posttransplant lymphoproliferative disease. *Int. J. Surg. Pathol.* 2010;18:278-285.

[118] Blaes AH, Cioc AM, Froelich JW, Peterson BA, Dunitz JM: Positron emission tomography scanning in the setting of post-transplant lymphoproliferative disorders. *Clin. Transplant* 2009;23:794-799.

[119] Gupta S, Fricker FJ, Gonzalez-Peralta RP, Slayton WB, Schuler PM, Dharnidharka VR: Post-transplant lymphoproliferative disorder in children: Recent outcomes and response to dual rituximab/low-dose chemotherapy combination. *Pediatr Transplant* 2010;14:896-902.

[120] Arita H, Izumoto S, Kinoshita M, Okita Y, Hashimoto N, Fujita T, Ichimaru N, Takahara S, Yoshimine T: Posttransplant lymphoproliferative disorders of the central nervous system after kidney transplantation: Single center experience over 40 years. Two case reports. *Neurol. Med. Chir.* (Tokyo) 2010;50:1079-1083.

[121] Stravodimou A, Cairoli A, Rausch T, Du Pasquier R, Michel P: PTLD burkitt lymphoma in a patient with remote lymphomatoid granulomatosis. *Case Rep. Med.* 2012;2012:239719.

[122] Banks CA, Meier JD, Stallworth CR, White DR: Recurrent posttransplant lymphoproliferative disorder involving the larynx and trachea: Case report and review of the literature. *Ann. Otol. Rhinol. Laryngol.* 2012;121:291-295.

[123] Lo RC, Chan SC, Chan KL, Chiang AK, Lo CM, Ng IO: Post-transplant lymphoproliferative disorders in liver transplant recipients: A clinicopathological study. *J. Clin. Pathol.* 2013;66:392-398.

[124] Khedmat H, Taheri S: Ultra-early onset post-transplantation lymphoproliferative disease. *Saudi J. Kidney Dis. Transpl.* 2013;24:1144-1152.

Biographical Sketch

Jan Styczynski, MD, PhD, is affiliated with Department of Pediatric Hematology and Oncology, Collegium Medicum, Nicolaus Copernicus University, Bydgoszcz, Poland, and appointed as professor in transplantology and pediatric hematology and oncology. His main scientific interest include: viral infections in transplantology, hematology and oncology; drug resistance in hematology and oncology; hematopoietic stem cell donor issues; and differences between children and adults in transplantology, hematology and oncology. He is the Secretary of Infectious Diseases Working Party (IDWP) of European Group for Blood and Marrow Transplantation (EBMT) from 2010, and Member of ECIL (European Conference on Infections in Leukemia) group from 2007. Member of American Society of Hematology, European Group for Blood and Marrow Transplantation and several national societies. He has published 40 papers over last 3 years.

Chapter VII

T-Cell Lymphoproliferative Disorders: The Role of the Epstein-Barr Virus

Jan Styczynski[*]
Department of Pediatric Hematology and Oncology, Collegium Medicum, Nicolaus Copernicus University, Bydgoszcz, Poland

Abstract

Post-transplant lymphoproliferative disorder (PTLD) comprises a spectrum of lymphoid proliferations ranging from polyclonal expansions to overt lymphomas, occurring both after solid organ and hematopoietic stem cell transplantation. The majority of PTLDs are of B-cell origin and are associated with EBV due to decreased T-cell immune surveillance. T-cell PTLDs are less common, ranging from 4 to 15% of PTLD cases with an infrequent association with EBV. According to the WHO classification, T-PTLD is defined as a monomorphic lesion that comprises all T-cell lymphomas as well as NK (natural killer) cell lymphomas, which can be found in non-transplanted patients. Since T-cell PTLD was first described in 1987, only 225 cases have been reported up to the beginning of 2014. A summary of reported cases indicates that T-PTLD is a heterogeneous group of different aberrant T-cell proliferations and represents a significant complication following transplantation, showing a uniformly poor prognosis. Among patients with T-PTLD, kidney recipients are the most common. Organ-specific incidence, however, is the highest following a heart transplant. EBV is present in approximately one-third of T-PTLDs, with peripheral T-cell lymphoma not otherwise specified (PTCL-NOS), being the most prevalent EBV-associated T-PTLD. A male predominance is observed in the EBV-positive group, particularly in the case of peripheral T-cell lymphoma. Immunosuppression is a major risk factor for T-PTLD development, and the use of calcineurin inhibitors might play a key role in lymphomagenesis. With a median post-transplant interval of 72 months, T-cell PTLDs are among the late-occurring PTLDs. Of the most common T-PTLD, anaplastic large cell

---

[*] Address for correspondence: Department of Pediatric Hematology and Oncology; Collegium Medicum; Nicolaus Copernicus University; ul. Curie-Sklodowskiej 9; 85-094 Bydgoszcz, Poland. E-mail: jstyczynski@cm.umk.pl.

lymphoma has the best prognosis, whereas peripheral T-cell lymphoma and hepatosplenic T-cell lymphoma have the worst prognosis. EBV-positive cases seem to have a longer survival than EBV-negative cases, suggesting a different pathogenetic mechanism.

Keywords: Epstein-Barr virus; post-transplant lymphoproliferative disorder; hematopoietic stem cell transplantation; solid organ transplantation; rituximab; reduction of immunosuppression

Abbreviations

ALCL	Anaplastic large cell lymphoma
ALK	Anaplastic lymphoma kinase
ATG	Anti-thymocyte globulin
BL	Burkitt lymphoma
CBT	Cord Blood Transplantation
CD	Cluster of differentiation
CHOP	Cyclophosphamide-Adriamycin-Vincristin-Prednisone
CMV	Cytomegalovirus
CNI	Calcineurin inhibitor
CNS	Central nervous system
CR	Complete remission
CT	Computed tomography
CTL	Cytotoxic T-cell
DLBCL	Diffuse large B-cell lymphoma
DLI	Donor Lymphocytes Infusion
DNA	Deoxyribonucleic acid
EBER	Epstein-Barr Virus-encoded RNA
EBMT	European Group for Blood and Marrow Transplantation
EBNA	Epstein-Barr Virus nuclear antigen
EBV	Epstein-Barr Virus nuclear antigen
ECIL	European Conference on Infections in Leukemia
CI	Confidence interval
GVHD	Graft-versus-host-disease
HD	Hodgkin Disease
HHV	Human Herpes Virus
HL	Hodgkin lymphoma
HLA	Human Leukocyte Antigen
HSC	Hematopoietic stem cell
HSCT	Hematopoietic stem cell transplantation
HSTCL	Hepatosplenic T-cell lymphoma
IM	Infectious mononucleosis
IS	Immunosuppressive
IVIG	Intravenous immunglobulin
LPD	Lymphoproliferative disorder

MMUD	Mismatched Unrelated Donor
MMFD	Mismatched Family Donor
MFD	Matched Family Donor
MUD	Matched Unrelated Donor
NAT	Nucleic acid testing
NHL	Non-Hodgkin lymphoma
NK-cell	Natural killer cell
PBL	Plasmablastic lymphoma
PBMC	Peripheral blood mononuclear cell
PCNSL	Primary central nervous system lymphoma
PCR	Polymerase chain reaction
PET	Positron emission tomography
PID	Primary immunodeficiency
PMBCL	Primary mediastinal B-cell lymphoma
PTCL	Peripheral T-cell lymphoma
PTLD	Post-transplant lymphoproliferative disorder
RI	Reduction of immunosuppression
SOT	Solid organ transplantation
TCL	T-cell leukemia
TCR	T-cell receptor
VCA	Viral capsid antigen
VEGF	Vascular endothelial growth factor
WHO	World Health Organization

Introduction

Lymphoproliferative Disorders

Lymphoproliferative disorders (LPD) refer to the clonal expansion of lymphatic system cells, classified according to the WHO system [1]. The following diseases can be regarded as examples of lymphoproliferative disorders: acute lymphoblastic leukemia, chronic lymphocytic leukemia, lymphomas, multiple myeloma, Waldenstrom's macroglobulinemia, Wiskott-Aldrich syndrome, autoimmune lymphoproliferative syndrome (ALPS), or post-transplant lymphoproliferative disorder.

Clinical Syndromes Associated with Epstein-Barr Virus Infection

The Epstein-Barr virus (EBV) is a widespread human herpesvirus infecting B-lymphocytes and also capable of infecting T cells and epithelial cells [2-4]. EBV was the first human virus implicated in oncogenesis and is associated with a heterogeneous group of malignant diseases.

Table 1. Clinical syndromes associated with EBV infection

Clinical syndromes associated with EBV infection
Primary syndromes [5-8]: 　1) Infectious mononucleosis 　2) Chronic active EBV infection 　3) X-linked lymphoproliferative syndrome EBV-associated tumors (reactivation syndromes): 　4) Lymphoproliferative disorders (LPD) in immunocompromised patients 　5) Burkitts lymphoma / NHL [9] 　6) Naso-pharyngeal carcinoma 　7) NK-cell leukemia/lymphoma [10] 　8) Hodgkin Disease (*de novo or after allo-HSCT*) [11] 　9) Hemophagocytic lymphohistiocytosis 　10) Angioimmunoblastic T-cell lymphoma [12] EBV-associated post-transplant diseases: 　11) Encephalitis / myelitis 　12) Pneumonia 　13) Hepatitis

EBV, Epstein-Barr virus; NHL, non-Hodgkin lymphoma; NK, natural killer; HSCT, hematopoietic stem cell transplantation.

The role of EBV in contributing to lymphomagenesis is especially well established in those lymphoproliferative diseases that arise in immunosuppressed individuals. EBV can give rise to both lytic and latent infections, and may cause a number of clinical syndromes and conditions (Table 1).

EBV-associated lymphoproliferative diseases (LPD) encompass a vast spectrum from reactive to neoplastic processes in the transformation and proliferation of lymphocytes spanning B, T, and NK cells, and are clinically complicated by the interaction between the biological properties of EBV-positive lymphocytes and the host immune status [13].

EBV-associated T- and NK-cell LPD (T/NK-LPD) was first incorporated into the 4th World Health Organization (WHO) classification of tumors of hematopoietic and lymphoid tissues, in which systemic EBV T-cell LPD of childhood and hydroa vacciniforme-like lymphoma are proposed as distinct entities [1, 14].

Based on their broad clinical manifestations, T-cell LPD have been described under various nosological terms, ranging from indolent (e.g., severe mosquito bite allergy and hydroa vacciniforme) to aggressive or fulminant forms (e.g., EBV-associated hemophagocytic lymphohistiocytosis (HLH), chronic active EBV disease (CAEBV) of the T/NK-cell type, fulminant EBV+ T-cell LPD of childhood, and fatal infectious mononucleosis) [13, 15-20].

Current understanding of these diseases is now evolving and has led to the recognition of a variety of EBV diseases, including B-cell LPD, T/NK-cell lymphoma, Burkitt lymphoma, classical Hodgkin lymphoma, aggressive NK-cell leukemia, and immunodeficiency-associated lymphoproliferative disorders such as post-transplant lymphoproliferative disease (PTLD).

T-LPD

Definition of EBV-Positive T-LPD

EBV-associated T/NK-cell lymphoproliferative disease (T/NK-LPD) is a systemic illness characterized by monoclonal proliferation of EBV-infected T or NK cells. Systemic EBV-positive T-cell LPD can be defined based on the following eligibility criteria: (1) illness or symptoms including fever, persistent hepatitis, lymphadenopathy, hepatosplenomegaly, hemophagocytosis, and interstitial pneumonia; (2) can occur shortly after primary EBV infection or in the setting of CAEBV; (3) monoclonal expansion of EBV-infected T cells with an activated cytotoxic phenotype in tissues or peripheral blood. This definition also includes the following exclusion criteria: other instances of overt leukemia and lymphoma, such as extranodal NK/T-cell lymphoma, aggressive NK-cell leukemia, and peripheral T-cell lymphoma [13]. According to the 2008 WHO classification, systemic T-cell LPD corresponds to the polymorphic and monomorphic groups of CAEBV infection [20]. With respect to their incidence, EBV-associated T/NK-cell lymphoproliferative disorders can be classified as frequent or rare.

Table 2. T-NK-cell lymphoproliferative diseases

Subtypes and classification			Diseases
T cell (lymphoma, leukemia) (CD3, CD4, CD8)	By development/marker		TdT+: ALL (Precursor T acute lymphoblastic leukemia/lymphoma), Prolymphocyte (Prolymphocytic)
			CD30+: Anaplastic large-cell lymphoma, Lymphomatoid papulosis type A
	Cutaneous	Mycosis fungoides +variants	Indolent: Mycosis fungoides, Pagetoid reticulosis, Granulomatous slack skin
			Aggressive: Sézary's disease, Adult T-cell leukemia/lymphoma
		Non-Mycosis fungoides	CD30-: Non-mycosis fungoides CD30− cutaneous large T-cell lymphoma, Pleomorphic T-cell lymphoma, Lymphomatoid papulosis type B
			CD30+: CD30+ cutaneous T-cell lymphoma
			Secondary cutaneous CD30+ large cell lymphoma, Lymphomatoid papulosis type A
	Other peripheral		Hepatosplenic, Angioimmunoblastic, Enteropathy-associated T-cell lymphoma, Peripheral T-cell lymphoma-not-otherwise-specified PTCL-NOS (Lennert lymphoma), Subcutaneous T-cell lymphoma
	By infection		HTLV-1 (human T-cell leukemia/lymphoma virus): Adult T-cell leukemia/lymphoma
NK cell/(mostly CD56)			Aggressive NK-cell leukemia, Blastic NK cell lymphoma
T or NK			EBV: Extranodal NK-T-cell lymphoma/Angiocentric lymphoma, Large granular lymphocytic leukemia

Adapted from: http://en.wikipedia.org/wiki/T-cell_lymphoma.

Frequent EBV-T/NK-LPD include: peripheral T-cell lymphoma not otherwise specified (PTCL NOS), angioimmunoblastic T-cell lymphoma, and extranodal nasal T/NK-cell lymphoma. Rare EBV-T/NK-LPD include: hepatosplenic T-cell lymphoma, nonhepatosplenic γδ-T-cell lymphoma, and enteropathy-type T-cell lymphoma [21] (Table 2).

EBV-Associated T/NK-LPD in Non-Immunocompromised Patients

In the analysis of 108 non-immunocompromised patients with EBV-positive T/NK-cell LPD (50 men and 58 women; median onset age: 8 years; age range: 1-50 years) evidenced by expansion of EBV+ T/NK cells in the peripheral blood, the T-cell type was diagnosed in 64 cases and the NK-cell type in 44 cases. EBV-infected cells in EBV+ T/NK-LPDs were immunophenotypically divided into CD4+ T cells, CD8+ T cells, γδ T cells, and NK cells, the variable proportions of which were observed in each of the clinical categories. Clinically, the patients were categorized into 4 groups: 80 cases of chronic active EBV disease, 15 of EBV-associated hemophagocytic lymphohistiocytosis, 9 of severe mosquito bite allergy, and 4 of hydroa vacciniforme. These clinical profiles were closely linked with the EBV-positive cell immunophenotypes. In a median follow-up period of 46 months, 47 patients (44%) died of severe organ-related complications. During the follow-up, 13 patients developed overt lymphoma or leukemia characterized by extranodal T/NK-cell lymphoma and aggressive NK-cell leukemia. 59 patients received hematopoietic stem cell transplantation, 66% of whom survived. Age >8 years at the onset of disease and liver dysfunction constituted risk factors for mortality, whereas patients who received transplantation had a better prognosis [13].

Systemic EBV-Positive T-Cell LPD in Children

Systemic Epstein-Barr virus (EBV)-positive T-cell lymphoproliferative disease (LPD) of childhood without an immunocompromised status is an extremely rare and distinct clinicopathological entity. The majority of such cases occur with an apparent primary EBV infection. Laboratory examinations present a markedly elevated white blood cell count and liver and renal function tests. Peripheral blood smears identify atypical lymphocytes with small azurophilic granules in the cytoplasm. Bone marrow aspiration reveals marked proliferation of small-sized lymphocytes with convoluted nuclei, which express EBER1, CD3, CD8 and cytotoxic granules. Monoclonal rearrangements of T-cell receptors can also be detected. So far, only 17 cases of this disease have been reported in children. The major clinicopathological features of systemic EBV-positive T-cell LPD of childhood are as follows: (a) clonal systemic proliferation of EBV-infected T-cells that appear morphologically innocuous with an activated cytotoxic phenotype; (b) a high prevalence in the Asian population, commonly affecting children and young adults; (c) a predilection for males; (d) the most commonly involved sites are the liver, spleen, lymph node and bone marrow, and the main clinical presentations are hepatosplenomegaly, fever and pancytopenia; (e) almost all cases have an aggressive clinical course, which results in high mortality. Cytological atypia of neoplastic cells in the peripheral blood in this disease is minimal, and thus the cytomorphological features of atypical lymphocytes are practically indistinguishable from those of infectious mononucleosis [22].

Chronic Active EBV (CAEBV) Infection

EBV-associated hemophagocytic lymphohistiocytosis (HLH), EBV-positive systemic T-cell lymphoproliferative disease (STLPD) of childhood, and chronic active EBV (CAEBV) infection may all develop after primary EBV infection. EBV-positive HLH and STLPD share similar clinicopathological findings and may constitute a continuous spectrum of acute EBV-associated T- or NK-cell proliferative disorders. The distinction of EBV-positive T-cell LPD from EBV-positive HLH may be difficult during routine diagnoses because of the technical limitations of clonality assessment [20]. CAEBV infection can be defined as: (1) persistent or recurrent symptoms related to EBV infection, lasting for more than three months; (2) high EBV genome levels in the affected tissues or peripheral blood; (3) a chronic illness that could not be explained by other known disease processes at diagnosis, and (4) no specific underlying immunological abnormality [23]. CAEBV infection is synonymous with chronic symptomatic EBV infection, and is almost always accompanied by varying degrees of lymphoproliferation. In the Asian population, CAEBV infection mainly involves T- or NK-cells. The EBV-infected T- or NK-cells may be polyclonal, oligoclonal, or monoclonal. As the disease progresses from a polyclonal lymphoproliferation to a monoclonal disease, histological atypia increases [20, 24]. EBV-positive cytotoxic T-cell lymphoma (EBV+ CTL) may develop during the clinical course of chronic active EBV-associated T/NK-cell lymphoproliferative disorder (CAEBV/TNK-LPD), despite multiagent chemotherapy and allogeneic stem cell transplantation. The immunophenotype of the EBV+ CTL is consistently a CD3/CD8 [25]. In Japan, T/NK-cell LPD may develop in patients treated for rheumatoid arthritis. Immunosuppressive treatment with the use of methotrexate is a risk factor for the development of T/NK-cell LPD, regardless of EBV status [26].

In terms of patient management, the clinician may use chemotherapy as the initial treatment when the patient is diagnosed with systemic T-cell LPD; however, in patients with EBV-positive HLH, the clinical selection of a therapeutic modality depends on the risk factors for EBV-positive HLH, which are as follows: a persistently high EBV genome copy number in the serum, an acute fulminant or CAEBV infection, an abnormal karyotype, and an association with hereditary disease [20,27,28]. Currently, successful therapies, such as conservative or mild treatments without etoposide, more aggressive therapies with etoposide, and very aggressive lifesaving measures, including hematopoietic stem cell transplantation, are administered to HLH patients, providing a survival rate greater than 75% [18, 29, 30].

T-PTLD

Post-Transplant Lymphoproliferative Disorder

Post-transplant lymphoproliferative disorders (PTLD) are broadly defined as a heterogeneous group of lymphoproliferative diseases that occur in the setting of acquired immune deficiency following allogeneic transplantation of either solid organs (SOT) or hematopoietic stem cells (HSCT). The incidence of lymphoproliferative disorders in transplant recipients is 30-50 times higher than in the general population and ranges from 2 to 10% [31]. PTLD comprises a spectrum of lymphoid proliferations ranging from polyclonal expansions to overt lymphomas [32]. In contrast to more than 90% of adult patients who are latently EBV-positive, pediatric and juvenile patients are more often EBV naive before transplantation and have their primary infection under immunosuppressive therapy, which puts them at a higher risk for PTLD manifestation [33-35]. The majority of PTLDs are of B-cell origin and are associated with EBV due to decreased T-cell immune surveillance (Figure 1).

PTLDs therefore refer to a spectrum of lymphoproliferative disorders which are associated with EBV reactivation in 60-70% of cases ranging from benign hyperplasia to life-threatening aggressive lymphomas [36, 37]. The clinical presentation of PTLD varies considerably and can be either disseminated or localized. Involvement is frequently extranodal and includes the transplanted organ itself and sanctuary sites such as the central nervous system [36, 38]. Morphologically, PTLDs can be subdivided into monomorphic, polymorphic, plasmacytic, or HL-like variants. There are two main types of high-grade lymphomas among monomorphic B-PTLDs: diffuse large B-cell lymphoma and Burkitt's lymphoma. On the other hand, in spite of lower frequency, T-PTLD manifest in a variety of aberrant T-cell proliferations. Most of B-PTLD is associated with EBV: over 90% in HSCT patients and over 70% in the SOT setting [4, 39-41].

T-cell or natural killer (NK)-cell post-transplant lymphoproliferative disorder (T/NK-PTLD) is a less common but severe complication after transplantation. T-cell PTLDs are ranging from 4% to 15% of all PTLD cases with an infrequent association with EBV [42]. Their incidence is more commonly reported in Asia; it may be as high as 40% in the Far East, probably due to the presence of human T-cell leukemia virus (HTLV-1) [31, 43]. Since T-cell PTLD was first described in 1987, up to the beginning of 2014 only 225 cases have been reported [32, 33, 42, 44-159]; they were mostly single case reports. In previously published papers, 130-163 cases in total were reviewed in detail by Swerdlow et al [160], Tiede et al [33], and Herreman et al [31].

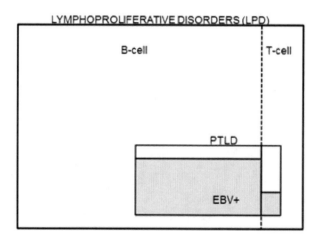

Figure 1. Relation between lymphoproliferative disorders (LPD) and posttransplant lymphoproliferative disorders (PTLD).

T-PTLD is defined as a monomorphic lesion that comprises all T-cell lymphomas as well as natural killer cell lymphomas, which can be found in non-transplanted patients [1]. Polymorphic T-PTLDs are usually excluded from this definition [1,161,162]. T cells do not usually express EBV receptor CD21; therefore, in most cases, the pathogenesis of monomorphic T-PTLD might not be based on an EBV infection alone [34,35]. T-cell PTLDs include a broad morphological spectrum of lesions, ranging from indolent oligoclonal expansions of T-cells (large granular lymphocytes) to aggressive T-cell lymphomas, consisting of intermediate to large-sized lymphoid cells.

Pathology

In non-transplanted immunocompetent patients, high-grade lymphomas are more frequently of B rather than of T lineage, indicating a different predisposition of these two lymphocytic differentiations to generate an aberrant clonal proliferation [33]. Also, primary immune disorders are frequently associated with EBV-positive B-cell lymphomas but rarely so with T-cell lymphomas [1]. A similar relationship is observed in PTLD [31,33].

The T-cell PTLDs are morphologically and immunophenotypically heterogeneous. The most frequent diagnoses include peripheral T-cell lymphoma not otherwise specified (PTCL, NOS) (19%), hepatosplenic T-cell lymphoma (HSTCL) (12%), and anaplastic large cell lymphoma (ALCL) (12%) - either ALK(+), ALK(-), systemic or primary cutaneous ALCL [31]. Other T-PTLD phenotypes include cutaneous T-cell lymphoma (CTCL; including mycosis fungoides, Sézary syndrome, and subcutaneous panniculitis-like T-cell lymphoma), adult T-cell leukemia/lymphoma (ATL), T-cell large granular lymphocytic leukemia (LGL), PTLD with NK (natural killer) cell phenotype, and T-PTLD with manifestation in the central nervous system [1].

Gene expression profiling indicated that the molecular basis of monomorphic PTLD is partially different from that of sporadic malignant lymphomas [163]. Furthermore, a transcriptosome analysis of PTCL-NOS and DLBCL patients has identified a molecular tumor signature profile that distinguishes these lymphomas [164]. Differences between PTLD and sporadic lymphomas defined by immunophenotype might be caused by many factors, such as viral infections, patient age, previous therapy, and immunosuppression.

Frequency of T-PTLD

The frequency of T-PTLD among all monomorphic PTLDs in a large single-center analysis was reported to be 5% (6 out of 117) [33]. A summary of published case reports indicate that T-PTLD occurs in patients of all ages, with known cases ranging from 1 to 83 years, and a median age of 44 years at diagnosis [31]. Approximately half of the identified T-PTLDs with known immunophenotype was either CD4+ (53%) or CD8+ (47%) [33].

With respect to the organ transplanted, most of the patients who developed T-cell PTLD had undergone a kidney transplant including two cases with additional pancreas transplantation (63%), followed by heart or heart and lung transplant including one patient who received a liver transplant 4 months after heart transplantation (19%), then liver (9%), hematopoietic or peripheral blood stem cell (7%), lung (1%) and multivisceral transplant (<1%) [31, 33].

This frequency is the obvious consequence of the fact that kidney transplantation is performed more often than any other organ transplantation. The same highest incidence is observed among B-PTLD patients. Interestingly, because of the large number of donor periportal lymphocytes, liver transplants are regarded to be more often associated with donor-derived PTLDs, mainly of polymorphic nature, while monomorphic B-PTLDs are more likely to be recipient-derived [33, 165, 166].

It is estimated that among kidney transplant recipients, children are at a higher risk for developing a PTLD because they are more frequently EBV-naive at the time of transplantation [34]. This is not the case with pediatric HSCT recipients [167]. Pediatric T-cell PTLD cases are very rare, and only 21 cases have been previously described in the literature [52]. Recent reviews of a large number of cases showed the rarity of T-PTLD in pediatric patients, as only 13% of pediatric/juvenile T-PTLDs were identified [31, 33]. Pediatric patients were diagnosed for PTCL, NOS (12 cases reported), ALCL (7 cases reported), and CTCL (2 cases reported) [33]. Both in B-PTLD and T-PTLD, young age was associated with a better survival [31, 33, 167].

T-PTLD after Hematopoietic Stem Cell Transplantation

T-PTLD is extremely rare after hematopoietic stem cell transplantation (HSCT), with 9 cases having been reported so far in the literature. Known T-PTLD cases comprised HSCT with bone marrow-derived cells in 6 cases, autologous HSCT with peripheral blood-derived cells in 2 cases, and HSCT with peripheral blood-derived cells after failed bone marrow transplantation in one patient [33, 53-58]. Hematopoietic stem cell transplantation was associated with early-onset T-PTLD, whereas late onset occurred after immunosuppression with steroids and azathioprine without the administration of calcineurin inhibitors [33]. In the hematopoietic stem cell transplantation setting, PTLD develops early in most cases, regardless of the immunophenotype. HSCT can thus be regarded as a predisposing risk factor for the development of early-onset T-PTLD, in comparison to SOT recipients.

Continuous immunosuppression is a risk factor for the development of late PTLD. As it normally does not apply to hematopoietic stem cell recipients, because immunosuppressive medication is usually withdrawn, T-PTLD cases are, in general, not found among HSCT patients. In this patient population, immunocompetence normalizes over time, in contrast to SOT recipients, who are at a risk for late PTLD, frequently EBV-negative.

PTLD is almost always of recipient origin following SOT, whereas it is almost exclusively donor-derived following HSCT. In contrast to SOT, cases of PTLD after allogeneic HSCT are almost exclusively of donor origin, since recipient lymphopoiesis is thought to be greatly diminished if not ablated by the conditioning regimen [168]. There are several cases described in literature, where PTLD after HSCT was recipient-derived [53,168-170]. PTLD in these cases was usually preceded by an autologous bone marrow reconstitution or mixed chimerism and developed late after transplantation (5-49 months). An unusual development of recipient-derived PTLD was the appearance of a B-cell clone during consolidation chemotherapy for T-cell leukemia, several months before stem cell transplantation [168].

Clinical Symptoms and Diagnosis of PTLD

T-cell PTLDs usually involve extranodal sites (93%). The most commonly reported extranodal sites include bone or bone marrow (25% and 56%, respectively), skin (24%), liver (24%), spleen (20%), lung or pleura (14%), peripheral blood (14%) and gastrointestinal tract (13%). Rarely, the brain, kidney, heart, pericardium, nose and pharynx can be affected. Graft involvement after solid organ transplantation was observed in 13% of cases [31].

The diagnosis of PTLD should be based on a biopsy with an analysis performed using histopathological criteria [1], based on immunohistochemical stainings, Epstein-Barr virus-encoded RNA (EBER) in situ hybridization and TCR $\alpha\beta\gamma\delta$ receptor analysis by PCR. Cases should be defined as EBV-positive if EBER is expressed in all tumor cells in which RNA is preserved.

In comparison to B-cell PTLDs, T-PTLD usually develops later following transplant. The median interval from transplant to diagnosis of T-PTLD was 72 months (range: 1-324 months) compared to 48 months (range 1-425 months) for all PTLD cases [171]. 90% of the patients with T-PTLD presented with disease onset later than 12 months after transplant, compared to 65% of monomorphic B-cell PTLD cases [171].

EBV-Positive T-PTLD

Approximately 72% of monomorphic B-cell PTLDs, and only 34-36.5% of T-cell PTLDs, are EBV-related, with peripheral T-cell lymphoma not otherwise specified (PTCL, NOS) being the most prevalent EBV-associated T-cell PTLD [31, 41]. A male predominance is observed, which is most striking in the EBV-positive group, particularly in PTCL, NOS. With a median post-transplant interval of 72 months, T-cell PTLDs are among the late-occurring PTLDs [31, 41].

The question arises of why in some cases EBV is responsible for the development of T-PTLD. In B-cell PTLD, EBV infects B-lymphocytes via CD21 followed by the expression of viral and cellular proteins and the induction of uncontrolled proliferation; this process might be facilitated by the lack of cytotoxic T-cells in immunosuppressed patients [7]. It has been suggested that a subset of T-cells may also express CD21 and can be infected by EBV [31, 172]. Alternatively, unidentified receptors may mediate EBV infection of T-cells. Magro et al suggested that a limited number of EBV-infected B cells could induce an excessive T-cell immune response as a result of the iatrogenic aberrations in T-cell regulatory function [31, 51]. Immunosuppressive drugs play a role in attenuating the regulatory T-cell population by controlling the emerging T-cell clones. A clonally restricted T-cell population may then undergo stepwise neoplastic transformation [31, 51].

EBV is most strongly associated with extranodal natural killer NK/T-cell lymphomas, nasal type (100% EBV+) and PTCL, NOS (39% EBV+), whereas cases of precursor T-lymphoblastic leukemia/lymphoma and T-cell large granular lymphocytic leukemia are EBV-negative, and so are most HSTCLs [31, 33].

The comparison of EBV-positive and EBV-negative T-PTLD cases revealed no significant difference regarding the time between transplantation and onset, thus contradicting the general assumption that EBV-negative PTLD arises later following transplant than EBV-positive PTLD [31, 41, 173]. The age of onset of EBV-negative and EBV-positive T-cell

PTLD was also similar in both groups (median 46 and 43 years, respectively). A notable difference, however, was the male/female ratio, which was very high in the EBV-positive group (13.3:1), compared to the EBV-negative group (3.2:1). Importantly, EBV-positive cases seemed significantly associated with longer median overall survival than EBV-negative cases (11 months vs. 6 months) [31].

Apart from EBV, several other viruses were associated with T-PTLD, including cytomegalovirus (CMV), human T-cell leukemia virus (HTLV), and human herpes virus-6 (HHV-6). The only T-PTLD subtype that was associated with a particular virus was adult T-cell leukemia/lymphoma (ATL). HTLV was positive (mainly seropositive) in seven out of eight ATL-PTLD cases; however, this virus was not systematically tested in most other cases [33].

Risk Factors for T-PTLD Development

The common rule that PTLD develops earlier after HSCT than after SOT is also confirmed in case of T-PTLD. The earliest T-PTLD manifestation (early-onset PTLD <12 months) was found after HSCT (median: 5 months; range: 2-43 months), which was significantly earlier than after kidney (1-324 months), heart (9-168 months), or liver (2-180 months) transplantation. Age less than 18 years or age more than 60 years were not recognized as risk factors [33].

Upon a retrospective evaluation of immunosuppressive drugs/drug combinations for T-PTLD manifestation, it was found that T-PTLD developed significantly earlier in patients who were treated with tacrolimus (alone or with other drugs) than in those patients who received azathioprine therapy (alone or with other drugs) [33]. These observations, based on reports compiled over 30 years, might not be applicable nowadays, since many new immunosuppressive compounds and regimens are currently in use, and old data may be out of value.

Therapy of T-PTLD

The overall recommendations for first-line treatment of B-cell PTLD are as follows: (i) anti-proliferative therapy with the use of anti-CD20 antibodies; (ii) reduction of immunosuppressive therapy, if possible; (iii) adoptive immunotherapy with in vitro-generated donor EBV cytotoxic T-cells, or an infusion of donor lymphocytes (DLI) to restore T-cell reactivity. The use of anti-CD20 monoclonal antibodies is generally recommended for both pre-emptive and symptomatic therapy , and this in spite of the lack of randomized trials in the HSCT setting. In the "era of rituximab", this is a recommendation of the highest priority, while other options should be taken into account when available or as a second-line therapy. The use of EBV-specific CTLs has been shown to be safe and efficacious in the HSCT setting, both prophylactically and in the treatment of established PTLD; however, there are disadvantages to this approach, related mainly to the availability of this product.

In general, therapy of T-PTLD varies from that of B-PTLD. Therapy regimens for T-PTLD were variable among cases reported over recent 30 years, as reviewed by Tiede et al [33]. Since most of the patients were after solid organ transplantation, therapy regimens were mainly based on reduction of immunosuppressive therapy, radiotherapy or chemotherapy, and corticosteroid administration. Combined therapy was often used and alterations to treatment protocols were frequent. Reduction of immunosuppression was the most often used approach, followed by chemotherapy and radiochemotherapy. Among patients treated solely with reduced immunosuppression with no additional therapy, 60% were alive after a median of 13 months. Chemotherapy alone was less efficient than other therapeutic strategies, and increased toxicities were observed after chemotherapy. Those reported patients who received no therapy due to their refusal or rapid progression of the disease, died due to disease progression or complications within a median of 3 weeks [33].

Treatment of all PTLDs after SOT involves reduction of immunosuppression (RI) to allow for the proliferation of cytotoxic T-cells if feasible, but durable remissions are uncommon with this approach alone and it inherently entails the risk of graft rejection. Localized disease may respond durably to surgical resection alone. Rituximab alone is not as effective in treating EBV+ lymphomas as in preventing its occurrence, but it can elicit responses in 35-70% of patients who fail to respond to reduction of immunosuppression alone [174]. For patients showing aggressive features at diagnosis, combination chemotherapy regimens such as R-CHOP (rituximab combined with cyclophosphamide, adiamycin, vincrictine, prednisolone) are commonly used with varying success. Response can be achieved in many patients, but treatment-related mortality has been reported to be as high as 50% due to frequent infectious complications [36,174]. PTLDs classically display type III latency patterns and immunotherapeutic strategies that generate EBV-specific T-cells have shown significant promise [37].

Reduction of immunosuppression is usually the first measure implemented in the SOT setting if PTLD occurs. This approach has shown benefit also in T-PTLD patients (mostly after SOT), as most patients with reduced immunosuppression survived [31, 33]. This is in contrast to B-PTLD cases, where monoclonal antibody treatment has recently become a well-tolerated standard of care [167, 175, 176], T-PTLD usually requires intensive chemotherapy and radiotherapy treatment. It seems that patients with T-PTLD may benefit from the addition of radiotherapy to chemotherapy and, similarly to B-PTLD, reduction of immunosuppression [33].

Therapeutically, reduction of immunosuppression remains a mainstay, and recent data have documented the importance of rituximab +/- combination chemotherapy. Therapy for primary CNS PTLD should be managed according to immunocompetent CNS paradigms. Finally, novel treatment strategies for PTLD have emerged, including adoptive immunotherapy and rational targeted therapeutics (e.g., anti-CD30 based therapy and downstream signaling pathways of latent membrane protein-2A) [41]. A successful therapy with bexarotene, a novel synthetic retinoid analog in the treatment of a combined kidney and pancreas transplant patient with Epstein-Barr virus (EBV) positive T-cell PTLD, has also been reported [88].

Donor lymphocyte infusion is an alternative treatment for EBV-associated LPDs. Owing to the fetal-maternal microchimerism tolerance, maternal lymphocyte infusion may possibly be effective without causing GVHD. In the study of 5 children with non-transplant-associated, EBV-positive T-cell LPD, requiring cytotherapy or hematopoietic stem cell transplantation, high doses of human leukocyte antigen-haploidentical maternal peripheral blood mononuclear cells ($>10^8$/kg/infusion) were infused 1-4 times. Symptoms of all 5 patients improved between 3 and 10 days after the infusion; thereafter, 3 cases showed complete remission for 6-18 months without further therapy and 2 had partial remission. During the period of observation, none of the patients developed obvious GVHD. The quantitative PCR analysis showed that in some patients maternal cells were eliminated or decreased after infusions, indicating the occurrence of the host-versus-graft reaction. This implies that high doses of mother's lymphocyte infusion may be an effective and safe treatment for non-transplant-associated EBV-positive T-cell LPD [177].

Survival and Prognostic Factors

In general, the overall survival is better in B-PTLD than in T-PTLD; it is better in EBV-positive cases than in EBV-negative ones; it is better in children than in adults. In the summary of reported cases, the median overall survival of all patients with T-PTLD was 6 months, ranging from 0 to 123 months, compared to 11 months in the case of monomorphic B-cell PTLD [171].

Pediatric patients had a significantly better overall survival than adult patients. The exception pertained to the LGL type, with 6 out of 7 adult patients remaining alive in the follow-up period of 4-36 months, median 18 months. All patients with LGL-PTLD were adults (median age: 48 years; range: 36-70 years); while none of the pediatric or juvenile patients had an LGL-PTLD [33].

Taking the immunophenotype into account, patients with CD4+ or CD8+ T-PTLD had a similar survival. On the other hand, hepatosplenic T-cell lymphoma (HSTCL-type) PTLD had an adverse prognosis and showed a significantly lower overall survival versus CTCL and LGL. All 19 reported patients died during the follow-up period, with 4 months median survival (range, 0.5-12 months). Infiltration of the central nervous system, bone marrow (in non HSCT patients), and graft (including HSCT patients) was associated with a poor prognosis [33]. The analyses of risk factors for overall survival have shown that major favorable prognostic factors were T-PTLD of the large granular lymphocytic leukemia subtype, anaplastic large cell lymphoma (ALCL), young age, and a combination of radiotherapy or radiochemotherapy and reduced immunosuppression. By contrast, PTCL-NOS, the hepatosplenic T-cell lymphoma subtype and cases with the involvement of bone marrow, the central nervous system, or graft had an adverse prognosis [31, 33].

Composite B-Cell and T-Cell Lineage PTLD

Post-transplant lymphoproliferative disorders harboring both B- and T-cell clones either concurrently or successively in the same patient are extremely rare and only a few cases have been reported in the literature so far [32, 51, 122, 155, 178-184]. EBV plays an important role in driving the proliferation. The lack of immune surveillance plays a major part in the proliferation of unchecked EBV-infected B cells as regards the pathogenesis of post-transplant lymphoproliferative disorders, with a subsequent development of B-cell lymphoproliferation [185]. The lack of immune surveillance possibly also affects T cells, which can lead to the subsequent emergence of T-cell clones [186].

In the analysis of B-cell PTLD samples for B- and T-cell clonality, T-cell subsets and EBV association, 50% of B-cell PTLDs showed evidence of monoclonal T-cell expansion, and among the T cells present in the tissue samples, CD8-positive cells predominated. B-cell PTLDs with the presence of a monoclonal T-cell population had a CD4:CD8 ratio of ≤0.4. There was no association between EBV and the presence of T-cell clones. T-cell clones were not identified in lymphomas other than B-cell PTLDs. Among 53.8% of the tested cases of EBV-positive B-cell PTLD with associated clonal expansion of T-cells, none had EBV-positive T cells. Thus, half of B-cell post-transplant lymphoproliferative disorders are associated with the clonal expansion of CD8-positive T cells, most of which do not amount to the coexistence of a T-PTLD [186].

An unusual composite B-cell and T-cell lineage PTLD of the lung with cutaneous manifestations of mycosis fungoides has been described in a 17-year-old male kidney transplant recipient who presented initially with dermatological symptoms and was found to have histological changes in the skin that were consistent with mycosis fungoides. Shortly after that diagnosis was made, imaging studies demonstrated EBV-negative monomorphic T-cell PTLD with a concomitant EBV-positive B-cell PTLD involving the same lesion of the lung. PCR analysis demonstrated clonal T-cell receptor gene rearrangements in both skin and lung biopsies. One clone was shared between the skin and the lung while a second clone was present only in the lung [155].

Another unique "composite" PTLD with two distinct components developing as a duodenal mass seventeen years after a combined kidney-pancreas transplant has been reported [32]. This PTLD consisted of two components, one of which was CD20 positive and EBV-negative monomorphic diffuse large B-cell lymphoma (DLBCL). The other component showed anaplastic morphology (ALCL), expressed some but not all T-cell markers, failed to express most B-cell markers except for PAX5, and was diffusely EBV-positive. This case is unique in a number of respects. These include the very lengthy period after transplant (17 years) before PTLD occurrence, the location (duodenum), and the apparently dichotomous components harboring EBV in an unexpected pattern, positive in the anaplastic "T-cell-like" cells and negative in the B-cell elements.

The analysis of cases reported in the literature that involved both B and T lineage either concurrently or successively shows that the duration of interval between organ transplant and the development of PTLD ranged from 42 days to 17 years [32, 155, 179-182]. The involved sites included the lymph node, skin, bone marrow, duodenum and spleen. In one case, the peripheral blood contained clonal proliferations of both B and T cells after bone marrow transplant [182]. Three cases developed T- and B-PTLD at different sites after either liver or kidney transplant [179-181]. In one case, a renal transplant recipient developed a cutaneous T-cell PTLD, followed by an EBV-associated PTLD with both B- and T-cell components [122].

Conclusion

PTLD is a heterogeneous disease; it may occur early, within the first year post-transplant, with the highest occurrence during the first 6 months after HSCT, or late, even up to 10 years after solid organ transplantation. Nearly 30% of the late-onset cases exhibit the biological pattern of EBV-negative malignant lymphoma, casting doubt on their correlation with EBV infection. Early-onset PTLDs are usually EBV-positive, histologically heterogeneous, including most polyclonal mononucleosis-like forms, and are associated with higher levels of EBV DNA copies in the peripheral blood [4]. EBV infection and transformation into B-PTLD is usually an early event after transplantation, occurring mostly within the first 12 months. By contrast, T-PTLD is usually EBV-negative and the relatively long latency between transplantation and T-PTLD onset may be explained by molecular events. T-cell PTLDs are less common, ranging from 4 to 15% of PTLD cases. EBV is present in approximately one-third of T-PTLDs. For the majority of B-PTLDs, a putative role of EBV has been proposed and accepted [187], whereas no direct role for EBV has been confirmed in T-PTLD. The pathogenesis of B-PTLD is mostly based on B lymphocytes infected by EBV. In general, T lymphocytes do not express the EBV receptor CD21; however, some T-PTLDs might show aberrant T cells, which are positive for CD21 and EBV [71]. Thus, this might be the explanation for the fact that about one-third of T-PTLDs were positive for EBV [31, 33].

In summary, T-PTLD is a heterogeneous group of different aberrant T-cell proliferations and represents a significant complication following transplantation, showing a uniformly poor prognosis. Immunosuppression is a major risk factor for T-PTLD development, which is usually late-occurring. Unfavorable prognostic factors include the hepatosplenic subtype and the involvement of bone marrow, the central nervous system, or graft. Hematopoietic stem cell transplantation is associated with early-onset T-PTLD, whereas a late onset was found to occur after long-lasting immunosuppression in SOT patients. EBV-positive cases seem to have a better survival rate than EBV-negative cases.

Glossary

Lymphoproliferative disorders (LPD):
Refer to clonal expansion of lymphatic system cells

PTLD:
Heterogenous group of EBV disease with neoplastic lymphoproliferation, developing after transplantation and caused by iatrogenic suppression of T-cell function. Diagnosis of neoplastic forms of EBV-PTLD should have at least two and ideally three of the following histological features: (i) disruption of underlying cellular architecture by a lymphoproliferative process; (ii) presence of monoclonal or oligoclonal cell populations as revealed by cellular and/or viral markers; (iii) evidence of EBV infection in many of the cells, that is, DNA, RNA or protein. Detection of EBV nucleic acid in blood is not sufficient for the diagnosis of EBV-related PTLD.

EBV-positive T-LPD:
EBV-associated T/NK-cell lymphoproliferative disease (T/NK-LPD) is a systemic illness characterized by monoclonal proliferation of EBV-infected T or NK cells. Systemic EBV-positive T-cell LPD can be defined based on following eligibility criteria: (1) illness or symptoms including fever, persistent hepatitis, lymphadenopathy, hepatosplenomegaly, hemophagocytosis, and interstitial pneumonia; (2) can occur shortly after primary EBV

infection or in the setting of CAEBV; (3) monoclonal expansion of EBV-infected T cells with an activated cytotoxic phenotype in tissues or peripheral blood.

Chronic active EBV (CAEBV) infection:
Defined as (1) persistent or recurrent symptoms related to EBV infection for more than three months; (2) high EBV genome levels in affected tissues or peripheral blood; (3) chronic illness that could not be explained by other known disease processes at diagnosis, and (4) no specific underlying immunological abnormality.

Summary Points List

- Most of B-PTLD is associated with EBV: over 90% in HSCT patients and over 70% in SOT setting. T-cell PTLDs are less common, ranging from 4-15% of all PTLD cases with an infrequent association with EBV ranging 30-35% of cases.
- Since T-cell PTLD was first described in 1987, up to the end of 2013, only 225 cases have been reported, including 9 cases after HSCT. Hematopoietic stem cell transplantation is associated with early-onset T-PTLD.
- In comparison to B-cell PTLDs, T-PTLD present usually later following transplant. The median interval from transplant to diagnosis of T-PTLD was 72 months compared to 48 months for all PTLD cases. 90% of the patients with T-PTLD presented with onset disease later than 12 months after transplant, compared to 65% of monomorphic B-cell PTLD.
- T-PTLD is usually EBV-negative and the relatively long latency between transplantation and T-PTLD onset may be explained by molecular events. The pathogenesis of B-PTLD is mostly based on B lymphocytes infected by EBV. Since some T-PTLD might show aberrant T cells, which are positive for CD21 and EBV, this might be the explanation that about one-third of T-PTLD were positive for EBV.
- Posttransplant lymphoproliferative disorders harbouring both B- and T-cell clones either concurrently or successively in the same patient are extremely rare and there are only a few cases reported in the literature so far. Half of B-cell post-transplant lymphoproliferative disorders are associated with clonal expansion of CD8-positive T cells, most of which do not amount to the coexistence of a T-PTLD.
- Prolonged immunosuppression is the most important risk factors for T-PTLD development.
- The major independent favorable prognostic factors are LGL-PTLD, young age at diagnosis, and the combination of radiotherapy/radiochemotherapy with reduced immunosuppression.

Future Issue List

- The frequency of composite B-cell and T-cell lineage PTLD is probably higher than expected. Clonality and detailed immunophenotype analyses can provide more

evidences. Composite B-cell and T-cell lineage PTLD might be the explanation for therapy failure in B-PTLD.
- The frequency of T-cell lineage PTLD after HSCT is probably higher than reported.

References

[1] Campo E, Swerdlow SH, Harris NL, Pileri S, Stein H, Jaffe ES: The 2008 WHO classification of lymphoid neoplasms and beyond: Evolving concepts and practical applications. *Blood* 2011;117:5019-5032.

[2] Kuppers R: B cells under influence: Transformation of B cells by Epstein-Barr virus. *Nat. Rev. Immunol.* 2003;3:801-812.

[3] Hassan R, White LR, Stefanoff CG, de Oliveira DE, Felisbino FE, Klumb CE, Bacchi CE, Seuanez HN, Zalcberg IR: Epstein-Barr virus (EBV) detection and typing by PCR: A contribution to diagnostic screening of EBV-positive burkitt's lymphoma. *Diagn. Pathol.* 2006; 1:17.

[4] Styczynski J, Einsele H, Gil L, Ljungman P: Outcome of treatment of Epstein-Barr virus-related post-transplant lymphoproliferative disorder in hematopoietic stem cell recipients: A comprehensive review of reported cases. *Transpl. Infect. Dis.* 2009; 11:383-392.

[5] Tierney RJ, Steven N, Young LS, Rickinson AB: Epstein-Barr virus latency in blood mononuclear cells: Analysis of viral gene transcription during primary infection and in the carrier state. *J. Virol.* 1994; 68:7374-7385.

[6] Decker LL, Klaman LD, Thorley-Lawson DA: Detection of the latent form of Epstein-Barr virus DNA in the peripheral blood of healthy individuals. *J. Virol.* 1996; 70: 3286-3289.

[7] Cohen JI: Epstein-Barr virus infection. *N. Engl. J. Med.* 2000;343:481-492.

[8] Crawford DH, Macsween KF, Higgins CD, Thomas R, McAulay K, Williams H, Harrison N, Reid S, Conacher M, Douglas J, Swerdlow AJ: A cohort study among university students: Identification of risk factors for Epstein-Barr virus seroconversion and infectious mononucleosis. *Clin. Infect. Dis.* 2006; 43:276-282.

[9] Siu LL, Chan JK, Kwong YL: Natural killer cell malignancies: Clinicopathologic and molecular features. *Histol. Histopathol.* 2002; 17:539-554.

[10] Heslop HE: Biology and treatment of Epstein-Barr virus-associated non-Hodgkin lymphomas. *Hematology Am. Soc. Hematol. Educ. Program* 2005: 260-266.

[11] Pallesen G, Hamilton-Dutoit SJ, Rowe M, Young LS: Expression of Epstein-Barr virus latent gene products in tumour cells of Hodgkin's disease. *Lancet* 1991;337:320-322.

[12] Anagnostopoulos I, Hummel M, Finn T, Tiemann M, Korbjuhn P, Dimmler C, Gatter K, Dallenbach F, Parwaresch MR, Stein H: Heterogeneous Epstein-Barr virus infection patterns in peripheral T-cell lymphoma of angioimmunoblastic lymphadenopathy type. *Blood* 1992; 80: 1804-1812.

[13] Kimura H, Ito Y, Kawabe S, Gotoh K, Takahashi Y, Kojima S, Naoe T, Esaki S, Kikuta A, Sawada A, Kawa K, Ohshima K, Nakamura S: EBV-associated T/NK-cell lymphoproliferative diseases in nonimmunocompromised hosts: Prospective analysis of 108 cases. *Blood* 2012; 119: 673-686.

[14] Jaffe ES: The 2008 WHO classification of lymphomas: Implications for clinical practice and translational research. *Hematology Am. Soc. Hematol. Educ. Program* 2009: 523-531.

[15] Quintanilla-Martinez L, Kumar S, Fend F, Reyes E, Teruya-Feldstein J, Kingma DW, Sorbara L, Raffeld M, Straus SE, Jaffe ES: Fulminant EBV(+) T-cell lymphoproliferative disorder following acute/chronic EBV infection: A distinct clinicopathologic syndrome. *Blood* 2000; 96: 443-451.

[16] Ishihara S, Yabuta R, Tokura Y, Ohshima K, Tagawa S: Hypersensitivity to mosquito bites is not an allergic disease, but an Epstein-Barr virus-associated lymphoproliferative disease. *Int. J. Hematol.* 2000; 72: 223-228.

[17] Iwatsuki K, Ohtsuka M, Harada H, Han G, Kaneko F: Clinicopathologic manifestations of Epstein-Barr virus-associated cutaneous lymphoproliferative disorders. *Arch. Dermatol.* 1997; 133: 1081-1086.

[18] Henter JI, Horne A, Arico M, Egeler RM, Filipovich AH, Imashuku S, Ladisch S, McClain K, Webb D, Winiarski J, Janka G: Hlh-2004: Diagnostic and therapeutic guidelines for hemophagocytic lymphohistiocytosis. *Pediatr. Blood Cancer* 2007; 48: 124-131.

[19] Kimura H, Hoshino Y, Kanegane H, Tsuge I, Okamura T, Kawa K, Morishima T: Clinical and virologic characteristics of chronic active Epstein-Barr virus infection. *Blood* 2001; 98: 280-286.

[20] Hong M, Ko YH, Yoo KH, Koo HH, Kim SJ, Kim WS, Park H: EBV-positive T/NK-cell lymphoproliferative disease of childhood. *Korean J. Pathol.* 2013; 47: 137-147.

[21] Carbone A, Gloghini A, Dotti G: EBV-associated lymphoproliferative disorders: Classification and treatment. *Oncologist* 2008; 13: 577-585.

[22] Yoshii M, Ishida M, Hodohara K, Okuno H, Nakanishi R, Yoshida T, Okabe H: Systemic Epstein-Barr virus-positive T-cell lymphoproliferative disease of childhood: Report of a case with review of the literature. *Oncol. Lett.* 2012; 4: 381-384.

[23] Okano M, Kawa K, Kimura H, Yachie A, Wakiguchi H, Maeda A, Imai S, Ohga S, Kanegane H, Tsuchiya S, Morio T, Mori M, Yokota S, Imashuku S: Proposed guidelines for diagnosing chronic active Epstein-Barr virus infection. *Am. J. Hematol.* 2005; 80: 64-69.

[24] Ohshima K, Kimura H, Yoshino T, Kim CW, Ko YH, Lee SS, Peh SC, Chan JK: Proposed categorization of pathological states of EBV-associated t/natural killer-cell lymphoproliferative disorder (LPD) in children and young adults: Overlap with chronic active EBV infection and infantile fulminant EBV T-LPD. *Pathol. Int.* 2008; 58: 209-217.

[25] Kato S, Miyata T, Takata K, Shimada S, Ito Y, Tomita A, Elsayed AA, Takahashi E, Asano N, Kinoshita T, Kimura H, Nakamura S: Epstein-Barr virus-positive cytotoxic T-cell lymphoma followed by chronic active Epstein-Barr virus infection-associated T/NK-cell lymphoproliferative disorder: A case report. *Hum. Pathol.* 2013; 44: 2849-2852.

[26] Kondo S, Tanimoto K, Yamada K, Yoshimoto G, Suematsu E, Fujisaki T, Oshiro Y, Tamura K, Takeshita M, Okamura S: Mature T/NK-cell lymphoproliferative disease and Epstein-Barr virus infection are more frequent in patients with rheumatoid arthritis treated with methotrexate. *Virchows Arch.* 2013; 462: 399-407.

[27] Imashuku S: Treatment of Epstein-Barr virus-related hemophagocytic lymphohistiocytosis (EBV-HLH); update 2010. *J. Pediatr. Hematol. Oncol.* 2011; 33: 35-39.
[28] Imashuku S, Kuriyama K, Sakai R, Nakao Y, Masuda S, Yasuda N, Kawano F, Yakushijin K, Miyagawa A, Nakao T, Teramura T, Tabata Y, Morimoto A, Hibi S: Treatment of Epstein-Barr virus-associated hemophagocytic lymphohistiocytosis (EBV-HLH) in young adults: A report from the HLH study center. *Med. Pediatr. Oncol.* 2003; 41: 103-109.
[29] Imashuku S, Teramura T, Tauchi H, Ishida Y, Otoh Y, Sawada M, Tanaka H, Watanabe A, Tabata Y, Morimoto A, Hibi S, Henter JI: Longitudinal follow-up of patients with Epstein-Barr virus-associated hemophagocytic lymphohistiocytosis. *Haematologica* 2004; 89: 183-188.
[30] Henter JI, Arico M, Egeler RM, Elinder G, Favara BE, Filipovich AH, Gadner H, Imashuku S, Janka-Schaub G, Komp D, Ladisch S, Webb D: Hlh-94: A treatment protocol for hemophagocytic lymphohistiocytosis. HLH study group of the histiocyte society. *Med. Pediatr. Oncol.* 1997; 28: 342-347.
[31] Herreman A, Dierickx D, Morscio J, Camps J, Bittoun E, Verhoef G, De Wolf-Peeters C, Sagaert X, Tousseyn T: Clinicopathological characteristics of posttransplant lymphoproliferative disorders of T-cell origin: Single-center series of nine cases and meta-analysis of 147 reported cases. *Leuk Lymphoma* 2013; 54: 2190-2199.
[32] La Fortune K, Zhang D, Raca G, Ranheim EA: A unique "composite" ptld with diffuse large B-cell and T-anaplastic large cell lymphoma components occurring 17 years after transplant. *Case Rep. Hematol.* 2013; 2013: 386147.
[33] Tiede C, Maecker-Kolhoff B, Klein C, Kreipe H, Hussein K: Risk factors and prognosis in T-cell posttransplantation lymphoproliferative diseases: Reevaluation of 163 cases. *Transplantation* 2013; 95: 479-488.
[34] Shroff R, Rees L: The post-transplant lymphoproliferative disorder-a literature review. *Pediatr. Nephrol.* 2004; 19: 369-377.
[35] Hussein K, Maecker-Kolhoff B, Klein C, Kreipe H: Transplant-associated lymphoproliferation. *Pathologe* 2011; 32: 152-158.
[36] Evens AM, Roy R, Sterrenberg D, Moll MZ, Chadburn A, Gordon LI: Post-transplantation lymphoproliferative disorders: Diagnosis, prognosis, and current approaches to therapy. *Curr. Oncol. Rep.* 2010; 12: 383-394.
[37] Roschewski M, Wilson WH: EBV-associated lymphomas in adults. *Best Pract. Res. Clin. Haematol.* 2012; 25: 75-89.
[38] Paya CV, Fung JJ, Nalesnik MA, Kieff E, Green M, Gores G, Habermann TM, Wiesner PH, Swinnen JL, Woodle ES, Bromberg JS: Epstein-Barr virus-induced posttransplant lymphoproliferative disorders. ASTS/ASTP EBV-PTLD task force and the mayo clinic organized international consensus development meeting. *Transplantation* 1999; 68: 1517-1525.
[39] Styczynski J, Reusser P, Einsele H, de la Camara R, Cordonnier C, Ward KN, Ljungman P, Engelhard D: Management of HSV, VZV and EBV infections in patients with hematological malignancies and after SCT: Guidelines from the second European Conference on Infections in Leukemia. *Bone Marrow Transplant.* 2009; 43: 757-770.

[40] Styczynski J, Gil L, Piatkowska M, Wlodarczyk Z: EBV-dependent post-transplant lymphoproliferative disorder after hematopoietic stem cell and solid organ transplantations: Similarities and differences. *Acta Haematol. Pol.* 2010; 41: 35-44.

[41] Al-Mansour Z, Nelson BP, Evens AM: Post-transplant lymphoproliferative disease (PTLD): Risk factors, diagnosis, and current treatment strategies. *Curr. Hematol. Malig. Rep.* 2013; 8: 173-183.

[42] Nelson BP, Nalesnik MA, Bahler DW, Locker J, Fung JJ, Swerdlow SH: Epstein-Barr virus-negative post-transplant lymphoproliferative disorders: A distinct entity? *Am. J. Surg. Pathol.* 2000; 24: 375-385.

[43] Vegso G, Hajdu M, Sebestyen A: Lymphoproliferative disorders after solid organ transplantation-classification, incidence, risk factors, early detection and treatment options. *Pathol. Oncol. Res.* 2011;17:443-454.

[44] Lippman SM, Grogan TM, Carry P, Ogden DA, Miller TP: Post-transplantation t cell lymphoblastic lymphoma. *Am. J. Med.* 1987; 82: 814-816.

[45] Gentile TC, Hadlock KG, Uner AH, Delal B, Squiers E, Crowley S, Woodman RC, Foung SK, Poiesz BJ, Loughran TP, Jr.: Large granular lymphocyte leukaemia occurring after renal transplantation. *Br. J. Haematol.* 1998;101:507-512.

[46] Hoshida Y, Li T, Dong Z, Tomita Y, Yamauchi A, Hanai J, Aozasa K: Lymphoproliferative disorders in renal transplant patients in japan. *Int. J. Cancer* 2001; 91:869-875.

[47] Kim JY, Kim CW, Ahn C, Bang YJ, Lee HS: Rapidly developing T-cell posttransplantation lymphoproliferative disorder. *Am. J. Kidney Dis.* 1999; 34:e3.

[48] Kwong YL, Lam CC, Chan TM: Post-transplantation lymphoproliferative disease of natural killer cell lineage: A clinicopathological and molecular analysis. *Br. J. Haematol.* 2000; 110: 197-202.

[49] Draoua HY, Tsao L, Mancini DM, Addonizio LJ, Bhagat G, Alobeid B: T-cell post-transplantation lymphoproliferative disorders after cardiac transplantation: A single institutional experience. *Br. J. Haematol.* 2004; 127: 429-432.

[50] Lundell R, Elenitoba-Johnson KS, Lim MS: T-cell posttransplant lymphoproliferative disorder occurring in a pediatric solid-organ transplant patient. *Am. J. Surg. Pathol.* 2004; 28: 967-973.

[51] Magro CM, Weinerman DJ, Porcu PL, Morrison CD: Post-transplant EBV-negative anaplastic large-cell lymphoma with dual rearrangement: A propos of two cases and review of the literature. *J. Cutan. Pathol.* 2007; 34 Suppl 1:1-8.

[52] Yang F, Li Y, Braylan R, Hunger SP, Yang LJ: Pediatric T-cell post-transplant lymphoproliferative disorder after solid organ transplantation. *Pediatr. Blood Cancer* 2008; 50:415-418.

[53] Au WY, Lie AK, Lee CK, Ma SK, Wan TS, Shek TW, Liang R, Kwong YL: Late onset post-transplantation lymphoproliferative disease of recipient origin following cytogenetic relapse and occult autologous haematopoietic regeneration after allogeneic bone marrow transplantation for acute myeloid leukaemia. *Bone Marrow Transplant.* 2001; 28:417-419.

[54] Awaya N, Adachi A, Mori T, Kamata H, Nakahara J, Yokoyama K, Yamada T, Kizaki M, Sakamoto M, Ikeda Y, Okamoto S: Fulminant Epstein-Barr virus (EBV)-associated T-cell lymphoproliferative disorder with hemophagocytosis following autologous

peripheral blood stem cell transplantation for relapsed angioimmunoblastic T-cell lymphoma. *Leuk Res.* 2006; 30: 1059-1062.
[55] Zutter MM, Durnam DM, Hackman RC, Loughran TP, Jr., Kidd PG, Ashley RL, Petersdorf EW, Martin PJ, Thomas ED: Secondary T-cell lymphoproliferation after marrow transplantation. *Am. J. Clin. Pathol.* 1990; 94: 714-721.
[56] Wang LC, Lu MY, Yu J, Jou ST, Chiang IP, Lin KH, Lin DT: T cell lymphoproliferative disorder following bone marrow transplantation for severe aplastic anemia. *Bone Marrow Transplant.* 2000; 26: 893-897.
[57] Yufu Y, Kimura M, Kawano R, Noguchi Y, Takatsuki H, Uike N, Ohshima K: Epstein-Barr virus-associated t cell lymphoproliferative disorder following autologous blood stem cell transplantation for relapsed hodgkin's disease. *Bone Marrow Transplant.* 2000; 26:1339-1341.
[58] Chang H, Kamel-Reid S, Hussain N, Lipton J, Messner HA: T-cell large granular lymphocytic leukemia of donor origin occurring after allogeneic bone marrow transplantation for B-cell lymphoproliferative disorders. *Am. J. Clin. Pathol.* 2005; 123: 196-199.
[59] Tsao L, Draoua HY, Mansukhani M, Bhagat G, Alobeid B: EBV-associated, extranodal nk-cell lymphoma, nasal type of the breast, after heart transplantation. *Mod. Pathol.* 2004; 17:125-130.
[60] Berho M, Viciana A, Weppler D, Romero R, Tzakis A, Ruiz P: T cell lymphoma involving the graft of a multivisceral organ recipient. *Transplantation* 1999; 68: 1135-1139.
[61] Thein M, Ravat F, Orchard G, Calonje E, Russell-Jones R: Syringotropic cutaneous T-cell lymphoma: An immunophenotypic and genotypic study of five cases. *Br. J. Dermatol.* 2004; 151: 216-226.
[62] Laffitte E, Venetz JP, Aubert JD, Duchosal MA, Panizzon RG, Pascual M: Mycosis fungoides in a lung transplant recipient with advanced ciclosporin nephropathy: Management with mechlorethamine and subsequent renal transplantation. *Dermatology* 2008; 217: 87-88.
[63] Roelandt PR, Maertens J, Vandenberghe P, Verslype C, Roskams T, Aerts R, Nevens F, Dierickx D: Hepatosplenic gammadelta T-cell lymphoma after liver transplantation: Report of the first 2 cases and review of the literature. *Liver Transpl.* 2009; 15:686-692.
[64] Williams KM, Higman MA, Chen AR, Schwartz CL, Wharam M, Colombani P, Arceci RJ: Successful treatment of a child with late-onset T-cell post-transplant lymphoproliferative disorder/lymphoma. *Pediatr. Blood Cancer* 2008; 50: 667-670.
[65] Sevmis S, Pehlivan S, Shabazov R, Karakayali H, Ozcay F, Haberal M: Posttransplant lymphoproliferative disease in pediatric liver transplant recipients. *Transplant. Proc.* 2009; 41:2881-2883.
[66] Costes-Martineau V, Delfour C, Obled S, Lamant L, Pageaux GP, Baldet P, Blanc P, Delsol G: Anaplastic lymphoma kinase (ALK) protein expressing lymphoma after liver transplantation: Case report and literature review. *J. Clin. Pathol.* 2002; 55: 868-871.
[67] Feher O, Barilla D, Locker J, Oliveri D, Melhem M, Winkelstein A: T-cell large granular lymphocytic leukemia following orthotopic liver transplantation. *Am. J. Hematol.* 1995; 49: 216-220.

[68] Amin A, Burkhart C, Groben P, Morrell DS: Primary cutaneous T-cell lymphoma following organ transplantation in a 16-year-old boy. *Pediatr. Dermatol.* 2009; 26: 112-113.

[69] George TI, Jeng M, Berquist W, Cherry AM, Link MP, Arber DA: Epstein-Barr virus-associated peripheral T-cell lymphoma and hemophagocytic syndrome arising after liver transplantation: Case report and review of the literature. *Pediatr. Blood Cancer* 2005; 44:270-276.

[70] Dockrell DH, Strickler JG, Paya CV: Epstein-Barr virus-induced T cell lymphoma in solid organ transplant recipients. *Clin. Infect. Dis.* 1998; 26: 180-182.

[71] Roncella S, Cutrona G, Truini M, Airoldi I, Pezzolo A, Valetto A, Di Martino D, Dadati P, De Rossi A, Ulivi M, Fontana I, Nocera A, Valente U, Ferrarini M, Pistoia V: Late Epstein-Barr virus infection of a hepatosplenic gamma delta T-cell lymphoma arising in a kidney transplant recipient. *Haematologica* 2000; 85: 256-262.

[72] Chen W, Huang Q, Zuppan CW, Rowsell EH, Cao JD, Weiss LM, Wang J: Complete absence of KSHV/HHV-8 in posttransplant lymphoproliferative disorders: An immunohistochemical and molecular study of 52 cases. *Am. J. Clin. Pathol.* 2009; 131: 632-639.

[73] Mandel L, Surattanont F, Dourmas M: T-cell lymphoma in the parotid region after cardiac transplant: Case report. *J. Oral Maxillofac. Surg.* 2001; 59: 673-677.

[74] Su IC, Lien HC, Chen CM: Primary brain T-cell lymphoma after kidney transplantation: A case report. *Surg. Neurol.* 2006;66 Suppl 2:S60-63.

[75] Lee LY, Harpaz N, Strauchen JA: Posttransplant CD30+ (Ki-1) anaplastic large cell lymphoma: A case report and review of the literature. *Arch. Pathol. Lab. Med.* 2003; 127: 349-351.

[76] Shiong YS, Lian JD, Lin CY, Shu KH, Lu YS, Chou G: Epstein-Barr virus-associated T-cell lymphoma of the maxillary sinus in a renal transplant recipient. *Transplant. Proc.* 1992; 24: 1929-1931.

[77] Sebire NJ, Malone M, Ramsay AD: Posttransplant lymphoproliferative disorder presenting as CD30+, ALK+, anaplastic large cell lymphoma in a child. *Pediatr. Dev. Pathol.* 2004; 7: 290-293.

[78] Katugampola RP, Finlay AY, Harper JI, Dojcinov S, Maughan TS: Primary cutaneous cd30+ T-cell lymphoproliferative disorder following cardiac transplantation in a 15-year-old boy with netherton's syndrome. *Br. J. Dermatol.* 2005;153:1041-1046.

[79] Urasaki E, Yamada H, Tokimura T, Yokota A: T-cell type primary spinal intramedullary lymphoma associated with human T-cell lymphotropic virus type i after a renal transplant: Case report. *Neurosurgery* 1996;38:1036-1039.

[80] Ross CW, Schnitzer B, Sheldon S, Braun DK, Hanson CA: Gamma/delta T-cell posttransplantation lymphoproliferative disorder primarily in the spleen. *Am. J. Clin. Pathol.* 1994;102:310-315.

[81] De Nisi MC, D'Amuri A, Lalinga AV, Occhini R, Biagioli M, Miracco C: Posttransplant primary cutaneous CD30 (Ki-1)-positive anaplastic large T-cell lymphoma. A case report. *Br. J. Dermatol.* 2005;152:1068-1070.

[82] Salama S: Primary "cutaneous" T-cell anaplastic large cell lymphoma, cd30+, neutrophil-rich variant with subcutaneous panniculitic lesions, in a post-renal transplant patient: Report of unusual case and literature review. *Am. J. Dermatopathol.* 2005; 27: 217-223.

[83] McMullan DM, Radovaneevic B, Jackow CM, Frazier OH, Duvic M: Cutaneous T-cell lymphoma in a cardiac transplant recipient. *Tex Heart Inst. J.* 2001;28:203-207.

[84] Tsurumi H, Tani K, Tsuruta T, Shirato R, Matsudaira T, Tojo A, Wada C, Uchida H, Ozawa K, Asano S: Adult T-cell leukemia developing during immunosuppressive treatment in a renal transplant recipient. *Am. J. Hematol.* 1992;41:292-294.

[85] Rolland SL, Seymour RA, Wilkins BS, Parry G, Thomason JM: Post-transplant lymphoproliferative disorders presenting as gingival overgrowth in patients immunosuppressed with ciclosporin. A report of two cases. *J. Clin. Periodontol.* 2004; 31: 581-585.

[86] Seckin D, Demirhan B, Oguz Gulec T, Arikan U, Haberal M: Posttransplantation primary cutaneous CD30 (Ki-1)-positive large-cell lymphoma. *J. Am. Acad. Dermatol.* 2001; 45:S197-199.

[87] Haldas J, Wang W, Lazarchick J: Post-transplant lymphoproliferative disorders: T-cell lymphoma following cardiac transplant. *Leuk Lymphoma* 2002;43:447-450.

[88] Tsai DE, Aqui NA, Vogl DT, Bloom RD, Schuster SJ, Nasta SD, Wasik MA: Successful treatment of T-cell post-transplant lymphoproliferative disorder with the retinoid analog bexarotene. *Am. J. Transplant.* 2005; 5: 2070-2073.

[89] Lucioni M, Ippoliti G, Campana C, Cavallini D, Incardona P, Viglio A, Riboni R, Vigano M, Magrini U, Paulli M: EBV positive primary cutaneous CD30+ large T-cell lymphoma in a heart transplanted patient: Case report. *Am. J. Transplant.* 2004; 4: 1915-1920.

[90] Stadlmann S, Fend F, Moser P, Obrist P, Greil R, Dirnhofer S: Epstein-Barr virus-associated extranodal NK/T-cell lymphoma, nasal type of the hypopharynx, in a renal allograft recipient: Case report and review of literature. *Hum. Pathol.* 2001; 32: 1264-1268.

[91] Kemnitz J, Cremer J, Gebel M, Uysal A, Haverich A, Georgii A: T-cell lymphoma after heart transplantation. *Am. J. Clin. Pathol.* 1990;94:95-101.

[92] Treaba D, Assad L, Goldberg C, Loew J, Reddy VB, Kluskens L, Gattuso P: Anaplastic T large cell lymphoma diagnosed by exfoliative cytology in a post renal transplant patient. *Diagn. Cytopathol.* 2002;27:35-37.

[93] Rodriguez-Gil Y, Palencia SI, Lopez-Rios F, Ortiz PL, Rodriguez-Peralto JL: Mycosis fungoides after solid-organ transplantation: Report of 2 new cases. *Am. J. Dermatopathol.* 2008; 30: 150-155.

[94] Steurer M, Stauder R, Grunewald K, Gunsilius E, Duba HC, Gastl G, Dirnhofer S: Hepatosplenic gammadelta-T-cell lymphoma with leukemic course after renal transplantation. *Hum. Pathol.* 2002; 33: 253-258.

[95] Pitman SD, Rowsell EH, Cao JD, Huang Q, Wang J: Anaplastic large cell lymphoma associated with Epstein-Barr virus following cardiac transplant. *Am. J. Surg. Pathol.* 2004; 28: 410-415.

[96] Ulrich W, Chott A, Watschinger B, Reiter C, Kovarik J, Radaszkiewicz T: Primary peripheral T cell lymphoma in a kidney transplant under immunosuppression with cyclosporine a. *Hum. Pathol.* 1989;20:1027-1030.

[97] Ng K, Trotter J, Metcalf C, Thatcher G, Marshall E: Extranodal Ki-1 lymphoma in a renal transplant patient. *Aust. N. Z. J. Med.* 1992;22:51-53.

[98] Albalate M, Octavio JG, Echezarreta G, Rivas C, Caramelo C, Marron B, Plaza JJ: Diffuse T-cell lymphoma in a kidney graft recipient 17 years after transplantation. *Nephrol. Dial. Transplant.* 1998;13:3242-3244.

[99] Guz G, Arican A, Karakayali H, Demirhan B, Bilgin N, Haberal M: Two renal transplants from one cadaveric donor: One recipient with simultaneous B cell lymphoma and Kaposi's sarcoma, and the other with T cell lymphoma. *Nephrol. Dial. Transplant.* 2000;15:1242-1244.

[100] Belhadj K, Reyes F, Farcet JP, Tilly H, Bastard C, Angonin R, Deconinck E, Charlotte F, Leblond V, Labouyrie E, Lederlin P, Emile JF, Delmas-Marsalet B, Arnulf B, Zafrani ES, Gaulard P: Hepatosplenic gammadelta T-cell lymphoma is a rare clinicopathologic entity with poor outcome: Report on a series of 21 patients. *Blood* 2003; 102:4261-4269.

[101] McGregor JM, Yu CC, Lu QL, Cotter FE, Levison DA, MacDonald DM: Posttransplant cutaneous lymphoma. *J. Am. Acad. Dermatol.* 1993;29:549-554.

[102] van Gorp J, Doornewaard H, Verdonck LF, Klopping C, Vos PF, van den Tweel JG: Posttransplant T-cell lymphoma. Report of three cases and a review of the literature. *Cancer* 1994; 73: 3064-3072.

[103] Pomerantz RG, Campbell LS, Jukic DM, Geskin LJ: Posttransplant cutaneous T-cell lymphoma: Case reports and review of the association of calcineurin inhibitor use with posttransplant lymphoproliferative disease risk. *Arch. Dermatol.* 2010;146:513-516.

[104] Audouin J, Le Tourneau A, Diebold J, Reynes M, Tabbah I, Bernadou A: Primary intestinal lymphoma of Ki-1 large cell anaplastic type with mesenteric lymph node and spleen involvement in a renal transplant recipient. *Hematol. Oncol.* 1989;7:441-449.

[105] Jenks PJ, Barrett WY, Raftery MJ, Kelsey SM, van der Walt JD, Kon SP, Breuer J: Development of human T-cell lymphotropic virus type i-associated adult T-cell leukemia/lymphoma during immunosuppressive treatment following renal transplantation. *Clin. Infect. Dis.* 1995; 21:992-993.

[106] Raftery MJ, Tidman MJ, Koffman G, Ogg CS, Macdonald DM, Cameron JS: Posttransplantation T cell lymphoma of the skin. *Transplantation* 1988; 46:475-477.

[107] Yurtsever H, Kempf W, Laeng RH: Posttransplant CD30+ anaplastic large cell lymphoma with skin and lymph node involvement. *Dermatology* 2003; 207:107-110.

[108] Garvin AJ, Self S, Sahovic EA, Stuart RK, Marchalonis JJ: The occurrence of a peripheral T-cell lymphoma in a chronically immunosuppressed renal transplant patient. *Am. J. Surg. Pathol.* 1988;12:64-70.

[109] Bartakke S, Abla O, Weitzman S: Successful use of alemtuzumab in a child with refractory peripheral T-cell posttransplant lymphoproliferative disorder. *J. Pediatr. Hematol. Oncol.* 2008; 30: 787-788.

[110] Michael J, Greenstein S, Schechner R, Tellis V, Vasovic LV, Ratech H, Glicklich D: Primary intestinal posttransplant T-cell lymphoma. *Transplantation* 2003; 75:2131-2132.

[111] Lye WC: Successful treatment of Epstein-Barr virus-associated T-cell cutaneous lymphoma in a renal allograft recipient: Case report and review of the literature. *Transplant. Proc.* 2000;32:1988-1989.

[112] Venizelos I, Tamiolakis D, Lambropoulou M, Nikolaidou S, Bolioti S, Papadopoulos H, Papadopoulos N: An unusual case of posttransplant peritoneal primary effusion

lymphoma with T-cell phenotype in a HIV-negative female, not associated with HHV-8. *Pathol. Oncol. Res.* 2005;11:178-181.

[113] Azhir A, Reisi N, Taheri D, Adibi A: Post transplant anaplastic large T-cell lymphoma. *Saudi J. Kidney Dis. Transpl.* 2009;20:646-651.

[114] Pascual J, Torrelo A, Teruel JL, Bellas C, Marcen R, Ortuno J: Cutaneous T cell lymphomas after renal transplantation. *Transplantation* 1992; 53:1143-1145.

[115] Ward HA, Russo GG, McBurney E, Millikan LE, Boh EE: Posttransplant primary cutaneous T-cell lymphoma. *J. Am. Acad. Dermatol.* 2001; 44:675-680.

[116] Jonveaux P, Daniel MT, Martel V, Maarek O, Berger R: Isochromosome 7q and trisomy 8 are consistent primary, non-random chromosomal abnormalities associated with hepatosplenic t gamma/delta lymphoma. *Leukemia* 1996;10:1453-1455.

[117] Peeters P, Sennesael J, De Raeve H, De Waele M, Verbeelen D: Hemophagocytic syndrome and T-cell lymphoma after kidney transplantation: A case report. *Transpl. Int.* 1997;10:471-474.

[118] Wu H, Wasik MA, Przybylski G, Finan J, Haynes B, Moore H, Leonard DG, Montone KT, Naji A, Nowell PC, Kamoun M, Tomaszewski JE, Salhany KE: Hepatosplenic gamma-delta T-cell lymphoma as a late-onset posttransplant lymphoproliferative disorder in renal transplant recipients. *Am. J. Clin. Pathol.* 2000;113:487-496.

[119] Mukai HY, Kojima H, Suzukawa K, Hori M, Komeno T, Hasegawa Y, Ninomiya H, Mori N, Nagasawa T: Nasal natural killer cell lymphoma in a post-renal transplant patient. *Transplantation* 2000;69:1501-1503.

[120] Bregman SG, Yeaney GA, Greig BW, Vnencak-Jones CL, Hamilton KS: Subcutaneous panniculitic T-cell lymphoma in a cardiac allograft recipient. *J. Cutan. Pathol.* 2005; 32: 366-370.

[121] Rajakariar R, Bhattacharyya M, Norton A, Sheaff M, Cavenagh J, Raftery MJ, Yaqoob MM: Post transplant T-cell lymphoma: A case series of four patients from a single unit and review of the literature. *Am. J. Transplant.* 2004;4:1534-1538.

[122] Euvrard S, Noble CP, Kanitakis J, Ffrench M, Berger F, Delecluse HJ, D'Incan M, Thivolet J, Touraine JL: Brief report: Successive occurrence of T-cell and B-cell lymphomas after renal transplantation in a patient with multiple cutaneous squamous-cell carcinomas. *N. Engl. J. Med.* 1992;327:1924-1926.

[123] Yasunaga C, Kasai T, Nishihara G, Matsuo K, Takeda K, Urabe M, Nakamoto M, Goya T: Early development of Epstein-Barr virus-associated T-cell lymphoma after a living-related renal transplantation. *Transplantation* 1998;65:1642-1644.

[124] Lee HK, Kim HJ, Lee EH, Kim SY, Park TI, Kang CS, Yang WI: Epstein-Barr virus-associated peripheral T-cell lymphoma involving spleen in a renal transplant patient. *J. Korean Med. Sci.* 2003;18:272-276.

[125] Waller EK, Ziemianska M, Bangs CD, Cleary M, Weissman I, Kamel OW: Characterization of posttransplant lymphomas that express T-cell-associated markers: Immunophenotypes, molecular genetics, cytogenetics, and heterotransplantation in severe combined immunodeficient mice. *Blood* 1993;82:247-261.

[126] Olesen LL, Molby L: [Malignant T-cell neoplasia during treatment with azathioprine and prednisone after kidney transplantation]. *Ugeskr. Laeger.* 1991;153:3410-3411.

[127] Williams NP, Buchner LM, Shah DJ, Williams W: Adult T-cell leukemia/lymphoma in a renal transplant recipient: An opportunistic occurrence. *Am. J. Nephrol.* 1994;14:226-229.

[128] Ravat FE, Spittle MF, Russell-Jones R: Primary cutaneous T-cell lymphoma occurring after organ transplantation. *J. Am. Acad. Dermatol.* 2006;54:668-675.

[129] Canoz O, Soyuer I, Taskapan H, Utas C: T cell extranodal lymphoma case involving pleura and pericardium in a renal transplant patient. *Clin. Nephrol.* 2001;55:416-418.

[130] Ghorbani RP, Shokouh-Amiri H, Gaber LW: Intragraft angiotropic large-cell lymphoma of T cell-type in a long-term renal allograft recipient. *Mod. Pathol.* 1996; 9:671-676.

[131] Khan WA, Yu L, Eisenbrey AB, Crisan D, al Saadi A, Davis BH, Hankin RC, Mattson JC: Hepatosplenic gamma/delta T-cell lymphoma in immunocompromised patients. Report of two cases and review of literature. *Am. J. Clin. Pathol.* 2001;116:41-50.

[132] Borisch B, Hennig I, Horber F, Burki K, Laissue J: Enteropathy-associated T-cell lymphoma in a renal transplant patient with evidence of Epstein-Barr virus involvement. *Virchows Arch. A Pathol. Anat. Histopathol.* 1992;421:443-447.

[133] Hacker SM, Knight BP, Lunde NM, Gratiot-Deans J, Sandler H, Leichtman AB: A primary central nervous system T cell lymphoma in a renal transplant patient. *Transplantation* 1992; 53: 691-692.

[134] Coyne JD, Banerjee SS, Bromley M, Mills S, Diss TC, Harris M: Post-transplant T-cell lymphoproliferative disorder/T-cell lymphoma: A report of three cases of T-anaplastic large-cell lymphoma with cutaneous presentation and a review of the literature. *Histopathology* 2004; 44: 387-393.

[135] Lin WC, Moore JO, Mann KP, Traweek ST, Smith C: Post transplant CD8+ gammadelta T-cell lymphoma associated with Human Herpes Virus-6 infection. *Leuk Lymphoma* 1999; 33:377-384.

[136] Gill RM, Ferrell LD: Vanishing bile duct syndrome associated with peripheral t cell lymphoma, not otherwise specified, arising in a posttransplant setting. *Hepatology* 2010; 51: 1856-1857.

[137] Francois A, Lesesve JF, Stamatoullas A, Comoz F, Lenormand B, Etienne I, Mendel I, Hemet J, Bastard C, Tilly H: Hepatosplenic gamma/delta T-cell lymphoma: A report of two cases in immunocompromised patients, associated with isochromosome 7q. *Am. J. Surg. Pathol.* 1997;21:781-790.

[138] Ichikawa Y, Iida M, Ebisui C, Fujio C, Yazawa K, Hanafusa T, Kouro T, Seki K, Nagano S: A case study of adult T-cell lymphoma in a kidney transplant patient. *Transplant. Proc.* 2000;32:1982-1983.

[139] Defossez-Tribout C, Carmi E, Lok C, Westeel PF, Chatelain D, Denoeux JP: [Cutaneous T-cell lymphoma following renal transplantation]. *Ann. Dermatol. Venereol.* 2003; 130: 47-49.

[140] Masuda M, Arai Y, Nishina H, Fuchinoue S, Mizoguchi H: Large granular lymphocyte leukemia with pure red cell aplasia in a renal transplant recipient. *Am. J. Hematol.* 1998; 57:72-76.

[141] Bustillo M, Perez Melon C, Otero Glz A, Esteban E, Armada E, Bello JA, Sastre JL: High grade lymphoma in a post-renal transplant patient. Description of a case and literature review. *Nephron* 2000; 84:189-191.

[142] Kaplan MA, Jacobson JO, Ferry JA, Harris NL: T-cell lymphoma of the vulva in a renal allograft recipient with associated hemophagocytosis. *Am. J. Surg. Pathol.* 1993; 17: 842-849.

[143] Jamali FR, Otrock ZK, Soweid AM, Al-Awar GN, Mahfouz RA, Haidar GR, Bazarbachi A: An overview of the pathogenesis and natural history of post-transplant T-cell lymphoma (corrected and republished article originally printed in leukemia & lymphoma, June 2007; 48(6): 1237 - 1241). *Leuk Lymphoma* 2007;48:1780-1784.

[144] Cooper SM, Turner GD, Hollowood K, Gatter K, Hatton C, Gray D, Russell-Jones R, Wojnarowska F: Primary cutaneous large cell CD30+ lymphoma in a renal transplant recipient. *Br. J. Dermatol.* 2003; 149:426-428.

[145] Hanson MN, Morrison VA, Peterson BA, Stieglbauer KT, Kubic VL, McCormick SR, McGlennen RC, Manivel JC, Brunning RD, Litz CE: Posttransplant T-cell lymphoproliferative disorders - an aggressive, late complication of solid-organ transplantation. *Blood* 1996; 88:3626-3633.

[146] Kumar S, Kumar D, Kingma DW, Jaffe ES: Epstein-Barr virus-associated T-cell lymphoma in a renal transplant patient. *Am. J. Surg. Pathol.* 1993; 17:1046-1053.

[147] Griffith RC, Saha BK, Janney CM, Ratner L, Brunt EM, Gajl-Peczalska KJ, Hanto DW: Immunoblastic lymphoma of T-cell type in a chronically immunosuppressed renal transplant recipient. *Am. J. Clin. Pathol.* 1990; 93:280-285.

[148] Labouyrie E, Morel D, Boiron JM, Dubus P, Montastruc M, Bloch B, Reiffers J, de Mascarel A, Merlio JP: Peripheral T-cell lymphoma in a chronically immunosuppressed renal transplant patient. *Mod. Pathol.* 1995;8:355-359.

[149] Jimenez-Heffernan JA, Viguer JM, Vicandi B, Jimenez-Yuste V, Palacios J, Escuin F, Gamallo C: Posttransplant CD30 (Ki-1)-positive anaplastic large cell lymphoma. Report of a case with presentation as a pleural effusion. *Acta Cytol.* 1997; 41: 1519-1524.

[150] Frias C, Lauzurica R, Vaquero M, Ribera JM: Detection of Epstein-Barr virus in posttransplantation t cell lymphoma in a kidney transplant recipient: Case report and review. *Clin. Infect. Dis.* 2000;30:576-578.

[151] Kim HK, Jin SY, Lee NS, Won JH, Park HS, Yang WI: Posttransplant primary cutaneous Ki-1 (CD30)+/CD56+ anaplastic large cell lymphoma. *Arch. Pathol. Lab. Med.* 2004; 128:e96-99.

[152] Kraus TS, Twist CJ, Tan BT: Angioimmunoblastic t cell lymphoma: An unusual presentation of posttransplant lymphoproliferative disorder in a pediatric patient. *Acta Haematol.* 2013; 131: 95-101.

[153] Hwang JY, Cha ES, Lee JE, Sung SH: Isolated post-transplantation lymphoproliferative disease involving the breast and axilla as peripheral T-cell lymphoma. *Korean J. Radiol.* 2013; 14: 718-722.

[154] Dalal P, Bichu P, Dhawan V, Ariyamuthu V, Malhotra K, Misra M, Khanna R: Post-transplant lymphoproliferative disorder - a case of late-onset T-cell lymphoma after failed renal transplant. *Adv. Perit. Dial.* 2012; 28:94-96.

[155] Mills KC, Sangueza OP, Beaty MW, Raffeld M, Pang CS: Composite B-cell and T-cell lineage post-transplant lymphoproliferative disorder of the lung with unusual cutaneous manifestations of mycosis fungoides. *Am. J. Dermatopathol.* 2012; 34:220-225.

[156] Mohapatra A, Viswabandya A, Samuel R, Deepti AN, Madhivanan S, John GT: Nk/T-cell lymphoma in a renal transplant recipient and review of literature. *Indian J. Nephrol.* 2011; 21: 44-47.

[157] Kfoury HK, Alghonaim M, AlSuwaida AK, Zaidi SN, Arafah M: Nasopharyngeal T-cell monomorphic posttransplant lymphoproliferative disorders and combined IgA

nephropathy and membranous glomerulonephritis in a patient with renal transplantation: A case report with literature review. *Transplant. Proc.* 2010; 42: 4653-4657.

[158] Caillard S, Porcher R, Provot F, Dantal J, Choquet S, Durrbach A, Morelon E, Moal V, Janbon B, Alamartine E, Pouteil Noble C, Morel D, Kamar N, Buchler M, Mamzer MF, Peraldi MN, Hiesse C, Renoult E, Toupance O, Rerolle JP, Delmas S, Lang P, Lebranchu Y, Heng AE, Rebibou JM, Mousson C, Glotz D, Rivalan J, Thierry A, Etienne I, Moal MC, Albano L, Subra JF, Ouali N, Westeel PF, Delahousse M, Genin R, Hurault de Ligny B, Moulin B: Post-transplantation lymphoproliferative disorder after kidney transplantation: Report of a nationwide french registry and the development of a new prognostic score. *J. Clin. Oncol.* 2013;31:1302-1309.

[159] Kinch A, Baecklund E, Backlin C, Ekman T, Molin D, Tufveson G, Fernberg P, Sundstrom C, Pauksens K, Enblad G: A population-based study of 135 lymphomas after solid organ transplantation: The role of Epstein-Barr virus, hepatitis c and diffuse large B-cell lymphoma subtype in clinical presentation and survival. *Acta Oncol.* 2013.

[160] Swerdlow SH: T-cell and nk-cell posttransplantation lymphoproliferative disorders. *Am. J. Clin. Pathol.* 2007; 127: 887-895.

[161] Leblond V, Sutton L, Dorent R, Davi F, Bitker MO, Gabarre J, Charlotte F, Ghoussoub JJ, Fourcade C, Fischer A, et al.: Lymphoproliferative disorders after organ transplantation: A report of 24 cases observed in a single center. *J. Clin. Oncol.* 1995; 13:961-968.

[162] Collins MH, Montone KT, Leahey AM, Hodinka RL, Salhany KE, Kramer DL, Deng C, Tomaszewski JE: Post-transplant lymphoproliferative disease in children. *Pediatr. Transplant.* 2001; 5:250-257.

[163] Vakiani E, Basso K, Klein U, Mansukhani MM, Narayan G, Smith PM, Murty VV, Dalla-Favera R, Pasqualucci L, Bhagat G: Genetic and phenotypic analysis of B-cell post-transplant lymphoproliferative disorders provides insights into disease biology. *Hematol. Oncol.* 2008;26:199-211.

[164] Mahadevan D, Spier C, Della Croce K, Miller S, George B, Riley C, Warner S, Grogan TM, Miller TP: Transcript profiling in peripheral T-cell lymphoma, not otherwise specified, and diffuse large B-cell lymphoma identifies distinct tumor profile signatures. *Mol. Cancer Ther.* 2005;4:1867-1879.

[165] Khedmat H, Taheri S: Early onset post transplantation lymphoproliferative disorders: Analysis of international data from 5 studies. *Ann. Transplant.* 2009;14:74-77.

[166] Capello D, Rasi S, Oreste P, Veronese S, Cerri M, Ravelli E, Rossi D, Minola E, Colosimo A, Gambacorta M, Muti G, Morra E, Gaidano G: Molecular characterization of post-transplant lymphoproliferative disorders of donor origin occurring in liver transplant recipients. *J. Pathol.* 2009;218:478-486.

[167] Styczynski J, Gil L, Tridello G, Ljungman P, Donnelly JP, van der Velden W, Omar H, Martino R, Halkes C, Faraci M, Theunissen K, Kalwak K, Hubacek P, Sica S, Nozzoli C, Fagioli F, Matthes S, Diaz MA, Migliavacca M, Balduzzi A, Tomaszewska A, Camara Rde L, van Biezen A, Hoek J, Iacobelli S, Einsele H, Cesaro S: Response to rituximab-based therapy and risk factor analysis in Epstein Barr virus-related lymphoproliferative disorder after hematopoietic stem cell transplant in children and adults: A study from the Infectious Diseases Working Party of the European Group for Blood and Marrow Transplantation. *Clin. Infect. Dis.* 2013;57:794-802.

[168] Kontny U, Boppana S, Jung A, Goebel H, Strahm B, Peters A, Dormann S, Werner M, Bader P, Fisch P, Niemeyer C: Post-transplantation lymphoproliferative disorder of recipient origin in a boy with acute T-cell leukemia with detection of B-cell clonality 3 months before stem cell transplantation. *Haematologica* 2005;90 Suppl:ECR27.

[169] Shapiro RS, McClain K, Frizzera G, Gajl-Peczalska KJ, Kersey JH, Blazar BR, Arthur DC, Patton DF, Greenberg JS, Burke B, et al.: Epstein-Barr virus associated b cell lymphoproliferative disorders following bone marrow transplantation. *Blood* 1988; 71:1234-1243.

[170] Zutter MM, Martin PJ, Sale GE, Shulman HM, Fisher L, Thomas ED, Durnam DM: Epstein-Barr virus lymphoproliferation after bone marrow transplantation. *Blood* 1988; 72:520-529.

[171] Dierickx D, Tousseyn T, Sagaert X, Fieuws S, Wlodarska I, Morscio J, Brepoels L, Kuypers D, Vanhaecke J, Nevens F, Verleden G, Van Damme-Lombaerts R, Renard M, Pirenne J, De Wolf-Peeters C, Verhoef G: Single-center analysis of biopsy-confirmed posttransplant lymphoproliferative disorder: Incidence, clinicopathological characteristics and prognostic factors. *Leuk Lymphoma* 2013;54:2433-2440.

[172] Fischer E, Delibrias C, Kazatchkine MD: Expression of CR2 (the C3dg/EBV receptor, CD21) on normal human peripheral blood t lymphocytes. *J. Immunol.* 1991; 146: 865-869.

[173] Rizvi MA, Evens AM, Tallman MS, Nelson BP, Rosen ST: T-cell non-hodgkin lymphoma. *Blood* 2006;107:1255-1264.

[174] DiNardo CD, Tsai DE: Treatment advances in posttransplant lymphoproliferative disease. *Curr. Opin. Hematol.* 2010;17:368-374.

[175] Czyzewski K, Styczynski J, Krenska A, Debski R, Zajac-Spychala O, Wachowiak J, Wysocki M: Intrathecal therapy with rituximab in central nervous system involvement of post-transplant lymphoproliferative disorder. *Leuk Lymphoma* 2013;54:503-506.

[176] Gil L, Styczynski J, Komarnicki M: Strategy of pre-emptive management of Epstein-Barr virus post-transplant lymphoproliferative disorder after stem cell transplantation: Results of european transplant centers survey. *Contemp. Oncol.* (Pozn) 2012;16:338-340.

[177] Wang Q, Liu H, Zhang X, Liu Q, Xing Y, Zhou X, Tong C, Zhu P: High doses of mother's lymphocyte infusion to treat EBV-positive T-cell lymphoproliferative disorders in childhood. *Blood* 2010;116:5941-5947.

[178] Hollingsworth HC, Stetler-Stevenson M, Gagneten D, Kingma DW, Raffeld M, Jaffe ES: Immunodeficiency-associated malignant lymphoma. Three cases showing genotypic evidence of both t- and b-cell lineages. *Am. J. Surg. Pathol.* 1994;18:1092-1101.

[179] Frankel AH, Thompson M, Vulliamy T, Williams G, Thomas JA, Crawford DH, Rees AJ, Lechler R: A T cell clone in association with an Epstein-Barr virus-related b cell lymphoma. *Transplantation* 1991;52:1108-1109.

[180] Nelson BP, Locker J, Nalesnik MA, Fung JJ, Swerdlow SH: Clonal and morphological variation in a posttransplant lymphoproliferative disorder: Evolution from clonal T-cell to clonal B-cell predominance. *Hum. Pathol.* 1998;29:416-421.

[181] Yin CC, Medeiros LJ, Abruzzo LV, Jones D, Farhood AI, Thomazy VA: EBV-associated b- and T-cell posttransplant lymphoproliferative disorders following primary EBV infection in a kidney transplant recipient. *Am. J. Clin. Pathol.* 2005;123:222-228.

[182] Chuhjo T, Yachie A, Kanegane H, Kimura H, Shiobara S, Nakao S: Epstein-Barr virus (EBV)-associated post-transplantation lymphoproliferative disorder simultaneously affecting both B and T cells after allogeneic bone marrow transplantation. *Am. J. Hematol.* 2003;72:255-258.

[183] Morovic A, Jaffe ES, Raffeld M, Schrager JA: Metachronous EBV-associated B-cell and T-cell posttransplant lymphoproliferative disorders in a heart transplant recipient. *Am. J. Surg. Pathol.* 2009; 33:149-154.

[184] Leon JE, Takahama Junior A, Vassallo J, Soares FA, de Almeida OP, Lopes MA: EBV-associated polymorphic posttransplant lymphoproliferative disorder presenting as gingival ulcers. *Int. J. Surg. Pathol.* 2011; 19:241-246.

[185] Baudouin V, Dehee A, Pedron-Grossetete B, Ansart-Pirenne H, Haddad E, Maisin A, Loirat C, Sterkers G: Relationship between CD8+ T-cell phenotype and function, Epstein-Barr virus load, and clinical outcome in pediatric renal transplant recipients: A prospective study. *Transplantation* 2004; 77:1706-1713.

[186] Ibrahim HA, Menasce LP, Pomplun S, Burke M, Bower M, Naresh KN: Presence of monoclonal T-cell populations in B-cell post-transplant lymphoproliferative disorders. *Mod. Pathol.* 2011; 24:232-240.

[187] Pasquale MA, Weppler D, Smith J, Icardi M, Amador A, Gonzalez M, Kato T, Tzakis A, Ruiz P: Burkitt lymphoma variant of post-transplant lymphoproliferative disease (PTLD). *Pathol. Oncol. Res.* 2002; 8:105-108.

Biographical Sketch

Jan Styczynski, MD, PhD, is affiliated with Department of Pediatric Hematology and Oncology, Collegium Medicum, Nicolaus Copernicus University, Bydgoszcz, Poland, and appointed as professor in transplantology and pediatric hematology and oncology. His main scientific interest include: viral infections in transplantology, hematology and oncology; drug resistance in hematology and oncology; hematopoietic stem cell donor issues; and differences between children and adults in transplantology, hematology and oncology. He is the Secretary of Infectious Diseases Working Party (IDWP) of European Group for Blood and Marrow Transplantation (EBMT) from 2010, and Member of ECIL (European Conference on Infections in Leukemia) group from 2007. Member of American Society of Hematology, European Group for Blood and Marrow Transplantation and several national societies. He has published 40 papers over last 3 years.

In: Epstein-Barr Virus (EBV)
Editor: Jan Styczynski

ISBN: 978-1-63117-476-6
© 2014 Nova Science Publishers, Inc.

Chapter VIII

Results of Therapy of EBV-Associated Post-Transplant Lymphoproliferative Disorder in Children and Adults with Anti-CD20 Antibodies after Hematopoietic Stem Cell Transplantation

Jan Styczynski[*]
Department of Pediatric Hematology and Oncology,
Collegium Medicum, Nicolaus Copernicus University, Bydgoszcz, Poland

Abstract

Epstein-Barr virus (EBV)–associated B-cell post-transplant lymphoproliferative disorder (PTLD) is a heterogenous group of EBV diseases with neoplastic lymphoproliferation, developing after hematopoietic stem cell (HSCT) or solid organ transplantation (SOT) resulting from outgrowth of EBV-infected B-cells and caused by iatrogenic suppression of T-cell function. Since the first report over 40 years ago, PTLD has remained one of the most morbid complications associated with transplantation. Before the current methods of anti-EBV therapy were introduced, the mortality from PTLD was >80%. The diagnosis of PTLD can be made at a probable or proven level. Probable PTLD is defined as significant lymphadenopathy or other end-organ disease accompanied by a high EBV DNA-emia, in the absence of other etiologic factors or established diseases. Proven EBV-PTLD is diagnosed when EBV is detected in a specimen obtained from an organ by biopsy or other invasive procedure, with a test with appropriate sensitivity and specificity together with symptoms and signs from the affected organ. Treatment options include manipulation of the balance between

---

[*] Corresponding author: Department of Pediatric Hematology and Oncology; Collegium Medicum, Nicolaus Copernicus University; ul. Curie-Sklodowskiej 9; 85-094 Bydgoszcz, Poland.
E-mail: jstyczynski@cm.umk.pl.

outgrowing EBV-infected B-cells and the EBV-cytotoxic T-lymphocyte response and targeting the B-cells with monoclonal antibodies or chemotherapy and other possible approaches. Therapy with anti-CD20 antibodies is currently regarded as the best available treatment for all transplant centers. The objective of this chapter is the analysis of differences in outcome of PTLD in children and adults after HSCT, treated with rituximab. Risk factor analysis for outcome of PTLD therapy was performed in 55 children and 89 adults after HSCT, treated with rituximab. Response to therapy was better in children than adults: 78% vs 64%. In children early response after 1 week of therapy and reduction of immunosuppression at PTLD diagnosis corresponded with a good prognosis, while involvement of extra-lymphoid tissue, initial plasma EBV DNA-emia>10^5 copies/mL and increase of EBV DNA-emia during therapy by 1 log were predictors of poor outcome. In adults, early response after 1 week of therapy, and reduction of immunosuppression was associated with improved outcome while age>30 years, initial plasma EBV DNA-emia>10^4 copies/mL and increase of EBV DNA-emia during therapy by 1 log predicted poor outcome.

Keywords: Epstein-Barr virus; post-transplant lymphoproliferative disorder; hematopoietic stem cell transplantation; solid organ transplantation; rituximab; reduction of immunosuppression; PTLD relapse

Abbreviations

ATG	Anti-thymocyte globulin
CBT	Cord Blood Transplantation
CD	Cluster of differentiation
CMV	Cytomegalovirus
CNI	Calcineurin inhibitor
CNS	Central nervous system
CR	Complete remission
CT	Computed tomography
CTL	Cytotoxic T-cell
DLBCL	Diffuse large B-cell lymphoma
DLI	Donor Lymphocytes Infusion
DNA	Deoxyribonucleic acid
EBER	Epstein-Barr Virus-encoded RNA
EBMT	European Group for Blood and Marrow Transplantation
EBNA	Epstein-Barr Virus nuclear antigen
EBV	Epstein-Barr Virus nuclear antigen
ECIL	European Conference on Infections in Leukemia
CI	Confidence interval
GVHD	Graft-versus-host-disease
HD	Hodgkin Disease
HLA	Human Leukocyte Antigen
HSC	Hematopoietic stem cell
HSCT	Hematopoietic stem cell transplantation
IS	Immunosuppressive

IVIG	Intravenous immunglobulin
MMUD	Mismatched Unrelated Donor
MMFD	Mismatched Family Donor
MFD	Matched Family Donor
MUD	Matched Unrelated Donor
NAT	Nucleic acid testing
NHL	Non-Hodgkin lymphoma
NK-cell	Natural killer cell
PCR	Polymerase chain reaction
PET	Positron emission tomography
PTLD	Post-transplant lymphoproliferative disorder
RI	Reduction of immunosuppression
SOT	Solid organ transplantation
WHO	World Health Organization

Introduction

Epstein-Barr virus (EBV)–associated B-cell post-transplant lymphoproliferative disorder (PTLD) is a heterogenous group of EBV diseases with neoplastic lymphoproliferation, developing after hematopoietic stem cell (HSCT) or solid organ transplantation (SOT) resulting from outgrowth of EBV-infected B-cells and caused by iatrogenic suppression of T-cell function. Since the first report over 40 years ago, PTLD has remained one of the most morbid complications associated with transplantation. Before the current methods of anti-EBV therapy were introduced, the mortality from PTLD was very high.

It was estimated for patients treated over 15 years ago that post-HSCT EBV-PTLD might affect approximately 4.3 in 1000 recipients (78 of 18,014 patients from 234 transplant centers) with an attributable mortality of 84.6% [1]. In the year 2014, EBV-PTLD is still a life-threatening complication, however several main therapeutic approaches have been used for the prevention and treatment of EBV-PTLD, published as the recommendations by the European Conference on Infections in Leukemia (ECIL) [2]. These guidelines include the administration of rituximab, reduction of immunosuppression (RI) or use of EBV-specific cytotoxic T-lymphocytes (EBV-CTL). Based on the analysis of summary of reported cases of outcome of treatment of EBV-related PTLD in HSCT recipients, treatment with rituximab seems to be the most promise approach [3]. Recent reports indicate that the use of rituximab in EBV-PTLD is efficacious, particularly for recipients of solid organ transplants (SOT) [4-7]. On the other hand, data for HSCT recipients are based mainly on limited series, anecdotal reports and a single summary of reported cases [3,8-13].

Within Infectious Diseases Working Group (IDWP) of European Group for Blood and Marrow Transplantation (EBMT) a multicenter, retrospective analysis of 4466 allogeneic HSCTs performed in 19 pediatric and adult EBMT transplant centers in Europe was conducted [14]. Finally 144 pediatric and adult patients who had been treated with rituximab for PTLD after allo-HSCT were analyzed, and the factors that might be associated with survival were taken into account. In final report, children and adults were pooled together as one group [14]. The results of therapy of nine patients have been also published previously as case series [15-19]. However, it has been suggested that these two age populations were different in outcome, so possibly risk factors and prognostic models could have also been different. To address this, another retrospective analysis was undertaken to find out differences between results of therapy of children and adults with EBV-PTLD treated with rituximab. Thus, the objective of this study is the analysis of the risk factors that might be associated with survival of patients, separately children and adults, who had been treated with rituximab for PTLD after allo-HSCT.

Patients and Methods

This multicenter, retrospective analysis is based on the total number of 2120 pediatric and 2346 adult patients undergoing allogeneic HSCTs which were performed in 19 pediatric and adult EBMT transplant centers in Europe. Centers volunteered the data on each of their patients who had been treated with rituximab between 1999 and 2011 for PTLD by completing a questionnaire specifically designed for the purpose. The inclusion criteria were: proven or probable PTLD diagnosis and rituximab treatment administered either alone or combined with other approaches. The clinical data were entered into a centralized database. The study was approved by the Institutional Review Board of the Medical College, Nicolaus Copernicus University, Bydgoszcz, Poland.

Definitions

Patients of 18 years old or less were defined as children. The diagnosis of EBV-related PTLD was defined as proven or probable according to published definition [2]. Proven PTLD was diagnosed when EBV was detected in a specimen obtained from an organ by biopsy or other invasive procedure, with a test with appropriate sensitivity and specificity together with symptoms and signs from the affected organ [2,3,14]. Probable PTLD was defined as significant lymphadenopathy or other end-organ disease accompanied by a high EBV DNA blood load, in the absence of other etiologic factors or established diseases [2,3,14]. PTLD occurring within the first 100 days after transplantation was defined as early onset disease. EBV DNA-emia was measured by quantitative or qualitative PCR, either in whole blood, plasma, serum or in PBMC-based (Peripheral Blood Mononuclear Cells) assays. Repeated PCR testing was done at local sites using the same methodology throughout the study period. EBV DNA levels were determined before the beginning of therapy and one week after each dose of rituximab. Reduction of immunosuppression (RI) was defined as a sustained decrease of at least 20% of the daily dose of immunosuppressive drugs with the exception of low-dose corticosteroid therapy, i.e., ≤ 0.2 mg/kg in patients <40 kg of body weight or ≤ 10 mg/day in patients with >40 kg of body weight [20]. Response to given treatment was assessed on clinical level as complete remission, partial response, stable or progressive disease, according to standard definition [21]. The virologic response was also assessed based on EBV DNA-emia reduction. Failure of PTLD treatment was defined by death due to PTLD [14]. The cause of death was reported as being related to PTLD or due to other causes [14].

Statistical Analysis

Descriptive statistics were used to show the patients' general characteristics. Respective analyzes were performed separately for children and for adults. Percentages were reported for categorical variables, median and ranges for continuous variables and overall survival (OS) was calculated from the date of PTLD diagnosis to the date of death from any cause or to the date of the latest follow-up. Death due to any cause was considered as an event. Survival from PTLD was analyzed in a competing risks framework. The time from the date of PTLD diagnosis to the date of death due to PTLD, death due to other causes or to the date of the latest follow-up was considered. PTLD-related death was considered as the event of interest, death due to other causes was considered as a competing event, and patients who did not develop an event were censored at their last follow-up. The probabilities of survival from PTLD were estimated by the Kaplan-Meier curves using the proper non-parametric method. Univariate comparisons were performed using the log-rank test [22,23].

The impact of the following variables was analyzed: age at transplant (>5 *vs* <5 years and >10 *vs* <10 years for children and >30 *vs* <30 years for adults), underlying diagnosis (malignant *vs* not malignant), stem cell source (peripheral blood (PB) *vs* bone marrow (BM) *vs* cord blood), acute GVHD at the time of PTLD diagnosis (≥grade II *vs* <grade II or absent), PTLD organ involvement (extranodal *vs* nodal), initial EBV DNA-emia ($\geq 10^4$ *vs* $<10^4$ genome copies/mL (gc/mL), and $\geq 10^5$ *vs* $<10^5$ gc/mL), RI upon PTLD diagnosis (yes *vs* no). Multivariate analysis for PTLD mortality was performed by using the Cox regression in order to estimate hazards and cause-specific hazards, respectively, including as candidates only variables that resulted statistically significant at 0.10 level from univariate analysis [24].

In order to analyze the influence of the viral load after 1 and 2 weeks on survival from PTLD, a landmark analysis was performed using data on only those patients who survived up to 1 and 2 weeks after PTLD diagnosis. Absolute and logarithmic changes from baseline at week 0 were analyzed. A P-value below 0.05 was regarded as statistically significant.

Results

Frequency of PTLD in Children

PTLD had been diagnosed in 55 cases, a median of 2.1 months after HSCT (range 0.2-81). Early onset of PTLD affected 40 patients (72.7%). Nine patients (16%) developed PTLD in the first month, whereas 10 patients (18%) were diagnosed later than 6 months after HSCT. PTLD was proven by biopsy in 31 cases (56.3%) and the remaining 24 (43.7%) cases were considered probable disease.

The overall EBV-PTLD frequency in the participating centers was 2.59 % (55/2120), and ranged from 0.88% in matched-family donor (MFD), 1.62% in mismatched family donor (MMFD), 3.47% in matched unrelated donor (MUD), and 7.62% in mismatched unrelated donor (MMUD) recipients (Table 1). Overall, the frequency of PTLD after alternative donor (MMFD or unrelated donor) allo-HSCT was 3.61% (HR=4.21, 95%CI=1.82-10.2, P<0.001) and the PTLD frequency after cord blood transplantation (CBT) was 3.14% (HR=3.14, 95%CI=1.01-12.9, P=0.035).

Frequency of PTLD in Adults

PTLD had been diagnosed in 89 cases, a median of 1.9 months after HSCT (range 0.5-42). Early onset of PTLD affected 71 patients (79.7%). Two patients (2.2%) developed PTLD in the first month, whereas 5 patients (5.6%) were diagnosed later than 6 months after HSCT. PTLD was proven by biopsy in 55 cases (61.8%) and the remaining 34 (38.2%) cases were considered probable disease.

The overall EBV-PTLD frequency in the participating centers was 3.79 % (89/2346), and ranged from 1.35% in matched-family donor (MFD), 25.0% in mismatched family donor (MMFD), 4.27% in matched unrelated donor (MUD), and 18.92% in mismatched unrelated donor (MMUD) recipients (Table 2). Overall, the frequency of PTLD after alternative donor (MMFD or unrelated donor) allo-HSCT was 5.99% (HR=4.65, 95%CI=2.58-8.49, P<0.001) and the PTLD frequency after cord blood transplantation (CBT) was 4.84% (HR=3.71, 95%CI=1.48-9.17, P=0.003).

Adults vs Children: Analysis of Risk Failure of Therapy

The overall EBV-PTLD frequency in adults was higher than in children (OR=1.48, p=0.023). This relationship was similar in all types of transplant: in matched-family donor (MFD; OR=1.54, p=0.347), in mismatched family donor (MMFD; OR=20.1, p=0.0001), in matched unrelated donor (MUD; OR=1.24, p=0.411), and in mismatched unrelated donor (MMUD; OR=2.83, p=0.0018) recipients. Also, the frequency of PTLD after alternative donor (MMFD or unrelated donor) allo-HSCT was higher among adults than children (OR=1.69, p=0.005) as well as after cord blood transplantation (CBT; OR=1.58, p=0.414).

Baseline Characteristics of Children

The median age at transplant of 55 patients with PTLD was 7.8 years (range, 0.3-16.8). Baseline disease, patient characteristics and univariate risk of survival from PTLD mortality are reported in Table 3. Clinically, 28 patients (51%) had extranodal PTLD involvement, including 8 (14.5%) with multiorgan (i.e., more than 2 systems) involvement.

Table 1. Frequency of PTLD and hazard risk related to type of transplant in children

	Allo-HSCT total	PTLD	Frequencies [%]	HR (95%CI)	P
MFD	792	7	0.88	1	
MMFD	431	7	1.62	1.85 (0.58-5.90)	0.267
MUD	661	23	3.47	4.04 (1.64-10.4)	0.001
MMUD	236	18	7.63	9.26 (3.60-24.7)	<0.001
TOTAL	2120	55	2.59	2.99 (1.30-7.20)	0.006

PTLD, Post-Transplant Lymphoproliferative Disorder; MFD, matched family donor; MMFD, mismatched family donor; MUD, matched unrelated donor; MMUD, mismatched unrelated donor; CI, confidence interval.

Table 2. Frequency of PTLD and hazard risk related to type of transplant in adults

	Allo-HSCT total	PTLD	Frequencies [%]	HR (95%CI)	p
MFD	1110	15	1.35	1	
MMFD	24	6	25.00	24.3 (7.44-77.3)	<0.001
MUD	1101	47	4.27	3.26 (1.75-6.12)	<0.001
MMUD	111	21	18.92	17.0 (8.07-36.1)	<0.001
TOTAL	2346	89	3.79	2.88 (1.62-5.21)	<0.001

PTLD, Post-Transplant Lymphoproliferative Disorder; MFD, matched family donor; MMFD, mismatched family donor; MUD, matched unrelated donor; MMUD, mismatched unrelated donor; CI, confidence interval.

Table 3. Baseline patient and disease characteristics with univariate analysis for children

Characteristics	Patients	Events	HR (95%CI)	100-days survival from PTLD diagnosis	P
Age, years					
<5	20	3	0.53 (0.14-1.95)	85.0±8.0	0.318
≥5	35	9		74.3±7.4	
Age, years					
<10	33	6	0.63 (0.20-1.95)	81.8±6.7	0.404
≥10	22	6		72.7±9.5	
Malignant disease					
No	21	3	0.51 (0.14-1.89)	85.7±7.6	.294
Yes	34	9		73.5±7.6	
Reduced Intensity Conditioning					
No	40	10	1.94 (0.42-8.84)	75.0±6.8	0.372
Yes	15	2		86.7±8.8	
Year of HSCT					
<2009	37	7	0.66 (0.21-2.07)	81.1±6.4	0.456
≥2009	18	5		72.2±10.6	
Donor					
Other	48	12	25.3 (0.02-317.0)	75.0±6.3	0.154
Family matched	7	0		100.0±0.0	
Donor type					
Mismatched	25	8	2.55 (0.77-8.47)	68.0±9.3	0.104
Matched	30	4		86.7±6.2	
Source					
Peripheral blood	32	8	1.33 (0.17-10.66)	75.0±7.7	0.786
Bone marrow	18	3	0.86 (0.09-8.25)	83.3±8.8	
Cord blood	5	1		80.0±17.9	
Anti-thymocyte Globulin use					
No	13	2	0.61 (0.13-2.79)	84.6±10.0	0.511

Table 3. (Continued)

Characteristics	Patients	Events	HR (95%CI)	100-days survival from PTLD diagnosis	P
Yes	42	10		76.2±6.6	
Donor EBV serology					
Negative	8	1	0.51 (0.06-3.95)	87.5±11.7	0.494
Positive	43	10		76.7±6.4	
Recipient EBV serology					
Negative	18	1	0.16 (0.02-1.29)	94.4±5.4	0.043
Positive	33	10		69.7±8.0	
PTLD onset					
≤2 months	29	5	0.58 (0.18-1.84)	82.8±7.0	0.337
>2 months	26	7		73.1±8.7	
PTLD onset					
Early (≤100 days)	40	10	0.48 (0.11-2.20)	75.0±6.8	0.323
Late (>100 days)	15	2		86.7±8.8	
Acute GVHD≥ II at PTLD diagnosis					
No	46	7	0.32 (0.08-1.24)	84.8±5.3	0.076
Yes	7	3		57.1±18.7	
Extensive chronic GVHD at PTLD diagnosis					
No	11	1	0.38 (0.02-6.10)	90.9±8.7	0.479
Yes	4	1		75.0±21.7	
Extranodal involvement					
No	27	2	0.19 (0.04-0.85)	92.6±5.0	0.013
Yes	28	10		64.3±9.1	
Multiorgan involvement					
No	47	8	0.31 (0.09-1.02)	83.0±5.5	0.036
Yes	8	4		50.0±17.7	
Level of PTLD diagnosis					
Probable	24	6	1.37 (0.44-4.25)	75.0±8.8	0.573
Proven	31	6		80.6±7.1	
Histology					
Polyclonal	5	0	0.04 (0.00-174.0)	100.0±0.0	0.334
Monoclonal/HD-like	23	4		82.6±7.9	
PTLD CD20 status					
Negative	1	0	0.05 (0.00-395.0)	100.0±0.0	0.692
Positive	27	4		85.2±6.8	
Initial EBVDNA-emia ≥10,000 gc/mL					
No	16	2	0.44 (0.10-2.01)	87.5±8.3	0.265
Yes	38	10		73.7±7.1	
Initial EBV DNA-emia ≥100,000 gc/mL					
No	28	3	0.28 (0.08-1.04)	89.3±5.8	0.037
Yes	26	9		65.4±9.3	
Initial EBV DNA-emia ≥1,000,000 gc/mL					
No	37	9	1.37 (0.37-5.04)	75.7±7.1	0.63

Characteristics	Patients	Events	HR (95%CI)	100-days survival from PTLD diagnosis	P
Yes	17	3		82.4±9.2	
Reduction of IS therapy					
No	21	8	3.63 (1.09-12.08)	61.9±10.6	0.021
Yes	34	4		88.2±5.5	
Chemotherapy					
No	42	7	0.43 (0.14-1.35)	83.3±5.8	0.125
Yes	13	5		61.5±13.5	
Donor Lymphocyte Infusion					
No	53	11	0.31 (0.04-2.40)	79.2±5.6	0.221
Yes	2	1		50.0±35.4	
Total Parenteral Nutrition					
No	33	3	0.17 (0.05-0.62)	90.9±5.0	0.002
Yes	19	9		52.6±11.5	
Bone marrow insufficiency					
No	24	3	0.37 (0.10-1.37)	87.5±6.8	0.111
Yes	28	9		67.9±8.8	
Platelet transfusion					
No	30	4	0.35 (0.11-1.17)	86.7±6.2	0.067
Yes	22	8		63.6±10.3	
Blood transfusion					
No	25	3	0.34 (0.09-1.26)	88.0±6.5	0.081
Yes	27	9		66.7±9.1	

PTLD, Post-Transplant Lymphoproliferative Disorder; HSCT, Hematopoietic Stem Cell Transplantation; GVHD, Graft-versus-Host-Disease; EBV, Epstein-Barr Virus; HD, Hodgkin Disease; IS, Immunosuppressive; CI, confidence interval

Baseline Characteristics of Adults

The median age at transplant of 144 patients with PTLD was 40.7 years (range, 18.1-68). Baseline disease, patient characteristics and univariate risk of survival from PTLD are reported in Table 4. Clinically, 3 patients (37%) had extranodal PTLD involvement, including 7 (7.8%) with multiorgan (i.e., more than 2 systems) involvement.

Table 4. Baseline patient and disease characteristics with univariate analysis for adults

Characteristics	Patients	Events	HR (95%CI)	100-days survival from PTLD diagnosis	p
Age, years					
<30	25	3	0.23 (0.07-0.75)	88.0±6.5	0.006
≥30	64	29		54.7±6.2	

Table 4. (Continued)

Characteristics	Patients	Events	HR (95%CI)	100-days survival from PTLD diagnosis	p
Malignant disease					
No	11	2	0.42 (0.10-1.74)	81.8±11.6	0.197
Yes	78	30		61.5±5.5	
Reduced Intensity Conditioning					
No	34	12	0.92 (0.45-1.88)	64.7±8.2	0.81
Yes	55	20		63.6±6.5	
Year of HSCT					
<2009	55	25	2.61 (1.13-6.05)	54.5±6.7	0.015
≥2009	34	7		79.4±6.9	
Donor					
Other	74	29	2.19 (0.67-7.19)	60.8±5.7	0.167
Family matched	15	3		80.0±10.3	
Donor type					
Mismatched	27	10	1.07 (0.51-2.26)	63.0±9.3	0.848
Matched	62	22		64.5±6.1	
Source					
Peripheral blood	76	28	0.83 (0.29-2.37)	63.2±5.5	0.353
Bone marrow	4	0	0.00 (0.00-183)	100.0±0.0	
Cord blood	9	4		55.6±16.6	
Anti-thymocyte Globulin use					
No	15	5	0.86 (0.33-2.25)	66.7±12.2	0.755
Yes	74	27		63.5±5.6	
Donor EBV serology					
Negative	13	5	1.10 (0.42-2.87)	61.5±13.5	0.845
Positive	67	24		64.2±5.9	
Recipient EBV serology					
Negative	6	4	2.46 (0.86-7.06)	33.3±19.2	0.07
Positive	78	26		66.7±5.3	
PTLD onset					
≤2 months	40	14	0.93 (0.46-1.88)	65.0±7.5	0.843
>2 months	49	18		63.3±6.9	
PTLD onset					
Early (≤100 days)	71	26	0.88 (0.36-2.15)	63.4±5.7	0.777
Late (>100 days)	18	6		66.7±11.1	
Acute GVHD≥ II at PTLD diagnosis					
No	79	27	0.48 (0.11-2.04)	65.8±5.3	0.292
Yes	3	2		33.3±27.2	
Extensive chronic GVHD at PTLD diagnosis					
No	11	4	1.25 (0.23-6.84)	63.6±14.5	0.788
Yes	7	2		71.4±17.1	

Characteristics	Patients	Events	HR (95%CI)	100-days survival from PTLD diagnosis	p
Extranodal involvement					
No	56	16	0.53 (0.27-1.07)	71.4±6.0	0.059
Yes	33	16		51.5±8.7	
Multiorgan involvement					
No	82	27	0.39 (0.15-1.02)	67.1±5.2	0.036
Yes	7	5		28.6±17.1	
Level of PTLD diagnosis					
Probable	34	8	0.50 (0.22-1.11)	76.5±7.3	0.168
Proven	55	24		56.4±6.7	
Histology					
Polyclonal	12	4	0.58 (0.20-1.66)	66.7±13.6	0.275
Monoclonal/HD-like	49	25		49.0±7.1	
PTLD CD20 status					
Negative	9	6	1.77 (0.71-4.37)	33.3±15.7	0.191
Positive	50	22		56.0±7.0	
Initial EBV DNA-emia ≥10,000 gc/mL					
No	17	2	0.27 (0.06-1.13)	88.2±7.8	0.046
Yes	68	26		61.8±5.9	
Initial EBV DNA-emia ≥100,000 gc/mL					
No	53	16	0.80 (0.38-1.69)	69.8±6.3	0.542
Yes	32	12		62.5±8.6	
Initial EBV DNA-emia ≥1,000,000 gc/mL					
No	69	20	0.56 (0.25-1.27)	71.0±5.5	0.139
Yes	16	8		50.0±12.5	
Reduction of IS therapy					
No	63	27	2.49 (0.96-6.48)	57.1±6.2	0.043
Yes	26	5		80.8±7.7	
Chemotherapy					
No	71	22	0.56 (0.26-1.18)	69.0±5.5	0.106
Yes	18	10		44.4±11.7	
Donor Lymphocyte Infusion					
No	80	30	1.98 (0.47-8.28)	62.5±5.4	0.321
Yes	9	2		77.8±13.9	
Total Parenteral Nutrition					
No	71	23	0.52 (0.24-1.13)	67.6±5.6	0.079
Yes	18	9		50.0±11.8	
Bone marrow insufficiency					
No	42	10	0.46 (0.22-0.97)	76.2±6.6	0.029
Yes	47	22		53.2±7.3	
Platelet transfusion					
No	52	11	0.31 (0.15-0.63)	78.8±5.7	0.001
Yes	37	21		43.2±8.1	

Table 4. (Continued)

Characteristics	Patients	Events	HR (95%CI)	100-days survival from PTLD diagnosis	p
Blood transfusion					
No	41	10	0.48 (0.23-1.02)	75.6±6.7	0.043
Yes	48	22		54.2±7.2	

PTLD, Post-Transplant Lymphoproliferative Disorder; HSCT, Hematopoietic Stem Cell Transplantation; GVHD, Graft-versus-Host-Disease; EBV, Epstein-Barr Virus; HD, Hodgkin Disease; IS, Immunosuppressive; CI, confidence interval.

Adults vs Children: Analysis of Therapy Risk Failure

In comparison of risk factors of therapy failure between adults and children (Table 5), following factors contributed to significantly better outcome in EBV-PTLD in children than in adult population: year of hematopoietic stem cell transplantation before 2009 (3.5-fold), matched donor HSCT (3.5-fold), recipient negative EBV serology (34-fold), absence of acute GVHD>II grade at diagnosis (2.9-fold), no extranodal involvement (5-fold), no multiorgan involvement (2.9-fold), proven PTLD diagnosis (3.2-fold), monoclonal/HD-like histology of PTLD (4.9-fold), positive PTLD CD20 status (4.5-fold), initial EBV DNA-emia <100,000 gc/mL (3.6-fold), initial EBV DNA-emia >1,000,000 gc/mL (4.6-fold), no Total Parenteral Nutrition at PTLD diagnosis (4.8-fold).

Table 5. Univariate analysis of therapy risk failure in adults in comparison to children

Characteristics	Children Patients	Children Events	Adults Patients	Adults Events	Odds ratio (95%CI)	p
Malignant disease						
No	21	3	11	2	1.33 (0.13-12.9)	0.999
Yes	34	9	78	30	1.74 (0.66-4.65)	0.553
Reduced Intensity Conditioning						
No	40	10	34	12	1.64 (0.54-5.03)	0.477
Yes	15	2	55	20	3.71 (0.68-26.5)	0.121
Year of HSCT						
<2009	37	7	55	25	3.57 (1.23-10.7)	0.016
≥2009	18	5	34	7	0.67 (0.15-3.07)	0.730
Donor						
Other	48	12	74	29	1.93 (0.81-4.68)	0.154
Family matched	7	0	15	3	undefined	0.522
Donor type						
Mismatched	25	8	27	10	1.25 (0.34-4.60)	0.928
Matched	30	4	62	22	3.58 (1.00-13.9)	0.049
Source						
Peripheral blood	32	8	76	28	1.75 (0.64-4.91)	0.332

Characteristics	Children Patients	Children Events	Adults Patients	Adults Events	Odds ratio (95%CI)	p
Bone marrow	18	3	4	0	0.0 (0.0-13.8)	0.999
Cord blood	5	1	9	4	3.20 (0.17-11.2)	0.580
Anti-thymocyte Globulin use						
No	13	2	15	5	2.75 (0.34-26.7)	0.395
Yes	42	10	74	27	1.84 (0.73-4.72)	0.229
Donor EBV serology						
Negative	8	1	13	5	4.38 (0.32-125)	0.335
Positive	43	10	67	24	1.84 (0.72-4.80)	0.237
Recipient EBV serology						
Negative	18	1	6	4	34.0 (1.77-1529)	0.006
Positive	33	10	78	26	1.15 (0.44-3.04)	0.928
PTLD onset						
≤2 months	29	5	40	14	2.58 (0.72-7.77)	0.174
>2 months	26	7	49	18	1.58 (0.50-5.11)	0.548
PTLD onset						
Early (≤100days)	40	10	71	26	1.73 (0.68-4.51)	0.296
Late (>100 days)	15	2	18	6	3.25 (0.44-29.1)	0.241
Acute GVHD≥ II at PTLD diagnosis						
No	46	7	79	27	2.89 (1.06-8.18)	0.036
Yes	7	3	3	2	2.67 (0.09-129)	0.979
Extensive chronic GVHD at PTLD diagnosis						
No	11	1	11	4	5.71 (0.41-168)	0.310
Yes	4	1	7	2	1.20 (0.0-52.9)	0.999
Extranodal involvement						
No	27	2	56	16	5.00 (1.03-34.47)	0.028
Yes	28	10	33	16	1.69 (0.54-5.42)	0.456
Multiorgan involvement						
No	47	8	82	27	2.39 (1.01-6.43)	0.050
Yes	8	4	7	5	2.50 (0.19-37.7)	0.608
Level of PTLD diagnosis						
Probable	24	6	34	8	0.92 (0.23-3.68)	0.855
Proven	31	6	55	24	3.23 (1.04-10.4)	0.042
Histology						
Polyclonal	5	0	12	4	undefined	0.260
Monoclonal/HD-like	23	4	49	25	4.95 (1.31-20.2)	0.014
PTLD CD20 status						
Negative	1	0	9	6	undefined	0.400
Positive	27	4	50	22	4.52 (1.22-18.1)	0.019
Initial EBV DNA-emia ≥10000 gc/mL						
No	16	2	17	2	0.93 (0.08-11.1)	0.999
Yes	38	10	68	26	1.73 (0.67-4.55)	0.303
Initial EBV DNA-emia ≥100000 gc/mL						
No	28	3	53	16	3.60 (1.05-17.4)	0.049
Yes	26	9	32	12	1.13 (0.34-3.83)	0.962

Table 5. (Continued)

Characteristics	Children Patients	Children Events	Adults Patients	Adults Events	Odds ratio (95% CI)	p
Initial EBV DNA-emia ≥1000000 gc/mL						
No	37	9	69	20	1.27 (0.47-3.50)	0.775
Yes	17	3	16	8	4.67 (1.07-31.4)	0.048
Reduction of IS therapy						
No	21	8	63	27	1.22 (0.40-3.78)	0.898
Yes	34	4	26	5	1.79 (0.36-9.23)	0.482
Chemotherapy						
No	42	7	71	22	2.24 (0.80-6.54)	0.143
Yes	13	5	18	10	2.00 (0.37-11.1)	0.564
Donor Lymphocyte Infusion						
No	53	11	80	30	2.29 (0.96-5.55)	0.063
Yes	2	1	9	2	0.29 (0.0-17.3)	0.470
Total Parenteral Nutrition						
No	33	3	71	23	4.79 (1.21-22.0)	0.020
Yes	19	9	18	9	1.11 (0.25-4.93)	0.862
Bone marrow insufficiency						
No	24	3	42	10	2.19 (0.47-11.4)	0.185
Yes	28	9	47	22	1.86 (0.63-5.56)	0.314
Platelet transfusion						
No	30	4	52	11	1.74 (0.44-7.34)	0.558
Yes	22	8	37	21	2.30 (0.68-7.88)	0.696
Blood transfusion						
No	25	3	41	10	2.37 (0.51-12.3)	0.340
Yes	27	9	48	22	1.69 (0.57-5.08)	0.577

Age As a Risk Factor

When age was taken into account as a risk factor of therapy failure, it has been shown that the survival from PTLD was worse with the increasing age (Table 6). Thus, it can be concluded that age is a continuous variable of poor outcome of therapy of PTLD with rituximab.

Treatment of Children

Patients were treated with a median of 3 doses of rituximab (range, 1-16), administered at dosage of 375 mg/m^2 at weekly intervals, except in 2 cases that were treated at 3-6 days intervals. Tapering off of immunosuppression was done in 34 cases. Chemotherapy was administered as a second line therapy because of a partial response, or stable or progressive disease to 13 patients (23.6%), including 6 out of 34 patients who had immunosuppression tapered and 7/21 without RI. Additional therapies included surgery in 3 cases and donor lymphocyte infusion (DLI) in 2 cases. In 30 patients antiviral agents were also used (mainly cidofovir), but it had no impact on survival from PTLD.

Treatment of Adults

Patients were treated with a median of 3 doses of rituximab (range, 1-16), administered at dosage of 375 mg/m^2 at weekly intervals, except in 4 cases that were treated at 3-6 days intervals, and a further single case that was treated every 10 days. Tapering off of immunosuppression was done in 26 cases. Chemotherapy was administered as a second line therapy because of a partial response, or stable or progressive disease to 18 patients (20.2%), including none out of 26 patients who had immunosuppression tapered and 18/63 without RI. Additional therapies included surgery in 1 case and donor lymphocyte infusion (DLI) in 9 cases. In 18 patients antiviral agents were also used (mainly cidofovir), but it had no impact on survival from PTLD.

Survival after PTLD in Children

Fourty-three (78.2%) patients survived after rituximab-based therapy, and 12 died due to PTLD. Only those who achieved a complete remission survived from PTLD. The overall survival from PTLD was 78.7±5.7% (Figure 1). PTLD resolved in 30 of 34 (82.3%) patients who received both rituximab and RI, and in 13 of 21 patients (61.9%) in whom immunosuppression tapering was not done (P=0.006). RI reduced the risk of death due to PTLD 3.6-fold in univariate analysis (Table 3). Despite chemotherapy as second line treatment, only 1 out of 7 patients without RI survived. No differences in PTLD mortality was found in proven vs probable PTLD categories both for patients with RI (1/18 vs 3/16, p=0.91) and without RI (5/13 vs 3/8, p=0.45).

Table 6. Age as a risk factor

Age groups	Patients	Events	Odds ratio (95%CI)	100-days survival from PTLD	P
Children, years					
<5	20	3	0.53 (0.14-1.95)	85.0±8.0	0.318
≥5	35	9		74.3±7.4	
Children, years					
<10	33	6	0.63 (0.20-1.95)	81.8±6.7	0.404
≥10	22	6		72.7±9.5	
All patients, years					
<18	54	11	0.50 (0.26-0.98)	78.2±5.0	0.040
≥18	90	33		64.0±5.1	
All patients, years					
<30	79	14	0.32 (0.19-0.62)	82.2±4.9	0.0003
≥30	65	30		53.6±5.1	
Adults, years					
<30	25	3	0.23 (0.07-0.75)	88.0±6.5	0.006
≥30	64	29		54.7±6.2	

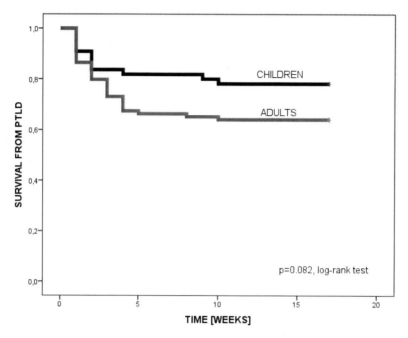

Figure 1. Survival from PTLD in children and adults.

There was no difference in PTLD mortality with respect to the type of transplant. The level of diagnosis expressed as proven or probable had no impact on PTLD mortality (p=0.57). Monomorphic vs polymorphic PTLD disease also had no difference in outcome (Table 3).

Factors predicting good outcome of PTLD therapy by univariate analysis in children were: nodal involvement only, initial EBV DNA-emia <10^5 gc/mL, recipient EBV negative serology, necessity of TPN at PTLD diagnosis and RI at PTLD diagnosis (Table 3). Reduction of immunosuppression was statistically not related to occurrence of acute GVHD at PTLD diagnosis (p=0.46).

Multivariate analysis for survival from PTLD was performed by using the significant prognostic factors identified in univariate analysis. Two variables remained that had prognostic significance for survival from PTLD: (i) nodal involvement only, (ii) RI at PTLD diagnosis (Table 7). A decreasing number of independent variables was associated with markedly different survival from PTLD; with 2, 1, or 0 factors the survival was 94%, 86% and 30%, respectively (P<0.0001) (Figure 2).

Table 7. Multivariate analysis of prognostic factors in children

Prognostic Factor	Survival from PTLD		
	Hazard Ratio	95% CI	P
Nodal involvement only vs extranodal involvement	5.7	1.2-26	0.024
Immunosuppression reduction upon PTLD diagnosis vs no reduction	4.3	1.3-14	0.017

PTLD, Post-Transplant Lymphoproliferative Disorder; Graft-versus-Host-Disease; CI, confidence interval.

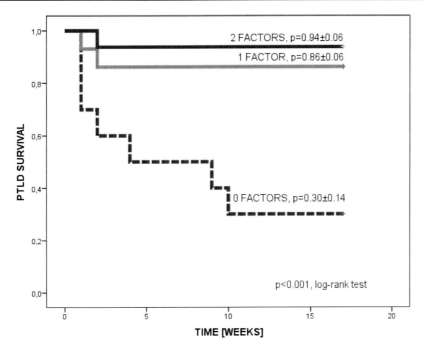

Figure 2. Pediatric 2-factors prognostic model.

This model maintained its predictivity when it was repeated in the two subgroups of patients with proven and probable diagnosis. Survival from PTLD in patients with proven diagnosis was 89%, 75% and 33% for 2, 1 or 0 factors, respectively (p=0.017), while in patients with probable diagnosis the survival from PTLD was 100%, 94% and 29% for 2, 1 or 0 factors, respectively (p<0.001).

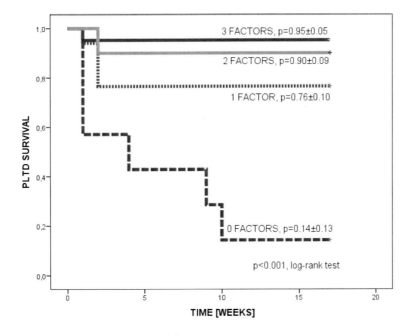

Figure 3. Pediatric 3-factors prognostic model.

Another prognostic model was prepared with the use of three factors. Apart from nodal involvement only, and RI at PTLD diagnosis, a third factor was taken into account: EBV DNA-emia at diagnosis <10^5 gc/mL (which was also significant in univariate analysis, Table 3). A decreasing number of independent variables was associated with markedly different survival from PTLD; with 3, 2, 1, or 0 factors the survival was 95%, 90%, 76% and 14%, respectively (P<0.0001) (Figure 3).

Since already one favorable factor is sufficient for probability of survival from PTLD in pediatric 3-factor model over 76%, it can be suggested that in case of EBV DNA-emia at diagnosis <10^5 gc/mL, reduction of immunosuppression might not be necessary.

Survival after PTLD in Adults

Fifty-seven (64%) patients survived after rituximab-based therapy, and 32 died due to PTLD. Only those who achieved a complete remission survived from PTLD. The overall survival from PTLD was 62.8±5.3% (Figure 1). PTLD resolved in 21 of 26 (81%) patients who received both rituximab and RI, and in 36 of 63 patients (57%) in whom immunosuppression tapering was not done (P=0.006). RI reduced the risk of death due to PTLD 2.5-fold in univariate analysis (Table 4). Despite chemotherapy as second line treatment, only 8/18 (44%) of the patients without RI survived. No differences in PTLD mortality was found in proven vs probable PTLD categories both for patients with RI (4/13 vs 1/13, p=0.32) and without RI (20/42 vs 7/21, p=0.41).

Mortality due to PTLD was lower in children than in adults (22% vs 36%, p=0.08). There were no differences in PTLD mortality with respect to the type of transplant. The level of diagnosis expressed as proven or probable had no impact on PTLD mortality in adults (p=0.16). Monomorphic vs polymorphic PTLD disease also had no difference in outcome in adults (Table 4).

Factors predicting good outcome of PTLD therapy by univariate analysis were: age <30 years, year of transplantation>2008, involvement of less than 2 systems, initial EBV DNA-emia <10^4 gc/mL, no bone marrow insufficiency (expressed as necessity of platelets or erythrocytes transfusion) and RI at PTLD diagnosis (Table 4). Reduction of immunosuppression was related to occurrence of acute GVHD at PTLD diagnosis (p=0.016).

Multivariate analysis for survival from PTLD was performed by using the significant prognostic factors identified in univariate analysis. Three variables remained that had prognostic significance for survival from PTLD: (i) age at transplant <30 years, (ii) initial EBV DNA-emia <10^4 gc/mL, (iii) RI at PTLD diagnosis (Table 8). A decreasing number of independent variables was associated with markedly different survival from PTLD; with 3, 2, 1 or 0 factors the survival was 100%, 92%, 79% and 38%, respectively (P<0.0001) (Figure 4).

This model maintained its predictivity when it was repeated in the two subgroups of patients with proven and probable diagnosis. Survival from PTLD in patients with proven diagnosis was 100%, 100%, 88% and 45% for 3, 2, 1 or 0 factors, respectively (p=0.023), while in patients with probable diagnosis the survival from PTLD was 100%, 87%, 65% and 34% for 3, 2, 1 or 0 factors, respectively (p=0.011).

Another prognostic model was prepared with the use of four factors. Apart from age at transplant <30 years, initial EBV DNA-emia <10^4 gc/mL, and RI at PTLD diagnosis, a fourth factor was taken into account: nodal involvement only (which was also significant in univariate analysis, Table 4). A decreasing number of independent variables was associated with markedly different survival from PTLD; with 4, 3, 2, 1, or 0 factors the survival was 100%, 89%, 86%, 55% and 25%, respectively (P<0.0001) (Figure 5).

Response to Therapy with Respect to Blood Viral Load in Children

Initial EBV DNA-emia was analyzed before the beginning of the therapy and a week after each dose of rituximab. A decrease of EBV DNA-emia improved the PTLD prognosis, while an increase of EBV DNA-emia after one or two weeks of therapy was predictor of poor response and increased the risk of death from PTLD by 6.4 and 2.0-fold in univariate analysis, respectively (Table 9).

Table 8. Multivariate analysis of prognostic factors in adults

Prognostic Factor	Survival from PTLD		
	Hazard Ratio	95% CI	P
Age <30 years vs ≥30 years	6.3	1.5-26	0.012
EBV DNA-emia <10,000 copies/mL at diagnosis	4.6	1.1-19	0.038
Immunosuppression reduction upon PTLD diagnosis vs no reduction	5.0	1.2-21	0.028

PTLD, Post-Transplant Lymphoproliferative Disorder; Graft-versus-Host-Disease; CI, confidence interval.

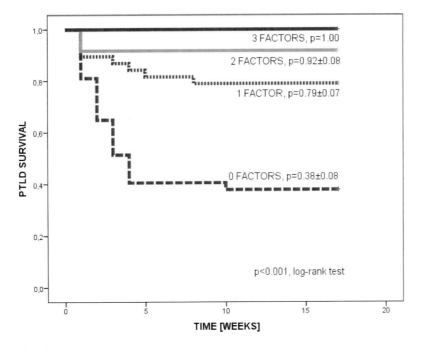

Figure 4. Adult 3-factors prognostic model.

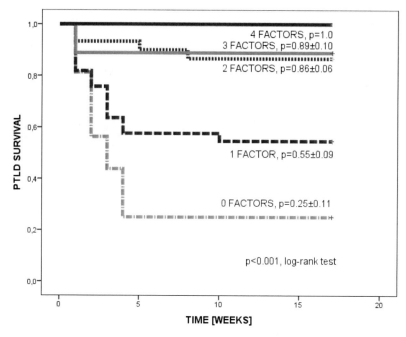

Figure 5. Adult 4-factors prognostic model.

Table 9. Hazards and survival from PTLD according to viral load response in children

Viral Load Response*	Patients	Events	HR (95% CI)	Survival from PTLD	P
Week 1					
Decreased	23	1	6.4 (0.79-52)	96±4%	0.041
Increased or stable	27	7	1.00	74±8%	
Week 2					
Decreased	35	4	2.0 (0.46-9.3)	88±5%	0.319
Increased or stable	14	3	1.00	78±11%	

Univariate HR by viral load variations at 1 and 2 weeks after beginning of rituximab therapy and cumulative incidence of survival from PTLD at 1 and at 2 weeks. Viral load was analyzed at 1 and 2 weeks in patients who were alive at each time-point (land-mark analysis). PTLD, Post-Transplant Lymphoproliferative Disorder; HR, Hazard Risk; CI, confidence interval.

* Logarithmic change in viral load was employed. Change in EBV DNA load of at least 1 log of magnitude was considered significant.

Response to Therapy with Respect to Blood Viral Load in Adults

Initial EBV DNA-emia was analyzed before the beginning of the therapy and a week after each dose of rituximab. A decrease of EBV DNA-emia improved the PTLD prognosis, while an increase of EBV DNA-emia after one or two weeks of therapy was predictor of poor response and increased the risk of death from PTLD by 5.7 and 4.8-fold in univariate analysis, respectively (Table 10).

Table 10. Hazards and survival from PTLD according to viral load response in adults

Viral Load Response*	Patients	Events	HR (95% CI)	Survival from PTLD	P
Week 1					
Decreased	25	2	5.7 (1.3-24.7)	92±5%	0.006
Increased or stable	52	20	1.00	61±6%	
Week 2					
Decreased	43	5	4.8 (1.7-13.3)	55±9%	0.001
Increased or stable	31	14	1.00	88±5%	

Univariate HR by viral load variations at 1 and 2 weeks after beginning of rituximab therapy and cumulative incidence of survival from PTLD at 1 and at 2 weeks. Viral load was analyzed at 1 and 2 weeks in patients who were alive at each time-point (land-mark analysis). PTLD, Post-Transplant Lymphoproliferative Disorder; HR, Hazard Risk; CI, confidence interval.

* Logarithmic change in viral load was employed. Change in EBV DNA load of at least 1 log of magnitude was considered significant.

Discussion

Epstein-Barr virus (EBV)-associated B-cell lymphoproliferation is a life-threatening complication after hematopoietic stem cell or solid organ transplantation resulting from outgrowth of EBV-infected B cells that would normally be controlled by EBV-cytotoxic T cells. During the past decade, new treatment options including manipulation of the balance between outgrowing EBV-infected B cells and the EBV cytotoxic T lymphocyte response and targeting the B cells with monoclonal antibodies or chemotherapy have helped to treat high-risk patients with lymphoproliferation [25]. The treatment of PTLD is a complex task requiring special considerations and supportive therapy. Antibody therapy based on targeting B cells is nowadays regarded as the most promising option, which is possible to use in all HSCT centers [2]. Rituximab, a chimeric mouse/human anti-CD20 monoclonal antibody, which binds to the surface and elicits the lysis of CD20-positive normal and malignant B-cells, has been a breakthrough in PTLD therapy. The antibody is generally well tolerated and rapidly induces the depletion of mature B-lymphocytes, reducing the compartment of EBV-infected cells, with an associated normalization of the viral load [26].

It was estimated for patients undergoing HSCT in the last decades of twentieth century, that post-HSCT EBV-PTLD caused mortality of 84.6% [1]. With the beginning of 21 century, new therapeutic strategies were introduced for patients with EBV-PTLD. As most cases of PTLD arise in donor- or recipient-derived B cells, basic strategy for prevention and treatment is to eliminate EBV-infected B cells [25]. Antibody therapy targets B cell-specific surface antigens present on the EBV-transformed malignant cells. The most widely used antibody is rituximab, a chimeric murine/human monoclonal anti-CD20 antibody. Rituximab has been used as prophylaxis of PTLD after HSCT, with good initial response rates over 50% for small groups of patients, with wide range of responses reflecting differences in the treated patient populations [25,27-29].

In the summary of reported cases of outcome of treatment of Epstein-Barr virus-related PTLD in HSCT recipients, it was shown that with current approaches the mortality from

EBV-PTLD can be significantly reduced [3]. The published literature and meeting abstracts assessed for the impact of different management strategies against EBV-PTLD. In this analysis of reported outcomes, preemptive use of rituximab and EBV-cytotoxic T lymphocytes (CTL) significantly reduced the risk of death due to EBV-PTLD in HSCT recipients with survival rates of 89.7% and 94.1%, respectively. Although it was difficult to estimate these effects more precisely because of the frequent use of combination therapies, treatment of established PTLD also reduced the risk of fatal outcome. However, the overall success rates were lower than after preemptive therapy, reaching 63% and 88.2% of total EBV DNA clearance with rituximab and CTL therapy, respectively [3]. Rituximab is administered as pre-emptive therapy in most transplant centers, although different approaches regarding indications for preemptive therapy are seen between centers [30]. Rituximab was shown also to be safe and effective when administered intrathecally in central nervous system involvement [31].

In this analysis of hematopoietic stem cell transplant setting, the frequency of PTLD was higher in adults than in children (3.79% vs 2.59%). This relationship was observed in all types of transplants, regardless on the type of donor: MFD (1.35% vs 0.88%), MMFD (25% vs 1.62%), MUD (4.27% vs 3.47%), MMUD (18.92% vs 7.63%), and also for HSCT with the use of cord blood as the stem cell source (4.84% vs 3.14%). Thus, these differences are multifactorial. Some explanations can include: lower rate of EBV infections in children, both donors and recipients; better tolerance of graft in children due to overall better immunologic tolerance; lower rate of GVHD in children, and possibly faster rate of immunological reconstitution in children disabling development of EBV-PTLD.

On the other hand, in solid organ transplant setting the frequency of PTLD is higher in childhood, regardless of the transplanted organ: the incidence is 2 to 3-fold, compared to adults. Pediatric patients are often EBV-seronegative, and PTLD might be induced by primary EBV infection [26,32].

With respect to outcome of therapy of EBV-PTLD based on the use of rituximab, several factors determined in univariate and multivariate analyses contributed to survival from PTLD. Although these factors were similar for both populations, final independent positive risk factors predicting good outcome of therapy found in multivariate analysis were different for childhood and adulthood. In pediatric populations two variables remained their independent prognostic significance for survival from PTLD: nodal involvement only, and RI at PTLD diagnosis. In adult patients, three variables remained that had prognostic significance for survival from PTLD: age at transplant <30 years, initial EBV DNA-emia $<10^4$ gc/mL, and RI at PTLD diagnosis. Consistent with PTLD in SOT recipients [33], by using these factors, risk-stratified survival prognostic models were developed - separately for children and for adults.

Thus, finally four risk factors needs more detailed discussion: age, extranodal involvement, EBV viremia and reduction of immunosuppression at PTLD diagnosis.

It was shown in this study, that age at transplant is a risk factor for therapy failure. In general, in HSCT setting of EBV-PTLD, age can be regarded as independent continuous variable. Children had better outcome than adults, younger children had better outcome than older ones, young adults (<30 years) had better outcome than those over 30 years at diagnosis. It is regarded that an increasing age is an adverse risk factor for the successful therapy of lymphomas [34,35].

Clinical manifestation limited to nodal involvement only reflects lower stage of the disease. PTLD may present with variable symptoms: fever, lymphadenopathy, weight loss, intestinal perforation and septic shock. Extranodal manifestations (liver, lung, intestines, kidney, tonsil, bone marrow and skin) are however, common. Central nervous system involvement may be as high as 30%, compared to only 1% among non-Hodgkin lymphomas of the non-transplanted population [36]. In SOT setting, PTLD may appear in the transplanted organ, the likelihood of which correlates with the time interval after transplantation: more cases appear in the graft within the first year after transplant [26]. Extra-nodal PTLD usually corresponds to disseminated type of the disease. As with the disseminated stage III and IV of lymphomas, a higher mortality rate can be expected in these patients compared to those with less advanced disease. An increasing age and extranodal involvement are usually regarded as adverse risk factors for the successful therapy of lymphomas [34,35].

Another factor that corresponds to initial stage of the disease might be EBV viremia. High EBV load, as defined by number of viral DNA genome copies in blood or serum (with cut-off value either 10^4 gc/mL or 10^4 gc/mL) might be a new factor (more stronger in adults, less in children), as far as response to therapy in PTLD is concerned. With the development of quantitative analysis of EBV DNA-emia, viral load can be regarded as a risk factor not only at diagnosis, but also as an initial response to rituximab-based therapy. An increase of EBV DNA-emia after 1-2 weeks of therapy with rituximab was related to poor prognosis (more stronger in adults, less in children, particularly after 2 weeks). This allows to propose a definition of early molecular response as a decrease of EBV DNA-emia after one- or two weeks of rituximab-based therapy [14].

Reduction of immunosuppression was shown to have beneficial effect in pre-emptive therapy of EBV DNA-emia and is also included in the ECIL recommendations [2,20,37]. Reduction of immunosuppressive therapy is recommended for all patients diagnosed with PTLD, whenever possible [2]. In baseline analysis of patients treated with rituximab, PTLD-associated mortality was significantly higher when immunosuppressive therapy was not reduced [14]. Acute GVHD≥grade II requires intensive immunosuppression, thus limiting the possibilities of RI. Advanced GVHD, both acute and chronic, is also influenced by significant immunologic impairment. It is also important that rituximab given for PTLD treatment, may decrease severity of GVHD [38,39]. Rituximab can also prevent systemic corticosteroid-requiring chronic GVHD after peripheral blood stem cell transplantation [40].

Additional, "second line" risk factors which could contribute to better survival from PTLD were: EBV DNA-emia at diagnosis <10^5 gc/mL in children, and nodal involvement only in adults. These factors, however, reflect *vice-versa* "first line" independent risk factors in children and adults.

There are also some pitfalls arising with the use of rituximab. Because CD20 expression is not confined to the malignant cells, normal B cells are also destroyed. This can be a significant concern in patients who are already immunosuppressed, and fatal viral infections have been reported after rituximab therapy [25,41]. Rituximab can deplete B cells for more than 6 months in these already immunosuppressed patients. An additional concern is that, when used as therapy, it does not restore the cellular immune response to EBV, which is a crucial requirement if EBV-mediated B-cell proliferation is to be controlled long-term [42]. This rather may not be a major problem in most HSCT recipients, in whom recovery of a donor-derived immune response should provide long-term protection, but it is a concern in solid organ transplant patients who remain on long-term immunosuppression. Another concern is that only one antigen is targeted and antigen-loss tumor cell variants may be selected [25].

Other therapeutic options are also possible in the treatment of EBV-PTLD in HSCT setting. Although it is difficult to estimate these effects more precisely because of the frequent use of combination therapies, a reduction of immunosuppression and/or donor lymphocyte infusion might also reduce the risk of death due to EBV-PTLD, with the response rates to these modalities estimated to be 56% and 41%, respectively. Finally, chemotherapy seems not to contribute to improved survival of patients with PTLD after HSCT and antiviral agents are not active against PTLD [3].

Conclusion

In this analysis of a large cohort of children and adults with EBV-related PTLD after HSCT, it has been shown, that the overall frequency of EBV-PTLD is higher in adults than in children. Therapy of EBV-PTLD with rituximab-based therapy results in better outcome in children than in adults.

This may be related to the use of rituximab-based therapy as first-line therapy, reduction of immunosuppression and improved supportive care measures. Survival from PTLD after rituximab-based therapy was 78% in children and 64% in adults, while only 15 years ago the mortality rate of this disease exceeded 84%. Multivariate analysis identified two variables predictive of good outcome in children and thee variables in adults. These include: nodal involvement only, and RI at PTLD diagnosis in pediatric population, while age at transplant <30 years, initial EBV DNA-emia <10^4 gc/mL, and RI at PTLD diagnosis in adult patients.

Strong adverse prognostic factors in PTLD patients after allo-HSCT, treated with rituximab, were identified. By using these factors, risk-stratified survival prognostic models were developed separately for children and for adults.

A decreasing number of independent variables was associated with markedly different survival from PTLD; with 2, 1, or 0 factors in children the survival was 94%, 86% and 30%, respectively, while with 3, 2, 1 or 0 factors in adults the survival was 100%, 92%, 79% and 38%, respectively.

Acknowledgments

The Author wish to thank to collaborators of the primary study on the use of rituximab in EBV-PTLD, namely: Simone Cesaro (Policlinico G.B. Rossi, Verona, Italy); Lidia Gil (Department of Hematology, Poznan University of Medical Sciences, Poznan, Poland); Gloria Tridello (Policlinico G.B. Rossi, Verona, Italy); Per Ljungman (Department of Hematology, Karolinska University Hospital and Division of Hematology, Department of Medicine Huddinge, Karolinska Institutet, Stockholm, Sweden); J. Peter Donnelly and Walter van der Velden (Department of Hematology, Radboud University Nijmegen Medical Centre, The Netherlands); Hamdy Omar (Department of Hematology, Karolinska University Hospital and Division of Hematology, Department of Medicine Huddinge, Karolinska Institutet,

Stockholm, Sweden and Department of Medicine, Suez Canal University, Egypt); Rodrigo Martino (Hospital Santa Creu i Sant Pau, Barcelona, Spain); Constantijn Halkes (Leiden University Hospital, The Netherlands); Maura Faraci (Department of Hematology-Oncology; Stem Cell Transplant Unit; G.Gaslini Children Research Institute, Genova, Italy); Koen Theunissen (Department of Hematology, Leuven, and Department of Hematology, Jessa Hospital and LOC, Hasselt, Belgium); Krzysztof Kalwak (Department of Pediatric Transplantology, Hematology and Oncology Medical University, Wroclaw, Poland); Petr Hubacek (Department of Pediatric Hematology and Oncology and Department of Medical Microbiology, University Hospital Motol, Prague, Czech Republic); Simona Sica (Universita Cattolica S. Cuore, Rome, Italy); Chiara Nozzoli (Bone Marrow Transplantation Unit, Careggi Hospital, Florence, Italy); Franca Fagioli (Onco-Ematologia Pediatrica, Torino, Italy); Susanne Matthes (St Anna Kinderspital, Vienna, Austria); Miguel A. Diaz (Niño Jesus Children`s Hospital, Madrid, Spain); Maddalena Migliavacca and Adriana Balduzzi (Clinica Pediatrica Università di Milano Bicocca, Ospedale San Gerardo, Monza, Italy); Agnieszka Tomaszewska (Institute of Hematology and Transfusion Medicine, Warsaw, Poland); Rafael de la Camara (Hospital de la Princesa, Madrid, Spain); Anja van Biezen and Jennifer Hoek (EBMT Data Office Leiden, Department of Medical Statistics & Bioinformatics, Leiden University Medical Centre, Leiden, The Netherlands); Simona Iacobelli (Centro Interdipartimentale di Biostatistica e Bioinformatica, Università di Roma "Tor Vergata", Italy); and Hermann Einsele (Department of Internal Medicine II, Julius Maximilian University of Würzburg, Germany).

Glossary

EBV DNA-emia Detection of EBV DNA in the blood.

Primary EBV infection EBV detected in a previously EBV-seronegative patient.

PTLD Heterogenous group of EBV disease with neoplastic lymphoproliferation, developing after transplantation and caused by iatrogenic suppression of T-cell function. Diagnosis of neoplastic forms of EBV-PTLD should have at least two and ideally three of the following histological features: (i) disruption of underlying cellular architecture by a lymphoproliferative process; (ii) presence of monoclonal or oligoclonal cell populations as revealed by cellular and/or viral markers; (iii) evidence of EBV infection in many of the cells, that is, DNA, RNA or protein. Detection of EBV nucleic acid in blood is not sufficient for the diagnosis of EBV-related PTLD.

Proven PTLD Level of PTLD diagnosis when EBV was detected in a specimen obtained from an organ by biopsy or other invasive procedure, with a test with appropriate sensitivity and specificity together with symptoms and signs from the affected organ.

Probable PTLD Level of PTLD diagnosis when significant lymphoadenopathy or other endorgan disease is accompanied by a high EBV DNA blood load, in the absence of other etiologic factors or established diseases.

Reduction of immunosuppression A sustained decrease of at least 20% of the daily dose of immunosuppressive drugs with the exception of low-dose corticosteroid therapy, i.e., ≤0.2 mg/kg in patients <40 kg of body weight or ≤10 mg/day in patients with >40 kg of body weight.

Prophylaxis of EBV DNA-emia (EBV reactivation) Any agents given to an asymptomatic patient to prevent EBV reactivation in seropositive patient (or when the donor is seropositive).

Pre-emptive therapy Any agents or EBV-specific T-cells given to an asymptomatic patient with EBV detected by a screening assay.

Treatment of EBV disease Agents or other therapeutic methods applied to a patient with EBV (proven or probable) disease.

Summary Points List

- The overall frequency of EBV-PTLD after HSCT is higher in adults (3.8%) than in children (2.6%). This relationship is observed in all types of transplants, regardless on the type of donor and source of hematopoietic stem cells.
- Therapy of EBV-PTLD with rituximab-based therapy results in better outcome in children than in adults. Survival from PTLD after rituximab-based therapy was 78% in children and 64% in adults, while only 15 years ago the mortality rate of this disease exceeded 84%.
- General factors contributing to current overall better survival: the use of rituximab-based therapy as first-line therapy, reduction of immunosuppression and improved supportive care measures.
- Factors predicting good outcome of EBV-PTLD after HSCT by multivariate analysis in children: nodal involvement only, and RI at PTLD diagnosis.
- Factors predicting good outcome of EBV-PTLD after HSCT by multivariate analysis in adults: age at transplant <30 years, initial EBV DNA-emia <10^4 gc/mL, and RI at PTLD diagnosis.
- Risk factor stratified survival prognostic models were developed separately for children and for adults. A decreasing number of independent variables was associated with markedly different survival from PTLD; with 2, 1, or 0 factors in children the survival was 94%, 86% and 30%, respectively, while with 3, 2, 1 or 0 factors in adults the survival was 100%, 92%, 79% and 38%, respectively.

Future Issue List

- The search for biomarkers related to PTLD in HSCT setting is necessary. Standard laboratory test results such as LDH, level of albumin, hemoglobin level or leukocyte count have been correlated with outcome of PLTD in SOT are not applicable to

HSCT, as these are influenced by many factors including conditioning, neutropenia and graft-versus-host disease.
- Randomized studies with the use of rituximab vs rituximab+other agents (e.g., steroids, reduction of immunosuppression) in pre-emptive therapy is necessary. Clinical and tissue-based studies with prospective evaluation of rituximab-based therapy and prognostic factor analyses in multicenter and multinational collaborations are warranted.

References

[1] Curtis, RE; Travis, LB; Rowlings, PA; Socie, G; Kingma, DW; Banks, PM; Jaffe, ES; Sale, GE; Horowitz, MM; Witherspoon, RP; Shriner, DA; Weisdorf, DJ; Kolb, HJ; Sullivan, KM; Sobocinski, KA; Gale, RP; Hoover, RN; Fraumeni, JF Jr; Deeg, HJ. Risk of lymphoproliferative disorders after bone marrow transplantation: A multi-institutional study. *Blood*, 1999, 94, 2208-2216.

[2] Styczynski, J; Reusser, P; Einsele, H; de, la, Camara, R; Cordonnier, C; Ward, KN; Ljungman, P; Engelhard, D. Management of HSV, VZV and EBV infections in patients with hematological malignancies and after SCT: Guidelines from the Second European Conference on Infections in Leukemia. *Bone Marrow Transplant*, 2009, 43, 757-770.

[3] Styczynski, J; Einsele, H; Gil, L; Ljungman, P. Outcome of treatment of Epstein-Barr virus-related post-transplant lymphoproliferative disorder in hematopoietic stem cell recipients: A comprehensive review of reported cases. *Transpl Infect Dis*, 2009, 11, 383-392.

[4] Green, M; Michaels, MG. Epstein-Barr virus infection and posttransplant lymphoproliferative disorder. *Am J Transplant*, 2013, 13 Suppl 3, 41-54: quiz 54.

[5] Wistinghausen, B; Gross, TG; Bollard, C. Post-transplant lymphoproliferative disease in pediatric solid organ transplant recipients. *Pediatr Hematol Oncol*, 2013, 30, 520-531.

[6] Mendizabal, M; Marciano, S; dos Santos Schraiber, L; Zapata, R; Quiros, R; Zanotelli, ML; Rivas, MM; Kusminsky, G; Humeres, R; Alves, de Mattos, A; Gadano, A; Silva, MO. Post-transplant lymphoproliferative disorder in adult liver transplant recipients: A south american multicenter experience. *Clin Transplant*, 2013, 27, E469-477.

[7] Colita, A; Moise, L; Arion, C; Popescu, I. Post-transplant lymphoproliferative disorders after solid organ transplantation in children. *Chirurgia (Bucur)*, 2012, 107, 431-437.

[8] McGuirk, JP; Seropian, S; Howe, G; Smith, B; Stoddart, L; Cooper, DL. Use of rituximab and irradiated donor-derived lymphocytes to control Epstein-Barr virus-associated lymphoproliferation in patients undergoing related haplo-identical stem cell transplantation. *Bone Marrow Transplant*, 1999, 24, 1253-1258.

[9] Doubrovina, E; Oflaz-Sozmen, B; Prockop, SE; Kernan, NA; Abramson, S; Teruya-Feldstein, J; Hedvat, C; Chou, JF; Heller, G; Barker, JN; Boulad, F; Castro-Malaspina, H; George, D; Jakubowski, A; Koehne, G; Papadopoulos, EB; Scaradavou, A; Small, TN; Khalaf, R; Young, JW; O'Reilly, RJ. Adoptive immunotherapy with unselected or EBV-specific T cells for biopsy-proven EBV+ lymphomas after allogeneic hematopoietic cell transplantation. *Blood*, 2012, 119, 2644-2656.

[10] Heslop, HE; Slobod, KS; Pule, MA; Hale, GA; Rousseau, A; Smith, CA; Bollard, CM; Liu, H; Wu, MF; Rochester, RJ; Amrolia, PJ; Hurwitz, JL; Brenner, MK; Rooney, CM. Long-term outcome of EBV-specific T-cell infusions to prevent or treat EBV-related lymphoproliferative disease in transplant recipients. *Blood*, 2010, 115, 925-935.

[11] De Pasquale, MD; Mastronuzzi, A; De Vito, R; Cometa, A; Inserra, A; Russo, C; De Ioris, MA; Locatelli, F. Unmanipulated donor lymphocytes for EBV-related PTLD after T-cell depleted hla-haploidentical transplantation. *Pediatrics*, 2012, 129, e189-194.

[12] Barker, JN; Doubrovina, E; Sauter, C; Jaroscak, JJ; Perales, MA; Doubrovin, M; Prockop, SE; Koehne, G; O'Reilly, RJ. Successful treatment of EBV-associated posttransplantation lymphoma after cord blood transplantation using third-party EBV-specific cytotoxic t lymphocytes. *Blood*, 2010, 116, 5045-5049.

[13] Faye, A; Quartier, P; Reguerre, Y; Lutz, P; Carret, AS; Dehee, A; Rohrlich, P; Peuchmaur, M; Matthieu-Boue, A; Fischer, A; Vilmer, E. Chimaeric anti-CD20 monoclonal antibody (rituximab) in post-transplant B-lymphoproliferative disorder following stem cell transplantation in children. *Br J Haematol*, 2001, 115, 112-118.

[14] Styczynski, J; Gil, L; Tridello, G; Ljungman, P; Donnelly, JP; van der Velden, W; Omar, H; Martino, R; Halkes, C; Faraci, M; Theunissen, K; Kalwak, K; Hubacek, P; Sica, S; Nozzoli, C; Fagioli, F; Matthes, S; Diaz, MA; Migliavacca, M; Balduzzi, A; Tomaszewska, A; Camara Rde, L; van Biezen, A; Hoek, J; Iacobelli, S; Einsele, H; Cesaro, S. Response to rituximab-based therapy and risk factor analysis in Epstein Barr virus-related lymphoproliferative disorder after hematopoietic stem cell transplant in children and adults: A study from the Infectious Diseases Working Party of the European Group for Blood and Marrow Transplantation. *Clin Infect Dis*, 2013, 57, 794-802.

[15] Hubacek, P; Cinek, O; Kulich, M; Zajac, M; Keslova, P; Formankova, R; Stary, J; Sedlacek, P. [EBV quantification in children after allogeneic hematopoietic stem cell transplantation]. *Cas Lek Cesk*, 2006, 145, 301-306.

[16] Reddiconto, G; Chiusolo, P; Fiorini, A; Farina, G; Laurenti, L; Martini, M; Marchetti, S; Fadda, G; Leone, G; Sica, S. Assessment of cellular origin and EBV status in a PTLD after double cord blood transplantation. *Leukemia*, 2007, 21, 2552-2554.

[17] Chiusolo, P; Metafuni, E; Cattani, P; Piccirillo, N; Santangelo, R; Manzara, S; Bellesi, S; De, Michele, T; Leone, G; Sica, S. Prospective evaluation of Epstein-Barr virus reactivation after stem cell transplantation: Association with monoclonal gammopathy. *J Clin Immunol*, 2010, 30, 894-902.

[18] Faraci, M; Lanino, E; Micalizzi, C; Morreale, G; Di, Martino, D; Banov, L; Comoli, P; Locatelli, F; Soresina, A; Plebani, A. Unrelated hematopoietic stem cell transplantation for cernunnos-xlf deficiency. *Pediatr Transplant*, 2009, 13, 785-789.

[19] Faraci, M; Caviglia, I; Morreale, G; Lanino, E; Cuzzubbo, D; Giardino, S; Di, Marco, E; Cirillo, C; Scuderi, F; Dallorso, S; Terranova, P; Moroni, C; Castagnola, E. Viral-load and B-lymphocyte monitoring of EBV reactivation after allogeneic hemopoietic SCT in children. *Bone Marrow Transplant*, 2010, 45, 1052-1055.

[20] Cesaro, S; Pegoraro, A; Tridello, G; Calore, E; Pillon, M; Varotto, S; Abate, D; Barzon, L; Mengoli, C; Carli, M; Messina, C. A prospective study on modulation of immunosuppression for epstein-barr virus reactivation in pediatric patients who underwent unrelated hematopoietic stem-cell transplantation. *Transplantation*, 2010, 89, 1533-1540.

[21] Cheson, BD; Pfistner, B; Juweid, ME; Gascoyne, RD; Specht, L; Horning, SJ; Coiffier, B; Fisher, RI; Hagenbeek, A; Zucca, E; Rosen, ST; Stroobants, S; Lister, TA; Hoppe, RT; Dreyling, M; Tobinai, K; Vose, JM; Connors, JM; Federico, M; Diehl, V. Revised response criteria for malignant lymphoma. *J Clin Oncol*, 2007, 25, 579-586.

[22] Kaplan, EL; Meier, P. Non parametric estimation for incomplete observations. *J Am Stat Assoc*, 1958, 53, 457-481.

[23] Peto, R; Peto, J. Asymptotically efficient rank invariant test procedures. *J R Stat Assoc*, 1972, 135, 185-198.

[24] Cox, DR. Regression model and life tables. *J R Stat Soc Ser B*, 1972, 34, 187-220.

[25] Heslop, HE, How i treat EBV lymphoproliferation. *Blood*, 2009, 114, 4002-4008.

[26] Vegso, G; Hajdu, M; Sebestyen, A. Lymphoproliferative disorders after solid organ transplantation-classification, incidence, risk factors, early detection and treatment options. *Pathol Oncol Res*, 2011, 17, 443-454.

[27] Kuehnle, I; Huls, MH; Liu, Z; Semmelmann, M; Krance, RA; Brenner, MK; Rooney, CM; Heslop, HE. CD20 monoclonal antibody (rituximab) for therapy of Epstein-Barr virus lymphoma after hemopoietic stem-cell transplantation. *Blood*, 2000, 95, 1502-1505.

[28] Brunstein, CG; Weisdorf, DJ; DeFor, T; Barker, JN; Tolar, J; van Burik, JA; Wagner, JE. Marked increased risk of Epstein-Barr virus-related complications with the addition of antithymocyte globulin to a nonmyeloablative conditioning prior to unrelated umbilical cord blood transplantation. *Blood*, 2006, 108, 2874-2880.

[29] van Esser, JW; Niesters, HG; van der Holt, B; Meijer, E; Osterhaus, AD; Gratama, JW; Verdonck, LF; Lowenberg, B; Cornelissen, JJ. Prevention of Epstein-Barr virus-lymphoproliferative disease by molecular monitoring and preemptive rituximab in high-risk patients after allogeneic stem cell transplantation. *Blood*, 2002, 99, 4364-4369.

[30] Gil, L; Styczynski, J; Komarnicki, M. Strategy of pre-emptive management of epstein-barr virus post-transplant lymphoproliferative disorder after stem cell transplantation: Results of European transplant centers survey. *Contemp Oncol* (Pozn), 2012, 16, 338-340.

[31] Czyzewski, K; Styczynski, J; Krenska, A; Debski, R; Zajac-Spychala, O; Wachowiak, J; Wysocki, M. Intrathecal therapy with rituximab in central nervous system involvement of post-transplant lymphoproliferative disorder. *Leuk Lymphoma*, 2013, 54, 503-506.

[32] Tsao, L; Hsi, ED. The clinicopathologic spectrum of posttransplantation lymphoproliferative disorders. *Arch Pathol Lab Med*, 2007, 131, 1209-1218.

[33] Evens, AM; David, KA; Helenowski, I; Nelson, B; Kaufman, D; Kircher, SM; Gimelfarb, A; Hattersley, E; Mauro, LA; Jovanovic, B; Chadburn, A; Stiff, P; Winter, JN; Mehta, J; Van Besien, K; Gregory, S; Gordon, LI; Shammo, JM; Smith, SE; Smith, SM. Multicenter analysis of 80 solid organ transplantation recipients with post-transplantation lymphoproliferative disease: Outcomes and prognostic factors in the modern era. *J Clin Oncol*, 2010, 28, 1038-1046.

[34] Larouche, JF; Berger, F; Chassagne-Clement, C; Ffrench, M; Callet-Bauchu, E; Sebban, C; Ghesquieres, H; Broussais-Guillaumot, F; Salles, G; Coiffier, B Lymphoma recurrence 5 years or later following diffuse large B-cell lymphoma: Clinical characteristics and outcome. *J Clin Oncol*, 2010, 28, 2094-2100.

[35] Diepstra, A; van Imhoff, GW; Schaapveld, M; Karim-Kos, H; van den Berg, A; Vellenga, E; Poppema, S. Latent Epstein-Barr virus infection of tumor cells in classical Hodgkin's lymphoma predicts adverse outcome in older adult patients. *J Clin Oncol*, 2009, 27, 3815-3821.

[36] Taylor, AL; Marcus, R; Bradley, JA. Post-transplant lymphoproliferative disorders (PTLD) after solid organ transplantation. *Crit Rev Oncol Hematol*, 2005, 56, 155-167.

[37] Cesaro, S; Murrone, A; Mengoli, C; Pillon, M; Biasolo, MA; Calore, E; Tridello, G; Varotto, S; Alaggio, R; Zanesco, L; Palu, G; Messina, C. The real-time polymerase chain reaction-guided modulation of immunosuppression enables the pre-emptive management of Epstein-Barr virus reactivation after allogeneic haematopoietic stem cell transplantation. *Br J Haematol*, 2005, 128, 224-233.

[38] Christopeit, M; Schutte, V; Theurich, S; Weber, T; Grothe, W; Behre, G. Rituximab reduces the incidence of acute graft-versus-host disease. *Blood*, 2009, 113, 3130-3131.

[39] Cutler, C; Miklos, D; Kim, HT; Treister, N; Woo, SB; Bienfang, D; Klickstein, LB; Levin, J; Miller, K; Reynolds, C; Macdonell, R; Pasek, M; Lee, SJ; Ho, V; Soiffer, R; Antin, JH; Ritz, J; Alyea, E. Rituximab for steroid-refractory chronic graft-versus-host disease. *Blood*, 2006, 108, 756-762.

[40] Cutler, C; Kim, HT; Bindra, B; Sarantopoulos, S; Ho, VT; Chen, YB; Rosenblatt, J; McDonough, S; Watanaboonyongcharoen, P; Armand, P; Koreth, J; Glotzbecker, B; Alyea, E; Blazar, BR; Soiffer, RJ; Ritz, J; Antin, JH. Rituximab prophylaxis prevents corticosteroid-requiring chronic GVHD after allogeneic peripheral blood stem cell transplantation: Results of a phase 2 trial. *Blood*, 2013, 122, 1510-1517.

[41] Suzan, F; Ammor, M; Ribrag, V. Fatal reactivation of cytomegalovirus infection after use of rituximab for a post-transplantation lymphoproliferative disorder. *N Engl J Med*, 2001, 345, 1000.

[42] Savoldo, B; Rooney, CM; Quiros-Tejeira, RE; Caldwell, Y; Wagner, HJ; Lee, T; Finegold, MJ; Dotti, G; Heslop, HE; Goss, JA. Cellular immunity to epstein-barr virus in liver transplant recipients treated with rituximab for post-transplant lymphoproliferative disease. *Am J Transplant*, 2005, 5, 566-572.

Biographical Sketch

Jan Styczynski, MD, PhD, is affiliated with Department of Pediatric Hematology and Oncology, Collegium Medicum, Nicolaus Copernicus University, Bydgoszcz, Poland, and appointed as professor in transplantology and pediatric hematology and oncology. His main scientific interest include: viral infections in transplantology, hematology and oncology; drug resistance in hematology and oncology; hematopoietic stem cell donor issues; and differences between children and adults in transplantology, hematology and oncology. He is the Secretary of Infectious Diseases Working Party (IDWP) of European Group for Blood and Marrow Transplantation (EBMT) from 2010, and Member of ECIL (European Conference on Infections in Leukemia) group from 2007. Member of American Society of Hematology, European Group for Blood and Marrow Transplantation and several national societies. He has published 40 papers over last 3 years.

Index

A

A20, 47, 74, 97, 102, 120
abdomen, 18, 155, 185
acetyltransferases, 102
acquired immunodeficiency syndrome (AIDS), 5, 10, 11, 15, 41, 43, 49, 52, 66, 67, 74, 78, 100, 104, 105, 107, 108, 115, 143, 144
activated B-cell, 45, 46, 51, 80, 94, 95, 98, 99, 101, 120
activation-induced cytidine deaminase (AICDA), 74, 94, 103
acute cerebral syndrome, 9
acute GVHD, 187, 243, 254, 256
acute lymphoblastic leukemia, 45, 209, 211
ACVBP, 188
acyclovir, 2, 16, 17, 91, 94, 162, 170, 189, 191, 202
adenopathy, 7, 8, 9, 185
adolescents, 1, 3, 4, 15, 18, 20, 198
adoptive immunotherapy, 153, 154, 162, 164, 165, 166, 172, 201, 218, 219
adriamycin, 13, 125
adults, v, 2, 7, 11, 13, 14, 15, 18, 19, 20, 24, 30, 41, 48, 56, 60, 61, 70, 78, 129, 132, 135, 136, 155, 178, 181, 182, 188, 190, 196, 203, 204, 205, 212, 220, 225, 226, 235, 237, 239, 240, 241, 243, 244, 245, 247, 250, 251, 252, 253, 254, 256, 257, 258, 259, 260, 261, 262, 264, 266, 268
Africa, 3, 5, 12, 14, 44, 50, 122
agglutinins, 15
Akt, 54, 69, 146
Ala, 74, 97
alanine, 74
Alaska, 12
alemtuzumab, 53, 85, 87, 180, 182, 191, 231
ALG, 182
alicia syndrome in the wonderland, 9

allogeneic HSCT, 54, 84, 89, 177, 180, 189, 192, 202, 216, 241, 242
allograft, 85, 127, 154, 160, 169, 177, 180, 181, 230, 231, 232, 233
allopurinol, 7
alloreactivity, 84
alternative, 53, 84, 90, 91, 97, 102, 117, 154, 163, 164, 180, 219, 243, 244
alternative donor, 180, 243, 244
America, 3, 4, 5, 13, 14, 31, 44, 45, 51, 66
amoxicillin, 7
ampicillin, 7
amygdale carcinoma, 10
anaplastic, 44, 45, 51, 63, 67, 74, 80, 82, 152, 207, 208, 211, 215, 220, 221, 226, 227, 228, 229, 230, 231, 232, 233, 234
anaplastic large cell lymphoma (ALCL), 44, 45, 51, 63, 67, 74, 80, 82, 208, 215, 216, 220, 221, 226, 229, 230, 231, 234
anaplastic lymphoma kinase (ALK), 51, 52, 67, 74, 80, 82, 160, 208, 215, 228, 229
angiocentric, 13, 211
angioimmunoblastic T-cell lymphoma, 210
animal model, 46, 56
Ann Arbor classification, 89
antibiotics, 7, 9
antibody, 10, 16, 32, 37, 38, 42, 53, 60, 68, 85, 87, 90, 91, 94, 96, 98, 100, 106, 125, 133, 134, 135, 136, 153, 160, 163, 165, 168, 171, 178, 180, 187, 199, 203, 219, 259, 266, 267
anti-CD20, 90, 125, 134, 171, 176, 186, 187, 189, 194, 199, 203, 218, 240, 259, 266
anti-CD3, 85, 175, 180, 182
anticonvulsants, 7
anti-D, 16
anti-EBNA, 16, 185
anti-EBV, 3, 14, 32, 35, 83, 159, 178, 180, 189, 190, 239, 241

Index

antigen-presenting cell, 85, 97
anti-lymphocyte antibodies, 175, 179, 183, 194
anti-lymphocytic therapy, 161
anti-metabolites, 182
anti-proliferative, 176, 186, 194, 218
antiretroviral therapy, 52, 76, 105, 143
anti-thymocyte globulin (ATG), 176, 180, 182, 192, 208, 240
anti-VCA, 16
antiviral agents, 57, 70, 167, 176, 186, 191, 193, 194, 253, 262
APC, 55
apoptosis, 34, 46, 47, 54, 58, 67, 69, 71, 73, 94, 95, 97, 98, 102, 103, 115, 119, 120, 122, 125, 138, 151, 154, 156, 165, 171
arginine butyrate, 57, 70, 91, 134, 162, 170, 171, 189, 201
arsenic trioxide, 57
artralgia, 9
Asia, 4, 13, 31, 35, 44, 45, 51, 80, 214
ataxia-telangiectasia, 10
ATR, 74, 100, 136
atypia, 49, 212, 213
atypic lymphocytes, 6, 7, 9, 15
AURK, 74
Aurora kinase, 74
autoimmune disease, 48, 74, 104, 109, 145
autoimmune hemolytic anemia, 17
autoimmune lymphoproliferative syndrome (ALPS), 209
autologous, 54, 69, 84, 91, 128, 134, 153, 164, 165, 172, 180, 189, 191, 203, 216, 227, 228
autologous CTLs, 54, 91, 153, 164, 165
autologous HSCT, 84, 180, 191, 216
azacytidine, 58
azathioprine, 87, 106, 182, 216, 218, 232

B

B2M, 74, 103
BACH, 74, 102
BAL, 178
BamA rightward transcripts (BART), 24, 26, 30, 33, 35, 74, 97, 98, 139
base pairs, 4
B-cell, v, vii, 10, 18, 41, 42, 43, 44, 45, 46, 47, 48, 49, 50, 51, 52, 53, 57, 60, 62, 63, 66, 67, 68, 69, 70, 73, 74, 75, 77, 79, 80, 81, 82, 83, 84, 85, 88, 90, 91, 92, 93, 94, 95, 96, 97, 98, 99, 100, 101, 102, 104, 105, 106, 107, 108, 109, 110, 111, 114, 115, 116, 119, 120, 121, 122, 123, 124, 125, 128, 133, 134, 135, 137, 139, 140, 141, 142, 143, 144, 145, 146, 147, 148, 149, 153, 154, 155, 156, 160, 161, 162, 163, 169, 170, 171, 179, 180, 181, 182, 183, 187, 191, 192, 199, 200, 207, 210, 214, 215, 216, 217, 218, 220, 221, 223, 226, 228, 232, 234, 235, 236, 237, 239, 241, 259, 261, 267
B-cell linker, 75
B-cell lymphoma, v, vii, 10, 18, 41, 43, 44, 48, 49, 50, 51, 52, 63, 67, 68, 69, 70, 73, 74, 77, 79, 80, 81, 82, 94, 95, 97, 99, 101, 104, 106, 121, 123, 139, 140, 141, 142, 143, 144, 145, 146, 148, 149, 160, 179, 214, 215, 221, 232, 235, 267
B-cell receptor (BCR), 54, 74, 94, 95, 98, 101, 109, 112, 115, 116, 119, 120, 125
Bcl2, 156, 162
betalacept, 87
bexarotene, 92, 135, 219, 230
BHRF, 74, 98
BIM, 47, 64, 75, 98, 139
biomarker, 35, 93
biopsy, 14, 29, 66, 68, 83, 88, 132, 146, 156, 157, 159, 166, 178, 185, 217, 236, 239, 242, 243, 244, 263, 265
BIRC, 75
bladder cancer, 10, 20
BLIMP1, 75, 140
BLNK, 75, 112
B-lymphocyte-induced maturation protein 1, 75
body cavity lymphoma (BCL), 47, 50, 73, 74, 75, 94, 95, 96, 97, 98, 100, 102, 103, 108, 114, 115, 116, 120, 136, 148, 149, 160
bone marrow, 10, 13, 14, 18, 51, 60, 83, 84, 88, 128, 129, 130, 131, 135, 136, 148, 195, 196, 200, 201, 212, 216, 217, 220, 221, 222, 226, 227, 228, 236, 237, 243, 256, 261, 263, 265, 266
Bortezomib, 57, 70, 91, 134, 164, 171
brain, 17, 19, 178, 195, 217, 229
brain tumor, 178
breast cancer, 10, 71
bronchoalveolar lavage, 178
BTG family, member (BTG), 75
BUB1, 75
BUB1 mitotic checkpoint serine/threonine kinase, 75
BUN, 185
Burkitt lymphoma (BL), 2, 5, 10, 11, 12, 13, 15, 18, 22, 30, 42, 43, 44, 47, 49, 50, 51, 57, 58, 66, 70, 71, 73, 75, 78, 80, 81, 82, 95, 98, 100, 105, 110, 112, 119, 121, 122, 134, 147, 149, 151, 160, 169, 204, 208, 210, 237
Burkitt-like, 10, 122

C

C3d fragment, 45
CAEBV, 13, 210, 211, 213, 223

Index

calcineurin inhibitors, 161, 172, 207, 216
calcium, 185
cancer, vii, viii, 2, 10, 11, 12, 20, 21, 22, 23, 25, 26, 29, 30, 31, 32, 33, 34, 35, 36, 37, 38, 39, 41, 42, 47, 48, 57, 59, 60, 61, 62, 63, 64, 66, 69, 70, 71, 78, 87, 98, 109, 117, 127, 130, 132, 134, 136, 137, 138, 139, 140, 142, 143, 144, 145, 146, 148, 149, 150, 151, 152, 164, 166, 167, 169, 170, 171, 172, 173, 186, 197, 203, 225, 227, 228, 229, 231, 235
cancer propagation, 47
capsomers, 4
cardiothoracic, 187
caspase inhibitor, 54
caspase recruitment domain family (CARD), 75
castleman-associated, 87, 112
cataracts, 9
CD10, 114, 160
CD138, 160
CD15, 82, 160
CD20, v, 60, 68, 125, 150, 153, 160, 163, 182, 185, 195, 218, 221, 239, 246, 249, 250, 251, 261, 267
CD3/bcl-6, 160
CD30, 44, 51, 67, 82, 83, 86, 160, 211, 219, 229, 230, 231, 234
CD34, 111, 182, 191
CD4+, 6, 50, 55, 143, 145, 173, 180, 183, 196, 212, 215, 220
CD52 monoclonal antibody, 180
CD8+, 6, 46, 48, 50, 51, 55, 56, 70, 145, 179, 180, 201, 212, 215, 220, 233, 237
CDC28 protein kinase regulatory subunit(CKS), 75
CDCA, 75
CDKs, 146, 165, 173
cell cycle, 46, 47, 94, 97, 102, 112, 113, 123, 153
cell cycle inhibitor, 47
cell infusion, 68, 136, 192, 266
cell lines, 26, 36, 39, 45, 53, 54, 57, 58, 69, 106, 109, 162, 165, 167, 189, 195
cell selection, 182
cellular FLICE-like inhibitory protein 2 (C-FLIP), 75, 120
cellular myelocytomatosis viral oncogene, 75
central nervous system (CNS), 7, 11, 17, 18, 44, 50, 66, 68, 75, 77, 87, 88, 92, 104, 105, 107, 110, 123, 135, 136, 155, 176, 187, 188, 192, 199, 200, 204, 208, 209, 214, 215, 219, 220, 222, 233, 236, 240, 260, 267
centromere protein (CENP), 75
cerebrospinal fluid, 178
cervico-uterine cancer, 10, 20
Chediak-Higashi syndrome, 10
chemokine (C-C motif) ligand (CCL), 75
chemokine (C-C motif) receptor (CCR), 75
chemokine (C-X-C motif) ligand (CXCL), 75
chemokine (C-X-C motif) receptor (CXCR), 75
chemoresponsiveness, 102
chemotherapeutic agents, 34, 60
chemotherapy, 13, 14, 31, 37, 42, 52, 53, 54, 57, 61, 89, 90, 92, 102, 103, 113, 117, 124, 125, 133, 134, 140, 154, 162, 163, 164, 166, 170, 171, 176, 186, 188, 191, 192, 193, 194, 196, 198, 199, 200, 203, 204, 213, 216, 219, 240, 247, 249, 252, 253, 256, 259, 262
chest, 18, 185
chest radiograph, 185
chicken-pox, 15
childhood, 3, 12, 17, 18, 30, 95, 132, 181, 192, 210, 212, 213, 225, 236, 260
children, v, 1, 2, 3, 4, 6, 8, 9, 10, 11, 12, 13, 16, 17, 18, 19, 20, 21, 24, 48, 60, 61, 70, 83, 85, 89, 128, 129, 136, 181, 182, 184, 188, 196, 198, 199, 200, 202, 203, 204, 205, 212, 216, 219, 220, 225, 235, 237, 239, 240, 241, 242, 243, 244, 245, 250, 251, 252, 253, 254, 256, 257, 258, 260, 261, 262, 263, 264, 265, 266, 268
chimeric, 53, 60, 69, 125, 203, 259
chimerism, 84, 216
CHL, 160, 161
CHOP, 75, 90, 125, 133, 151, 153, 162, 163, 166, 170, 176, 188, 192, 200, 208
chromosomal abnormalities, 148, 161, 170, 232
chromosomal breaks, 161
chronic active EBV infection, 210
chronic antigenic stimulation, 42, 50
chronic fatigue syndrome, 9
chronic lymphocytic leukemia, 45, 63, 69, 142, 209
chronic mononucleosis, 8, 9
chronic sequelaé, 58
cidofovir, 53, 57, 68, 191, 253
CIITA, 75, 102, 103, 142
cisplatin, 14, 31, 54
Class II, 75
    major histocompatibility complex, 75, 84
    transactivator, 75, 97, 142
class switch recombination (CSR), 75, 94, 99, 100
clathrin-ALK, 52
clearance, 57, 192, 193, 260
clonality, 88, 160, 213, 221, 223, 236
cluster of differentiation (CD), 4, 13, 53, 75, 133, 134, 142, 152, 153, 172, 176, 208, 224, 227, 232, 236, 240
C-MYC, 47, 51, 64, 75, 97, 98, 102, 103, 108, 110, 114, 115, 116, 119, 122, 156
CNV, 75
cognitive dysfunction, 178, 195

common variable immunodeficiency (CVID), 10, 75, 106
comparative genomic hybridization (CGH), 75, 116, 117, 140
compartment, 42, 46, 158, 159, 169, 259
competitive PCR, 158
complement, 5, 10, 45, 95, 107
complement system, 45
complete blood count, 185
complete remission, 32, 36, 52, 164, 165, 176, 187, 192, 193, 194, 203, 208, 220, 240, 242, 253, 256
composite, 220, 221, 223, 226, 234
computed tomography (CT), 14, 29, 30, 75, 87, 159, 176, 185, 208, 240
conditioning, 60, 179, 181, 182, 188, 191, 197, 198, 216, 245, 248, 250, 265, 267
confidence interval, 208, 240, 244, 245, 247, 250, 254, 257, 258, 259
cord blood, 60, 78, 84, 128, 129, 165, 172, 175, 180, 182, 198, 208, 240, 243, 244, 260, 266, 267
Cord Blood Transplantation, 129, 172, 180, 198, 208, 240, 243, 244, 266, 267
corticosteroid, 125, 219, 242, 261, 264, 268
creatinine, 185
CREBBP, 75, 102
cryptorchidism, 9
CTLA, 75, 87
CTLA-4, 87
cumulative incidence, 85, 184, 258, 259
cutaneous tumors, 10, 20
CXCL13, 86
cyclin, 31, 37, 47, 64, 75, 97, 109
cyclin A, 47
cyclin D1, 31, 37, 47, 64
cyclin-dependent kinase inhibitor (CDKN), 75
cyclophosphamide, 75, 90, 106, 125, 151, 163, 166, 171, 176, 208, 219
Cyclophosphamide-Adriamycin-Vincristin-Prednisone, 75, 176, 208
cyclosporin, 67, 87, 132, 182
cytarabine, 188
cytokine, 33, 37, 47, 50, 91, 113, 118, 128, 135, 149, 150, 183
cytology, 178, 230
cytomegalovirus (CMV), 6, 7, 42, 50, 75, 84, 85, 86, 112, 131, 147, 175, 176, 182, 183, 189, 194, 198, 201, 202, 208, 218, 240, 268
cytotherapy, 172, 219
cytotoxic T-cell, 176, 208, 240
cytotoxic T-lymphocytes (CTL), 11, 14, 49, 51, 54, 75, 83, 86, 98, 103, 110, 118, 120, 164, 172, 176, 178, 180, 182, 187, 189, 208, 213, 240, 241, 260

D

DAP-K, 75, 116, 119
deacetylation, 97
death, 43, 55, 75, 77, 105, 113, 119, 150, 164, 184, 185, 187, 189, 242, 243, 253, 256, 257, 258, 260, 262
death-associated protein kinase, 75, 119, 150
deletion, 26, 117, 183
deoxyribonucleic acid, 75, 176, 208, 240
deoxyribozymes, 30, 34
depletion, 13, 53, 83, 84, 127, 175, 179, 182, 187, 190, 192, 194, 198, 259
dermatomyositis, 13
diet, 2, 16, 17
differential diagnosis, 185
diffuse large B-cell lymphoma (DLBCL), 44, 45, 49, 50, 51, 52, 62, 66, 67, 75, 79, 80, 81, 82, 98, 99, 100, 101, 102, 103, 104, 105, 107, 108, 113, 114, 115, 116, 117, 121, 122, 139, 140, 142, 160, 208, 215, 221, 240
disomy, 78, 117
distribution, 1, 2, 3, 17, 30, 137
DNA, 1, 3, 4, 11, 12, 22, 25, 29, 30, 32, 33, 34, 35, 36, 37, 38, 41, 42, 45, 46, 57, 58, 59, 75, 85, 86, 88, 91, 94, 100, 102, 103, 116, 117, 119, 125, 130, 131, 136, 141, 155, 156, 157, 158, 159, 162, 164, 166, 167, 168, 169, 176, 177, 185, 190, 192, 193, 208, 222, 224, 240, 242, 250, 257, 258, 259, 260, 261, 263
DNA repair, 46
DNA sequences, 45
donor, vii, 14, 48, 54, 60, 83, 84, 85, 91, 118, 129, 165, 175, 176, 177, 179, 180, 181, 182, 183, 186, 189, 190, 192, 194, 198, 200, 201, 205, 208, 215, 216, 218, 219, 228, 231, 235, 237, 240, 243, 244, 245, 246, 247, 248, 249, 250, 251, 252, 253, 259, 260, 261, 262, 264, 265, 266, 268
Donor Lymphocytes Infusion (DLI), 176, 186, 189, 194, 208, 218, 240, 253
donor origin, 84, 129, 179, 216, 228, 235
donor-related, 182
double-stranded, 4, 24, 30, 35, 47, 58, 64, 75, 117, 155, 166
doubling time, 50, 158
Downey cells, 15
doxorubicin, 57, 151, 166
Duncan disease, 11
duodenum, 221
dyspnea, 178

E

E1A binding protein p300 (EP300), 75, 102, 141
early antigen, 16, 30, 32, 185
early B-cell factor (EBF), 75
early lesions, 48, 49, 79, 92, 160, 161, 178, 180
early onset, 113, 180, 193, 204, 242
early PTLD (E-PTLD), 75, 79, 80, 81, 90, 92, 114, 160, 175, 183, 194
early response, 88, 132, 240
Eastern Cooperative Oncology Group (ECOG), 75, 89, 92
EBCL, 43, 48, 49, 51, 52
EBER ISH, 88, 122
EBI, 75
EBMT, 205, 208, 237, 240, 241, 242, 263, 268
EBV, v, vii, viii, 1, 2, 3, 4, 5, 6, 7, 8, 9, 10, 11, 12, 13, 14, 15, 16, 17, 19, 20, 21, 22, 23, 24, 25, 26, 29, 30, 31, 32, 33, 34, 35, 36, 37, 38, 39, 41, 42, 43, 44, 45, 46, 47, 48, 49, 50, 51, 52, 53, 54, 55, 56, 57, 58, 61, 62, 63, 64, 65, 66, 68, 69, 70, 73, 74, 75, 78, 79, 80, 81, 82, 83, 85, 86, 87, 88, 89, 90, 91, 92, 93, 94, 95, 96, 97, 98, 99, 100, 101, 103, 104, 105, 106, 107, 108, 109, 110, 111, 112, 113, 114, 115, 116, 117, 118, 119, 120, 121, 122, 123, 124, 125, 126, 127, 129, 130, 131, 134, 136, 137, 138, 139, 142, 143, 144, 145, 146, 147, 148, 150, 151, 152, 153, 154, 155, 156, 157, 158, 159, 160, 161, 162, 163, 164, 165, 166, 167, 168, 169, 170, 171, 172, 173, 175, 176, 177, 178, 179, 180, 181, 182, 183, 184, 185, 186, 187, 188, 189, 190, 191, 192, 193, 194, 195, 196, 197, 198, 199, 200, 201, 204, 207, 208, 209, 210, 211, 212, 213, 214, 215, 216, 217, 218, 219, 220, 221, 222, 223, 224, 225, 226, 227, 228, 230, 236, 237, 239, 240, 241, 242, 243, 244, 246, 247, 248, 249, 250, 251, 252, 254, 256, 257, 258, 259, 260, 261, 262, 263, 264, 265, 266, 267
EBV DNA-emia, 177, 183, 185, 187, 190, 192, 239, 242, 243, 246, 249, 250, 251, 252, 254, 256, 257, 258, 260, 261, 262, 263, 264
EBV hepatitis, 178, 179
EBV-1, 2, 3, 4, 183
EBV-2, 3, 4, 183
EBV-associated tumors, 11, 21, 46, 110, 210
EBV-CTL, 153, 162, 164, 165, 166, 178, 180, 182, 183, 187, 189, 190, 241
EBV-lymphoblastoid, 165
EBV-naïve, 48
EBV-peptide, 165
EBV-TL, 159
ECIL, 176, 185, 190, 205, 208, 237, 240, 241, 261, 268

ECOG performance status, 89
ECT and RLD domain containing E3 ubiquitin protein ligase, 76
effector cell, 179
elderly, 45, 51, 63, 100, 103, 104, 107, 108, 143, 145
electron microscopy, 2, 11
ELISA, 32
encephalitis, 64, 96, 177, 178, 184, 195, 210
end-organ diseases, 177, 184
endoscopy, 29, 159, 185
Enhancer of zeste homolog 2 (EZH2), 75, 102, 140, 141
enteritis, 178, 179, 195
epidemiology, vii, 3, 21, 67, 95, 128, 129, 154, 155, 175, 193, 198
epigenetic aberrations, 119
episomal, 12, 13, 45, 156
epithelium, 1, 5, 6, 7, 11, 15, 20, 96, 101
Epstein-Barr Virus nuclear antigen (EBNA), 4, 5, 7, 10, 11, 12, 16, 34, 43, 46, 47, 51, 56, 57, 64, 75, 97, 99, 100, 101, 136, 151, 156, 165, 176, 208, 240
Epstein-Barr Virus-encoded RNA (EBER), 22, 23, 24, 26, 30, 31, 33, 35, 38, 44, 47, 64, 75, 81, 88, 91, 98, 100, 101, 106, 121, 122, 156, 160, 176, 185, 208, 217, 240
erythrocytes, 15, 16, 256
escaping of apoptosis, 58
eskimos, 14
etoposide, 98, 203, 213
Europe, 3, 4, 5, 31, 45, 51, 107, 241, 242
European Conference on Infections in Leukemia, 176, 185, 195, 205, 208, 226, 237, 240, 241, 265, 268
European Group for Blood and Marrow Transplantation, 205, 208, 237, 240, 241, 268
Eustachian tube, 14, 31
ex vivo, 91, 137, 164, 165, 189, 190
extracellular signal regulated kinase (ERK), 47, 75
extra-lymphoid, 187, 240
extranodal, 13, 25, 75, 79, 82, 89, 93, 103, 104, 107, 108, 110, 123, 152, 169, 185, 187, 211, 212, 214, 217, 228, 230, 233, 243, 244, 246, 247, 249, 250, 251, 254, 260, 261
extranodal nasal-type NK/T-cell lymphom (ENKTCL), 75, 123
eyelids, 7, 9

F

FANCL, 76, 117
Fanconi anemia, 76
Fc receptor, 90

FDA, 164
FDG-PET, 87, 159
female, 218, 232
fetal-maternal, 219
first line, 92, 162, 163, 194, 261
FK506, 165, 172
Florid follicular hyperplasia (FFH), 76, 79, 82, 170
flow cytometry, 153, 185
fludarabine, 191
Fluoro-deoxy-glucose (FDG), 76, 87, 132, 159, 169
fluorothymidine (FLT), 76, 88, 132
fluorouracil, 14, 31
follicular hyperplasia, 76, 79, 82, 170
Forkhead box protein P (FOXP), 76
Forssman antigen, 16
foscarnet, 57, 191
Fragile site (FRA), 76, 117
French, 129, 135, 184, 198, 235
frequency, viii, 3, 6, 8, 22, 44, 45, 49, 51, 52, 107, 115, 116, 145, 180, 181, 185, 198, 214, 215, 223, 224, 243, 244, 245, 260, 262, 264
fulminant, 7, 10, 107, 178, 185, 210, 213, 225, 227
functional B-cell receptor, 54, 115

G

gains of chromosomes, 161
Gal-1, 165
galectin-1, 165, 173
gammaglobulins, 17
ganciclovir, 57, 58, 70, 71, 91, 94, 134, 162, 167, 170, 171, 189, 191, 201, 202
ganglionary growth, 6
ganglions, 8
gastric carcinoma, 10, 22, 23, 24, 25, 26, 113, 147
gastro-intestinal, 92, 107, 123, 185
gastrointestinal tract, 13, 154, 217
gemcitabine, 31, 57
gene, 10, 13, 14, 23, 24, 26, 29, 31, 32, 34, 35, 37, 42, 43, 45, 46, 47, 48, 50, 57, 58, 62, 63, 64, 68, 69, 70, 76, 95, 97, 98, 100, 101, 102, 103, 105, 109, 111, 112, 113, 116, 117, 119, 120, 121, 123, 136, 138, 139, 140, 142, 144, 146, 147, 148, 150, 152, 156, 168, 173, 183, 215, 221, 224
gene expression profiling (GEP), 76, 112, 113, 114, 139, 152
general population, 2, 14, 20, 74, 80, 94, 103, 104, 105, 106, 114, 115, 116, 124, 126, 177, 213
genome, 1, 2, 4, 7, 10, 12, 14, 20, 22, 24, 25, 31, 33, 35, 42, 43, 44, 45, 46, 47, 59, 67, 86, 95, 96, 102, 109, 112, 118, 119, 141, 149, 156, 213, 223, 243, 261

germinal center (GC), 42, 62, 76, 80, 81, 94, 95, 97, 98, 99, 100, 101, 102, 106, 110, 115, 116, 120, 122, 125, 136, 137, 145, 150, 160, 243, 246, 249, 250, 251, 252, 254, 256, 260, 261, 262, 264
germinal center B-cell (GCB), 76, 80, 95, 101, 103, 110, 113, 114, 115, 120, 137, 140, 145
Gianotti-Crosti syndrome, 9, 11, 18
glycine, 46, 76
glycine-alanine, 46
glycoprotein, 4, 6, 34, 56, 76, 155
GM-CSF, 76, 92
gold standard, 31, 35, 61, 88, 176, 187, 193, 194
gp350, 2, 6, 11, 16, 17, 34, 39, 56, 57, 70, 93, 96, 97, 136, 155
Graft-versus-host disease (GVHD), 14, 48, 54, 76, 84, 85, 164, 176, 180, 182, 185, 186, 187, 189, 192, 208, 219, 240, 246, 247, 248, 250, 251, 260, 261, 265, 268
gram-negative, 94
granuloma, 13, 14
granzyme, 13
guardian of the genome, 46
Guillain-Barre syndrome, 9

H

head, 14, 29, 30, 32, 37, 39, 87, 152, 185
headache, 6
hearing impairment, 9
heart, 48, 60, 84, 93, 132, 161, 177, 181, 184, 192, 202, 207, 215, 217, 218, 228, 230, 237
hematopoietic stem cell (HSC), v, vii, 44, 48, 60, 65, 68, 76, 78, 83, 84, 86, 94, 111, 129, 130, 164, 170, 175, 176, 177, 179, 188, 192, 195, 196, 197, 198, 201, 205, 207, 208, 210, 212, 213, 216, 219, 222, 223, 224, 227, 235, 237, 239, 240, 241, 247, 250, 259, 260, 264, 265, 266, 268
hematopoietic stem cell transplantation (HSCT), v, viii, 48, 53, 54, 60, 65, 76, 78, 83, 84, 85, 91, 164, 175, 176, 177, 179, 180, 181, 182, 184, 185, 186, 187, 188, 189, 190, 191, 192, 193, 194, 195, 197, 198, 201, 207, 208, 210, 212, 213, 214, 216, 218, 219, 220, 221, 223, 224, 239, 240, 241, 243, 244, 245, 247, 248, 250, 259, 260, 261, 262, 264, 266
hemolytic anemia, 96
hemophagocytic lymphohistiocytosis, 19, 210, 212, 213, 225, 226
hemophagocytosis, 19, 211, 222, 227, 233
hepatic cell cancers, 10
hepatitis, 7, 9, 10, 15, 18, 96, 148, 177, 178, 179, 183, 184, 192, 210, 211, 222, 235
hepatitis B, 18, 192
hepatitis C, 148, 183, 235

Index

hepatosplenic, 76, 80, 82, 160, 208, 211, 212, 215, 220, 222, 228, 229, 230, 231, 232, 233
hepatosplenic T-cell lymphoma (HSTCL), 76, 80, 82, 208, 215, 220
hepatosplenomegaly, 7, 8, 96, 154, 155, 211, 212, 222
HERC, 76
herpes viruses, 4, 177
herpesvirus family, 154, 177
hes-1, 47
heterophilic antibodies, 9, 16
HHV-8, 13, 50, 112, 229, 232
high-dose methotrexate, 200
highly active antiretroviral therapy, 66, 105, 143
high-risk patients, vii, 89, 90, 159, 168, 181, 185, 194, 259, 267
histiocyte-rich, 44, 51, 67
histiocytes, 51
histochemistry, 185
histological evaluation, 33, 185
histone, 39, 47, 57, 70, 76, 97, 102, 141
histone acetyltransferase, 76, 102
histone deacetylase 1, 47
histone methyltransferase (HMT), 76, 102
HL-like, 49, 82, 128, 161, 170, 214
Hodgkin Disease, 12, 208, 210, 240, 247, 250
Hodgkin lymphoma (HL), 10, 11, 13, 14, 18, 43, 44, 45, 49, 51, 59, 60, 61, 62, 63, 65, 66, 69, 76, 79, 80, 82, 87, 100, 101, 105, 107, 109, 113, 114, 116, 123, 125, 128, 139, 140, 141, 142, 145, 148, 150, 151, 160, 161, 170, 176, 180, 188, 204, 208, 210, 214, 224, 261
host-versus-graft, 220
HTLV-1, 211, 214
Human Herpes Virus (HHV), vii, 5, 12, 13, 30, 42, 50, 76, 112, 176, 208, 218, 229, 232, 233
Human Immunodeficiency Virus (HIV), 11, 14, 15, 41, 43, 44, 49, 50, 52, 66, 67, 74, 76, 80, 96, 104, 105, 108, 109, 110, 111, 112, 115, 117, 122, 124, 137, 143, 144, 150, 232
human La protein, 22, 47
Human Leukocyte Antigen (HLA), 48, 54, 55, 76, 84, 91, 96, 97, 118, 119, 129, 149, 153, 164, 165, 167, 172, 175, 176, 180, 183, 191, 192, 194, 195, 208, 219, 240, 266
hydroa vacciniforme, 210, 212
hydroxyldaunorubicin, 90
hygiene, 3, 4
hyperbilirubinemia, 8
hypermutation, 78, 94, 99, 100, 102, 114, 115, 120, 137, 141, 148
hyperpyrexia, 178
hypersensitivity syndrome, 7
hypogammaglobulinemia, 18, 53, 78, 106, 163
hypotonia, 9

I

IARC, 30, 62, 65, 127
IAR-LPD, 76, 106
iatrogenic, 83, 108, 117, 119, 120, 121, 124, 180, 217, 222, 239, 241, 263
IDWP, 205, 237, 241, 268
IFI, 76, 113
IFN-alpha, 91
IgA, 12, 14, 32, 37, 95, 234
IgG, 16, 32, 37, 83, 95, 96, 97, 183, 192
IgH, 76, 122
IgM, 16, 83, 94, 95, 96
IgV, 76, 115, 116
IL-15, 56
IL2-inducible T-cell kinase (ITK), 76, 109
immortalization, 2, 7, 46, 47, 63, 64, 97, 151, 157
immune escape, 47, 98, 117
immune function, 50, 107, 179
immune reconstitution, 179
immune suppression, 50, 120, 121, 184, 188, 193
immune system, viii, 17, 18, 42, 46, 51, 58, 59, 60, 61, 83, 85, 95, 97, 103, 105, 112, 114, 121, 123, 124, 125, 137, 154, 165, 177
immunglobulin, 76, 177, 208, 241
immunity, 6, 10, 16, 17, 22, 42, 52, 56, 59, 61, 63, 67, 69, 83, 84, 89, 106, 107, 120, 128, 137, 141, 145, 157, 166, 168, 178, 180, 182, 183, 189, 190, 201, 268
immunoblasts, 79, 85, 160
immunoblasts-like cells, 85
immunochemotherapy, 151, 164
immunocompetence, 54, 216
immunocompetent host, 41, 49, 51, 58, 79, 96, 111, 112, 114, 115, 117, 156
immunocompromised, vii, viii, 10, 12, 15, 30, 43, 44, 48, 58, 62, 73, 78, 104, 105, 108, 110, 114, 117, 118, 126, 156, 157, 177, 178, 210, 212, 233
immunoglobulin, 32, 38, 51, 76, 78, 115, 141, 148, 169, 187, 202
immunoglobulin heavy chain, 76
immunoglobulin variable chain, 76, 115
immunoglobulins, 176, 185, 186, 194
immunohistochemistry, 88, 148, 153
immunomodulatory agent (IA), 63, 76, 104, 106, 109, 149, 202
immunomodulatory agent-related lymphoproliferative disorder, 76, 106
immunophenotype, 45, 51, 161, 213, 215, 216, 220, 223

immunosuppressive, 15, 52, 53, 54, 78, 83, 84, 87, 89, 90, 103, 106, 110, 112, 114, 121, 125, 127, 131, 142, 150, 161, 165, 172, 175, 177, 179, 181, 183, 186, 192, 194, 202, 208, 213, 214, 216, 217, 218, 219, 230, 231, 240, 242, 247, 250, 261, 264
immunosuppressive therapy, 52, 84, 89, 161, 165, 175, 177, 181, 186, 192, 194, 202, 214, 218, 219, 261
immunotherapy, 23, 26, 52, 54, 58, 60, 61, 68, 69, 91, 111, 146, 153, 154, 162, 163, 164, 165, 166, 172, 176, 186, 191, 194, 201, 218, 219, 265
In situ hybridization (ISH), 33, 61, 76, 81, 88, 137, 217, 121
in vivo, 22, 26, 54, 55, 58, 63, 96, 101, 131, 146, 168, 175, 190, 191, 192, 194
inclusion bodies, 15
index-of-suspicion, 87
Indoleamine-2,3-dioxygenase (IDO), 76, 103, 113, 114, 127
infectious mononucleosis (IM), v, vii, 1, 2, 3, 4, 6, 7, 8, 9, 11, 15, 16, 17, 19, 20, 21, 23, 24, 30, 42, 48, 56, 60, 61, 70, 73, 76, 78, 79, 82, 93, 95, 96, 100, 101, 107, 110, 113, 132, 133, 134, 136, 137, 138, 141, 154, 157, 160, 167, 168, 176, 177, 178, 179, 180, 189, 208, 210, 212, 224
influenza, 18, 19, 77, 96
ING4, 47
ING5, 47
inhibitors, 53, 54, 56, 57, 70, 102, 161, 165, 172, 182, 207, 216
intention-to-treat, 56
interferon (IFN), 24, 47, 55, 64, 66, 76, 91, 98, 107, 111, 112, 113, 118, 120, 133, 134, 176, 186, 193, 194, 200
interferon regulatory factor (IRF), 76, 139
interferon-induced protein with tetratricopeptide repeats 3 (IFIT), 76, 113
interferon-α, 47
interleukin, 47, 76, 134, 135, 149, 165
interleukin 10, 47
interleukin-6, 134, 135, 165
international prognostic index (IPI), 76, 89, 103
interstitial pneumonia, 14, 211, 222
interval, 79, 83, 92, 93, 125, 126, 192, 194, 207, 208, 217, 221, 223, 240, 244, 245, 247, 250, 254, 257, 258, 259, 261
intestine, 48, 60, 83, 177, 181, 183
intrathecal, 177, 188, 199, 236, 267
intravenous immunoglobulin (IVIG), 176, 177, 186, 187, 193, 194, 208, 241

J

Janus activated kinase, 47
jaws, 2, 12

K

karyotype, 161, 213
Ki-1, 51, 229, 230, 231, 234
kidney, 48, 60, 65, 70, 84, 85, 93, 129, 132, 133, 136, 177, 181, 184, 190, 192, 198, 204, 207, 215, 216, 217, 218, 219, 221, 227, 229, 230, 231, 232, 233, 234, 235, 236, 261
killer cell lectin-like receptor subfamily D (KLRD), 76
kissing disease, 1, 5, 19, 78

L

lactate dehydrogenase (LDH), 76, 87, 89, 92, 185, 204, 264
laryngeal tumors, 10, 20
late PTLD, 155, 175, 183, 193, 194, 216
latency, 5, 6, 7, 10, 12, 13, 22, 23, 31, 32, 33, 35, 42, 43, 46, 47, 52, 56, 57, 73, 76, 81, 88, 96, 97, 98, 99, 100, 108, 109, 110, 111, 112, 119, 120, 122, 125, 143, 156, 157, 162, 196, 219, 222, 223, 224
latency 0, 42, 43
latency I, 5, 7, 22, 43, 96, 156, 224
latency II, 13, 31, 35, 43, 81, 108
latency III, 81, 108
latency membrane protein (LMP), 5, 7, 10, 11, 12, 43, 46, 47, 51, 54, 55, 56, 57, 76, 88, 97, 99, 100, 110, 156
latent EBV virus, 189
LCK, 76, 112
LCP, 76
leader protein, 77, 97, 100
leiomyosarcoma, 11, 203
leukemia, 13, 17, 45, 46, 49, 60, 62, 63, 69, 70, 77, 78, 82, 139, 140, 142, 152, 176, 185, 195, 197, 205, 208, 209, 210, 211, 212, 214, 215, 216, 217, 218, 220, 226, 228, 230, 231, 232, 233, 234, 236, 237, 240, 241, 265, 266, 268
leukoplakia, 11, 14, 15, 30, 96
lifestyle, 44
lipopolysaccharide (LPS), 77, 94
liver, 9, 19, 36, 48, 51, 60, 68, 84, 85, 86, 92, 111, 121, 123, 127, 129, 130, 131, 132, 135, 149, 150, 154, 177, 181, 183, 185, 191, 192, 201, 202, 203, 204, 212, 215, 216, 217, 218, 221, 228, 229, 235, 261, 265, 268

liver function tests, 185
LMP1, 22, 23, 26, 31, 34, 37, 39, 46, 47, 65, 81, 91, 97, 98, 100, 108, 109, 110, 111, 113, 114, 115, 119, 120, 121, 122, 123, 138, 139, 146, 150, 151, 156, 183
loss of heterozygosity (LOH), 76, 117
low-risk patients, 181
lung, 21, 25, 26, 37, 38, 48, 60, 64, 71, 84, 92, 123, 131, 132, 158, 169, 177, 178, 181, 183, 192, 202, 215, 217, 221, 228, 234, 261
lung biopsy, 178
lymphadenopathy, 8, 14, 18, 96, 154, 155, 184, 211, 222, 224, 239, 242, 261
lymphoblastoid cell line (LCL), 45, 47, 55, 76, 106, 109, 110, 112, 113, 146, 165
lymphocryptovirus, 4
lymphocytes, viii, 1, 2, 4, 5, 6, 7, 9, 10, 11, 12, 15, 19, 22, 24, 26, 30, 41, 42, 43, 45, 46, 47, 48, 49, 50, 51, 52, 53, 54, 56, 58, 59, 64, 65, 66, 68, 69, 83, 85, 91, 96, 99, 108, 116, 120, 124, 130, 134, 136, 137, 139, 142, 144, 145, 148, 150, 151, 157, 158, 159, 160, 162, 164, 167, 168, 172, 176, 178, 182, 185, 186, 189, 194, 197, 201, 209, 210, 212, 215, 216, 217, 218, 222, 223, 236, 241, 259, 260, 265, 266
lymphocytosis, 7, 8, 15
lymphoepithelial-like, 178
lymphoid interstitial pneumonitis, 11
lymphoid tissue, 6, 20, 45, 65, 77, 80, 82, 83, 96, 107, 127, 169, 181, 210
lymphoma, vii, viii, 2, 5, 10, 11, 12, 13, 14, 15, 17, 18, 22, 23, 25, 30, 32, 35, 42, 43, 44, 45, 48, 49, 50, 51, 52, 53, 57, 59, 60, 61, 62, 63, 64, 65, 66, 67, 68, 69, 70, 71, 73, 74, 75, 76, 77, 78, 79, 80, 81, 82, 86, 87, 89, 90, 92, 94, 95, 97, 99, 100, 101,103, 104, 105, 106, 107, 109, 110, 111, 112, 114, 115, 116, 119, 120, 121, 122, 123, 124, 125, 126, 127, 128, 129, 130, 132, 133, 134, 136, 137, 139, 140, 141, 142, 143, 144, 145, 146, 147, 148, 149, 150, 151, 152, 160, 161, 162, 164, 166, 167, 168, 169, 170, 172, 177, 180, 181, 199, 200, 201, 202, 203, 204, 207, 208, 209, 210, 211, 212, 213, 214, 215, 217, 218, 220, 221, 222, 224, 225, 226, 227, 228, 229, 230, 231, 232, 233, 234, 235, 236, 237, 240, 241, 266, 267, 268
lymphomagenesis, 41, 73, 74, 79, 95, 100, 101, 103, 105, 106, 111, 119, 122, 125, 136, 143, 151, 152, 171, 207, 210
lymphoproliferative disorder (LPD), v, vii, 5, 10, 11, 12, 13, 14, 18, 23, 41, 42, 43, 49, 50, 58, 60, 65, 66, 68, 69, 73, 74, 75, 76, 77, 78, 79, 82, 88, 99, 100, 104, 106, 108, 110, 126, 127, 128, 129, 130, 131, 132, 133, 134, 135, 136, 138, 143, 144, 145, 146, 147, 148, 149, 150, 151, 153, 156, 167, 168, 169, 170, 171, 172, 173, 175, 176, 177, 195, 196, 197, 198, 199, 200, 201, 202, 203, 204, 207, 208, 209, 210, 211, 212, 213, 214, 219, 220, 221, 222, 223, 224, 225, 226, 227, 228, 229, 230, 231, 232, 233, 234, 235, 236, 237, 239, 240, 241, 244, 245, 247, 250, 254, 257, 258, 259, 265, 266, 267, 268
lymphoreticular system, 1, 20
LYN, 54, 77, 112
Lyn/Syk pathway, 54
lysis, 5, 191, 259
lytic activation, 47, 57, 70, 134
lytic cycle, 7, 43, 47, 57, 58, 59, 62, 73, 91, 97, 99, 101, 111, 138

M

magnetic resonance imaging (MRI), 14, 29, 30, 77, 87, 159
major histocompatibility complex (MHC), 46, 51, 55, 75, 77, 84, 103, 109, 136, 142, 155, 173
malaria, 12, 44
male, 14, 35, 207, 217, 218, 221
malignant, vii, viii, 2, 10, 11, 14, 15, 19, 25, 33, 37, 44, 50, 51, 56, 59, 60, 62, 69, 73, 74, 78, 79, 80, 81, 86, 90, 91, 104, 113, 124, 147, 151, 156, 170, 209, 215, 222, 232, 236, 243, 245, 248, 250, 259, 261, 267
MALT, 77, 82, 105
management, v, vii, viii, 14, 21, 29, 37, 38, 52, 61, 65, 67, 83, 86, 92, 130, 131, 133, 164, 168, 169, 170, 175, 177, 183, 186, 188, 192, 193, 195, 197, 199, 201, 203, 213, 226, 228, 236, 260, 265, 267, 268
mandibles, 12
Mantle Cell Lymphoma, 164
MAPK, 47, 77, 97, 102, 118
maribavir, 189, 201
matched family donor, 85, 180, 209, 241, 244, 245
matched related donors, 180
maternal, 219
Mdm2, 47
MDR, 13
measles, 15
memory cells, 88, 99, 100, 101, 110
meningoencephalitis, 9, 178, 179
meta-analysis, 25, 90, 103, 122, 127, 226
metaphysitis, 9
metastasis, 14, 46, 64
methotrexate, 13, 14, 74, 104, 106, 144, 176, 177, 182, 188, 200, 213, 225
methotrexate-associated, 13, 74, 104, 106, 144
methyltransferases, 102

metisazone, 17
metronidazole, 17
metronomic, 188
MGMT, 77, 119, 150
microchimerism, 219
microenvironment, 31, 58, 59, 62, 73, 103, 105, 111, 113, 119, 120, 121, 123, 125, 126, 142, 144, 145, 147, 150
micrognathia, 9
microRNA, 21, 29, 30, 33, 34, 35, 36, 38, 39, 77, 139, 141, 142
microsatellite instability (MSI), 77, 116, 117, 120
miR, 21, 103
miRNA, 77, 103, 139
mismatched family donor, 85, 180, 209, 241, 243, 244, 245
mismatched unrelated donor, 85, 180, 209, 241, 243, 244, 245
mitogen activated protein kinase, 47
mitotic activity, 45
mixed cellularity, 11
Mixed lineage leukemia (MLL), 77
MK-2206, 54, 69
molecular response, 261
molecular studies, 185
monitoring, 34, 38, 130, 131, 153, 157, 158, 159, 161, 166, 168, 169, 181, 182, 183, 185, 190, 201, 202, 266, 267
monoclonal antibodies, 42, 52, 106, 135, 182, 189, 218, 240, 259
monocytes, 86, 158
monocytosis, 9
monomorphic, 23, 48, 49, 77, 79, 80, 82, 87, 88, 91, 93, 100, 104, 108, 114, 117, 121, 123, 128, 138, 147, 156, 160, 161, 163, 170, 178, 180, 188, 192, 207, 211, 214, 215, 216, 217, 220, 221, 223, 234, 254, 256
monomorphic post-transplant lymphoproliferative disorder (M-PTLD), 23, 77, 79, 80, 90, 92, 100, 111, 112, 113, 123, 138
mononucleosis-like, 60, 82, 160, 180, 222
monotest, 15, 16
monotherapy, 53, 90, 153, 162, 163, 166, 187, 188, 203
mortality, 48, 50, 85, 86, 89, 90, 92, 154, 155, 161, 163, 183, 186, 187, 188, 203, 212, 219, 239, 241, 243, 244, 253, 254, 256, 259, 261, 262, 264
mosquito bite allergy, 210, 212
mTOR, 53, 54, 68, 165, 182
mucocutaneous ulcer, 108
mucosa-associated lymphoid tissue, 82
multicenter, 56, 65, 134, 135, 165, 171, 172, 180, 187, 193, 199, 241, 242, 265, 267

multidrug resistant, 13
multifactorial, 260
multiorgan, 184, 244, 246, 247, 249, 250, 251
multiorgan failure, 184
multiple myeloma, 57, 60, 91, 164, 209
multivariate analysis, 260, 264
multivisceral, 84, 181, 215, 228
MUM, 77, 160
MUM-1/IRF4, 160
muromonab, 53
Murphy system, 89
myalgia, 8, 9, 96
MYC, 47, 110, 116, 122, 140, 151, 156, 161
mycophenolate mofetil, 87, 182
mycosis fungoides, 211, 215, 221, 234
myelitis, 9, 177, 184, 210
myeloablative, 179, 181, 191
myeloma, 49, 57, 60, 82, 91, 160, 164, 209
myeloproliferative diseases, 8, 10
myxovirus, 77

N

nasopharyngeal carcinoma, v, vii, 2, 3, 10, 12, 14, 21, 22, 23, 26, 29, 30, 31, 35, 36, 37, 38, 39, 42, 61, 63, 69, 70, 93, 136, 177
nasopharyngectomy, 32, 36
NAT, 22, 36, 136, 137, 138, 139, 140, 141, 150, 151, 177, 185, 209, 224, 241
natural killer cell, 11, 21, 49, 59, 77, 82, 110, 177, 209, 214, 224, 227, 232, 241
natural killer cell group, 77
neck, 14, 29, 30, 32, 37, 39, 185
negative predictive value, 159
neoantigens, 116
neurological impairments, 178
neutropenia, 7, 17, 265
NK-cell, 77, 80, 82, 86, 101, 103, 110, 118, 121, 123, 127, 151, 177, 192, 209, 210, 211, 212, 213, 228, 235, 241
NK-cell leukemia/lymphoma, 210
NKG, 77
Nm23-H1, 46, 64
nodular sclerosing, 11, 142
Non-Hodgkin lymphoma (NHL), 11, 18, 22, 41, 43, 44, 45, 49, 50, 51, 54, 55, 56, 60, 77, 80, 101, 105, 129, 143, 177, 202, 209, 210, 236, 241
non-keratinizing carcinoma, 12
NOS, 77, 80, 82, 123, 207, 211, 212, 215, 216, 217, 220
nose, 39, 123, 217
NPM-ALK, 52
nuclear bodies, 46, 63, 70

nuclear factor (NF), 45, 47, 51, 67, 77, 97, 102, 108, 115, 119, 120, 122, 123, 138, 140, 141, 145, 149, 150, 151, 156
nucleic acid testing, 185
nucleocapsid, 4, 96, 155, 166
Nucleoporin 37kDa, 77
NUP37, 77, 109
nursery, 3

O

O6-methylguanine-DNA methyltransferase, 77, 119, 150
OAS, 77, 113
occult bleeding, 185
OKT3, 85, 175, 183, 194
oligoadenylate synthetase (OS), 77, 163, 243
oligonucleotides, 34
oncogenesis, vii, 2, 58, 103, 109, 110, 122, 138, 140, 156, 209
oncovin, 90, 166
organomegaly, 185
ORI, 77, 97
origin of replication, 97
oropharyngeal, 1, 3, 6, 7, 8, 9, 11, 20, 31, 37, 137
overall response rate (ORR), 91, 163, 189
overall survival, 89, 93, 103, 108, 163, 184, 186, 187, 218, 220, 243, 253, 256

P

p16INK4A, 47
p300, 47, 75
p53, 46, 47, 63, 64, 78, 151
pain, 6, 8, 9, 17, 18, 155
pancreas, 60, 93, 129, 177, 198, 215, 219, 221
panniculitis, 13, 82, 215
paralysis, 9, 18
parotid carcinoma, 10
parthenolide, 58, 71
partial response, 89, 91, 162, 163, 192, 194, 242, 252, 253
pathogenesis, v, vii, viii, 5, 21, 22, 26, 36, 42, 58, 61, 62, 64, 66, 73, 74, 79, 87, 92, 94, 98, 100, 102, 103, 105, 108, 109, 110, 112, 114, 120, 121, 122, 123, 126, 127, 137, 138, 139, 141, 142, 143, 144, 145, 149, 150, 152, 177, 179, 180, 214, 220, 222, 223, 234
Paul-Bunnell test, 2, 15
PAX, 77, 114, 115
PAX5, 98, 102, 221
PD-L1, 55, 56, 147

pediatric, viii, 16, 48, 56, 68, 83, 84, 85, 90, 93, 128, 130, 131, 132, 148, 150, 151, 155, 169, 175, 178, 181, 182, 183, 184, 188, 191, 192, 196, 197, 199, 202, 203, 205, 207, 214, 216, 220, 227, 228, 234, 237, 239, 241, 242, 255, 256, 260, 262, 263, 265, 266, 268
pelvis, 185
perforation, 155, 261
pericardium, 217, 233
peripheral blood, 2, 6, 7, 24, 29, 32, 38, 46, 60, 84, 85, 86, 92, 119, 123, 125, 130, 136, 139, 145, 157, 158, 168, 185, 187, 189, 203, 211, 212, 213, 215, 216, 217, 219, 221, 222, 223, 224, 228, 236, 242, 243, 261, 268
peripheral blood mononuclear cell (PBMC), 77, 130, 158, 168, 209, 219, 242
Peripheral T-cell lymphoma (PTCL), 49, 77, 80, 82, 123, 207, 209, 211, 212, 215, 216, 217, 220, 234
phagocytic system, 6
pharynx, 9, 20, 217
phase, 1, 6, 17, 31, 32, 34, 55, 56, 57, 70, 89, 90, 91, 97, 98, 132, 133, 134, 135, 136, 161, 162, 163, 164, 166, 170, 171, 172, 187, 189, 199, 200, 201, 268
phenotype, 10, 13, 43, 44, 58, 83, 100, 116, 122, 136, 137, 143, 160, 161, 211, 212, 215, 223, 232, 237
PI3K/mTOR, 54
PIM, 77, 114, 115
Pim-1 oncogene, 77
plant extract, 58
plasma, 23, 32, 35, 37, 38, 42, 46, 47, 49, 50, 79, 82, 86, 91, 94, 95, 99, 100, 101, 102, 122, 130, 135, 136, 138, 158, 159, 160, 168, 178, 179, 186, 240, 242
plasma cells, 23, 42, 94, 95, 99, 100, 101, 138, 160, 178
plasmablastic lymphoma (PBL), 22, 73, 77, 80, 81, 103, 105, 121, 122, 127, 151, 157, 209
plasmacytic, 49, 60, 77, 79, 80, 82, 153, 154, 160, 166, 167, 180, 214
plasmacytic hyperplasia (PH), 49, 77, 79, 160, 180, 197, 198, 226
plasmodium falciparum, 12
platelets, 20, 185, 256
pleura, 123, 217, 233
PLK, 77
PLWHA, 49, 50
PMBCL, 77, 101, 209
pneumonia, 14, 177, 178, 184, 195, 210, 211, 222
pneumonitis, 9, 11, 178, 179

polyclonal, 6, 10, 12, 49, 50, 52, 60, 79, 80, 89, 105, 107, 114, 144, 160, 165, 175, 183, 194, 207, 213, 222, 246, 249, 251

polycomb group, 102

polymerase chain reaction (PCR), 2, 21, 77, 86, 88, 130, 131, 137, 158, 159, 168, 169, 177, 178, 181, 185, 190, 199, 200, 209, 217, 220, 221, 224, 241, 242, 268

polymorphic, 48, 49, 60, 77, 79, 81, 82, 85, 91, 100, 104, 108, 114, 123, 151, 156, 160, 161, 178, 180, 192, 211, 214, 216, 237, 254, 256

polymorphisms, 90, 101, 118, 119, 120, 149, 150, 183

population, 2, 3, 4, 12, 14, 20, 21, 29, 32, 41, 51, 54, 61, 67, 74, 79, 80, 85, 94, 95, 101, 103, 104, 105, 106, 114, 115, 116, 124, 126, 127, 142, 145, 148, 155, 158, 163, 177, 184, 187, 212, 213, 216, 217, 221, 235, 250, 261, 262

positive predictive value, 159

positron emission tomography (PET), viii, 77, 87, 132, 169, 177, 185, 199, 209, 241

post-perfusion syndrome, 9

posttransplant lymphoproliferative disorder (PTLD), v, viii, 43, 48, 49, 52, 53, 54, 55, 56, 57, 60, 68, 69, 74, 77, 79, 80, 81, 82, 83, 84, 85, 86, 87, 88, 89, 90, 91, 92, 93, 94, 97, 98, 99, 100, 101, 104, 105, 106, 108, 109, 110, 111, 112, 113, 114, 115, 116, 117, 118, 119, 120, 121, 123, 124, 125, 126, 127, 128, 129, 130, 131, 132, 133, 134, 135, 136, 144, 147, 148, 151, 153, 154, 155, 156, 157, 158, 159, 160, 161, 162, 163, 164, 165, 166, 167, 169, 170, 171, 175, 176, 177, 178, 179, 180, 181, 182, 183, 184, 185, 186, 187, 188, 189, 190, 191, 192, 193, 194, 195, 196, 197, 198, 199, 200, 202, 203, 204, 207, 209, 210, 213, 214, 215, 216, 217, 218, 219, 220, 221, 222, 223, 224, 226, 227, 229, 231, 232, 234, 236, 237, 239, 240, 241, 242, 243, 244, 245, 246, 247, 248, 249, 250, 251, 252, 253, 254, 255, 256, 257, 258, 259, 260, 261, 262, 263, 264, 265, 266, 268

post-transplant period, 48, 177

P-PTLD, 77, 79, 80, 88, 90, 91, 92, 100, 108, 113, 114, 115, 123

pRb, 47

PRDM, 77

predictivity, 255, 256

prednisone, 17, 90, 106, 125, 151, 163, 166, 171, 232

pre-emptive treatment, 164, 181

preparative regimen, 182

prevention, vii, viii, 2, 16, 17, 20, 69, 91, 93, 94, 130, 161, 162, 164, 165, 168, 169, 172, 175, 179, 180, 186, 190, 191, 193, 195, 200, 201, 202, 241, 259, 267

primary, 3, 4, 6, 7, 9, 10, 11, 13, 14, 15, 19, 30, 31, 32, 33, 34, 37, 41, 42, 43, 44, 46, 48, 50, 56, 58, 61, 62, 65, 66, 69, 74, 77, 80, 82, 83, 85, 86, 87, 90, 94, 96, 97, 99, 101, 104, 105, 106, 107, 109, 110, 112, 113, 124, 125, 131, 135, 136, 137, 142, 144, 154, 155, 157, 165, 175, 177, 178, 179, 181, 183, 184, 193, 194, 198, 203, 209, 210, 211, 212, 213, 214, 215, 219, 222, 224, 229, 230, 231, 232, 233, 234, 236, 260, 262, 263

primary central nervous system lymphoma (PCNSL), 50, 66, 77, 105, 209

primary effusion lymphoma, 13, 87, 112, 232

primary immunodeficiency (PID), 10, 44, 48, 65, 74, 77, 104, 106, 107, 124, 125, 144, 198, 209

primary mediastinal B-cell lymphoma, 209

primary syndromes, 210

probable, 67, 239, 242, 243, 244, 246, 249, 251, 253, 254, 255, 256, 263, 264

prognosis, viii, 2, 12, 14, 17, 20, 30, 31, 35, 39, 45, 51, 60, 74, 84, 85, 86, 89, 90, 92, 93, 103, 108, 115, 119, 121, 126, 127, 136, 140, 153, 155, 160, 161, 178, 184, 192, 197, 207, 212, 220, 222, 226, 240, 257, 258, 261

prognostic model, 187, 242, 255, 256, 257, 258, 260, 262, 264

programmed cell death ligand 1, 55

programmed death ligand (PDL), 77, 103, 113

progression, 22, 32, 33, 35, 47, 89, 90, 91, 102, 108, 116, 117, 123, 124, 153, 156, 161, 163, 166, 182, 187, 219

proliferation, 6, 12, 26, 34, 43, 44, 45, 46, 50, 51, 52, 53, 54, 58, 60, 68, 79, 81, 83, 85, 91, 92, 94, 98, 99, 102, 103, 105, 107, 108, 109, 111, 113, 114, 115, 121, 153, 154, 156, 162, 166, 167, 179, 180, 183, 210, 211, 212, 215, 217, 219, 220, 222, 261

ProMACE-CytaBOM, 188

promyelocytic leukemia, 46, 70

prophylactic, 34, 36, 94, 162, 176, 189, 191, 192, 194

protease 7, 46

proteasome inhibitor, 57, 91, 164

protein kinase C, 45

protein nucleoside diphosphate kinase, 46

protein tyrosine kinase, 45, 76

proteins, 5, 6, 7, 10, 26, 29, 34, 43, 46, 47, 55, 57, 58, 61, 62, 64, 73, 74, 81, 84, 88, 96, 97, 98, 101, 103, 105, 108, 110, 111, 112, 113, 118, 119, 120, 121, 122, 125, 146, 153, 156, 217

proteinuria, 9

proto-oncogene, 51, 102, 119, 137, 192

proven, 56, 68, 87, 93, 124, 165, 239, 242, 243, 244, 246, 249, 250, 251, 253, 254, 255, 256, 263, 264, 265

psychiatric symptoms, 178
pyothorax, 11, 13, 45, 63
pyothorax-associated lymphomas, 13

R

radiochemotherapy, 219, 220, 223
radiotherapy, 14, 31, 32, 36, 37, 38, 92, 219, 220, 223
rapamycin, 53, 68, 160, 165, 182
Ras homolog family member H (RHOH), 77, 102
rash, 8, 19
R-CHOP, 151, 219
reactivation, 31, 42, 56, 70, 83, 85, 86, 98, 106, 112, 131, 144, 147, 154, 155, 157, 172, 177, 181, 182, 183, 184, 185, 190, 191, 193, 197, 198, 199, 201, 202, 210, 214, 264, 266, 268
reactivation syndromes, 210
recipient, 48, 54, 55, 60, 83, 84, 85, 91, 118, 126, 129, 147, 151, 175, 179, 181, 182, 183, 184, 190, 192, 193, 194, 200, 203, 216, 221, 227, 228, 229, 230, 231, 232, 233, 234, 236, 237, 246, 248, 250, 251, 254, 259
recipient origin, 129, 179, 183, 192, 216, 227, 236
reconstitution, 53, 66, 179, 180, 182, 196, 201, 216, 260
recurrence, 34, 186, 267
recurrent parotiditis, 9
reduced-intensity conditioning (RIC), 181, 182
reduction of immunosuppression (RIS), 52, 77, 89, 90, 92, 93, 111, 113, 114, 124, 125, 176, 180, 187, 194, 208, 219, 240, 241, 256, 260, 262, 264, 265
Reed-Sternberg cells (RS), 11, 12, 77, 79, 123, 129, 137, 144, 151, 200, 201, 236
refractory PTLD, 192
regimens, 60, 91, 92, 106, 128, 132, 150, 153, 161, 162, 164, 166, 170, 179, 182, 188, 195, 218, 219
regulatory T-cells, 113, 121, 150
reinfection, 184, 193
rejection, 52, 53, 60, 85, 87, 89, 91, 92, 118, 124, 154, 160, 165, 177, 187, 188, 219
relapse, 90, 102, 163, 171, 176, 187, 188, 192, 202, 203, 227, 240
relapsed PTLD, 192
replication, 5, 6, 7, 11, 15, 16, 31, 32, 35, 37, 42, 43, 46, 52, 55, 59, 69, 77, 78, 91, 94, 96, 97, 101, 111, 120, 137, 156, 158, 162, 167, 172, 189, 191
residual disease, 38, 162
responders, 90, 187
retinoid, 92, 135, 219, 230
Reye syndrome, 9
rheumatoid arthritis, 144, 213, 225

ribonucleic acid (RNA), 7, 21, 22, 23, 24, 26, 29, 30, 33, 34, 38, 47, 64, 75, 77, 81, 88, 100, 105, 139, 142, 156, 157, 159, 185, 217, 222, 263
ribosomal protein L22, 22, 47
RIG-I, 24, 47, 64
risk factors, 44, 48, 62, 65, 83, 84, 85, 87, 126, 135, 136, 143, 144, 155, 175, 179, 180, 182, 183, 184, 191, 193, 194, 197, 212, 213, 218, 220, 223, 224, 227, 242, 250, 260, 261, 267
rituximab, viii, 53, 60, 66, 68, 86, 89, 90, 92, 113, 124, 125, 129, 130, 131, 132, 133, 134, 151, 153, 154, 155, 162, 163, 164, 166, 170, 171, 176, 182, 184, 186, 187, 188, 190, 191, 192, 193, 194, 195, 196, 199, 200, 201, 203, 204, 208, 218, 219, 235, 236, 240, 241, 242, 252, 253, 256, 257, 258, 259, 260, 261, 262, 264, 265, 266, 267, 268
RUNX3, 47

S

saliva, 1, 3, 5, 6, 11, 14, 17, 19, 20, 31, 95, 96, 101
salivary gland lymph epithelial carcinoma, 10
sanctuary sites, 214
screening, 29, 30, 31, 32, 33, 35, 39, 146, 157, 158, 159, 185, 190, 191, 224, 264
second line, 194, 252, 253, 256, 261
second transplant, 176, 192, 194
secondary, vii, 8, 34, 42, 43, 44, 52, 67, 81, 99, 109, 124, 163, 184, 193, 211, 228
senescence, 46
sensitivity, 32, 35, 66, 86, 157, 158, 159, 239, 242, 263
sensitization, 57
sepsis, 178, 186
septic shock, 185, 261
seronegative, 157, 164, 181, 183, 190, 260, 263
seropositive, 3, 41, 155, 157, 177, 182, 183, 189, 190, 218, 264
serostatus, 182
serum, 15, 16, 19, 32, 35, 37, 38, 89, 158, 185, 203, 204, 213, 242, 261
serum electrolytes, 185
severe combined immunodeficiency (SCID), 48, 66, 77, 106, 109, 146, 147
Sézary syndrome, 82, 215
SH2D1A, 48, 65
SH3-binding domain protein (SH3BP), 78
shift, 192
signaling pathways, 33, 47, 54, 56, 59, 109, 115, 219
single nucleotide polymorphism (SNP), 78, 116, 149
skin, 7, 8, 13, 18, 48, 123, 154, 211, 217, 221, 231, 261
small bowel, 164, 181, 183, 197

small intestine, 48, 83, 181
small lymphocytic lymphoma, 45, 82
small SH2 binding protein, 48
smooth muscle tumors, 44, 178, 195
solid organ transplantation (SOT), v, vii, viii, 48, 52, 53, 54, 56, 78, 83, 84, 85, 91, 116, 133, 135, 136, 148, 155, 163, 164, 168, 171, 175, 176, 177, 179, 180, 181, 182, 183, 184, 185, 186, 187, 188, 189, 190, 191, 192, 193, 194, 195, 197, 198, 199, 200, 203, 204, 208, 209, 213, 214, 216, 217, 218, 219, 221, 222, 223, 227, 235, 239, 240, 241, 259, 260, 261, 264, 265, 267, 268
Somatic hypermutation (SHM), 78, 94, 95, 99, 100, 102, 114, 115, 120, 141, 148
specificity, 32, 33, 35, 55, 86, 94, 158, 159, 239, 242, 263
spindle cell tumors, 179
spleen, 7, 9, 51, 59, 78, 123, 212, 217, 221, 229, 231, 232
Spleen tyrosine kinase (SYK), 54, 69, 78, 112
splenic rupture, 7
squamous cell carcinoma, 12, 45
standardization, 158, 185, 195
stem cell, vii, 44, 48, 53, 60, 65, 68, 76, 78, 83, 84, 86, 128, 129, 130, 131, 134, 147, 164, 170, 172, 176, 177, 178, 182, 188, 189, 192, 194, 195, 196, 197, 198, 199, 200, 201, 203, 205, 207, 208, 210, 212, 213, 215, 216, 219, 222, 223, 224, 227, 228, 235, 236, 237, 239, 240, 241, 243, 250, 259, 260, 261, 263, 265, 266, 267, 268
steroids, 17, 216, 265
stimulation, 42, 44, 50, 84, 85, 87, 101, 105, 109, 112, 115, 116, 120, 172, 179, 180, 183
STLPD, 213
strains, 5, 101, 111
sulphates, 7
supportive therapy, 259
suppressor, 6, 46, 49, 61, 64, 102, 117, 144, 151, 192
surgery, 14, 19, 29, 39, 71, 92, 176, 177, 182, 186, 193, 194, 252, 253
survival, viii, 31, 38, 45, 46, 47, 54, 63, 65, 67, 69, 73, 79, 89, 92, 93, 95, 97, 98, 101, 103, 108, 109, 112, 116, 119, 120, 122, 127, 135, 136, 140, 141, 142, 148, 163, 164, 171, 184, 186, 187, 189, 200, 201, 208, 213, 216, 218, 220, 222, 235, 241, 243, 244, 245, 246, 247, 248, 249, 250, 252, 253, 254, 255, 256, 257, 258, 259, 260, 261, 262, 264
survivin, 109, 146, 165, 173
syphilis, 15

T

T/NK-cell, 43, 80, 82, 160, 180, 181, 210, 211, 212, 213, 222, 224, 225
tacrolimus, 87, 132, 165, 172, 182, 183, 203, 218
TCD, 182, 190
T-cell, v, 25, 43, 44, 48, 49, 50, 51, 53, 54, 55, 56, 63, 67, 68, 69, 70, 78, 79, 80, 82, 84, 87, 88, 91, 92, 93, 100, 101, 103, 106, 107, 108, 110, 113, 114, 119, 120, 121, 123, 124, 127, 131, 134, 135, 136, 145, 151, 160, 161, 164, 169, 172, 175, 178, 179, 182, 183, 186, 189, 190, 191, 192, 194, 195, 197, 200, 202, 207, 209, 210, 211, 212, 213, 214, 215, 216, 217, 218, 219, 220, 221, 222, 223, 224, 225, 226, 227, 228, 229, 230, 231, 232, 233, 234, 235, 236, 237, 239, 241, 263, 266
T-cell leukemia (TCL), 78, 82, 209, 211, 214, 215, 216, 218, 230, 231, 232, 236
T-cell receptor (TCR), 78, 88, 108, 123, 209, 212, 217, 221
telomerase reverse transcriptase (TERT), 78, 97, 120
testis, 13, 18
third party, 165, 195
thrombocytopenia, 7, 17, 96
thrombocytopenic purpura, 9
thymidine kinase, 57, 162, 167, 189
thymoma, 10
TIA, 13, 78, 121
time to treatment failure, 163
tiredness, 17
titer, 32, 35, 125
tolerance, 91, 219, 260
tongue, 15, 31, 37, 137
tonsillitis, 7, 185
Total Body Irradiation, 60, 182
Total Parenteral Nutrition, 247, 249, 250, 252
toxicity, 34, 56, 90, 125, 163, 164, 186
TP53, 78, 97, 116, 122
transactivation, 47
transaminasemia, 8
transaminases, 7
transcriptosome, 215
transformation, 3, 12, 23, 26, 33, 34, 41, 44, 45, 46, 47, 50, 63, 85, 97, 107, 109, 111, 112, 113, 120, 138, 151, 156, 180, 210, 217, 222, 224
Transforming growth factor (TGF), 78, 103
translation, 33
translocations, 10, 95, 100, 102, 103, 122
transplant registry, 184
transverse myelitis, 9
treatment, v, viii, 2, 12, 13, 14, 16, 17, 30, 31, 32, 34, 36, 41, 51, 52, 53, 56, 57, 58, 60, 62, 67, 68, 83, 86, 88, 89, 90, 91, 92, 93, 94, 102, 103, 106, 107,

109, 111, 113, 124, 125, 126, 127, 128, 130, 132, 133, 134, 135, 144, 153, 154, 156, 158, 159, 161, 162, 163, 164, 166, 167, 170, 171, 172, 173, 176, 181, 183, 185, 186, 187, 188, 189, 191, 192, 194, 195, 197, 198, 199, 200, 201, 203, 204, 213, 218, 219, 224, 225, 226, 227, 228, 230, 231, 232, 236, 240, 241, 242, 252, 253, 256, 259, 261, 262, 264, 265, 266, 267
treatment strategies, 30, 34, 58, 62, 91, 92, 93, 158, 181, 219, 227
treatment-related mortality, 90, 183, 219
Treg, 78, 121
trisomy, 161, 232
TTF, 114, 115, 163
tumor necrosis factor (TNF), 47, 78, 103, 106, 118, 149
tumor necrosis factor receptor, 47
tumorigenesis, 26, 33, 38

U

ubiquitin, 46, 76
UD, 78, 117, 180, 198, 244, 245
ulcers, 178, 195, 237
umbillical cord blood (UCB), 78, 84
unrelated donor, vii, 85, 177, 180, 209, 241, 243, 244, 245
upper airway, 8
uric acid, 185
USP7, 46
UTR, 33, 78, 98

V

vaccination, 16, 17, 34, 58, 61, 93
vaccinia, 56, 70, 78, 136
valganciclovir, 162, 171
vascular endothelial growth factor (VEGF), 78, 97, 98, 111, 120, 146, 209
Viral Capsid Antigen (VCA), 11, 14, 16, 30, 32, 37, 78, 101, 185, 209
viral latency, 47, 73, 125, 157, 196
viral load, 49, 50, 68, 85, 86, 90, 91, 106, 119, 125, 130, 131, 132, 149, 153, 154, 157, 158, 159, 161, 164, 166, 168, 169, 181, 185, 186, 189, 190, 195, 202, 204, 243, 257, 258, 259, 261
viral sepsis, 178
viral syndromes, 178
virion, 4, 155, 166, 172, 189
virus-carrying cells, 46
VRK, 78
V-set and immunoglobulin domain containing (VSIG), 78
V-yes-1, 77

W

Waldeyer chain, 6
weakness, 17, 18
weight loss, 261
WHIM, 78, 106
WHO classification, 48, 51, 66, 80, 82, 107, 160, 180, 196, 224, 225
Wiskott-Aldrich syndrome, 10, 20, 48, 65, 209
Wnt signaling pathways, 47
World Health Organization (WHO), 11, 12, 13, 17, 29, 31, 35, 42, 45, 48, 49, 51, 54, 58, 61, 62, 63, 65, 66, 74, 78, 79, 80, 82, 83, 86, 88, 95, 103, 104, 107, 114, 123, 127, 151, 154, 157, 160, 163, 164, 169, 170, 177, 178, 180, 181, 184, 185, 188, 190, 192, 196, 199, 207, 209, 210, 211, 212, 213, 215, 216, 218, 219, 221, 224, 225, 241, 242, 243, 252, 253, 256, 258, 259, 261, 266

X

X chromosome, 78, 114
XIAP, 54, 69
X-linked lymphoproliferative syndrome, 23, 210
XLP, 48, 78, 106, 107

Z

Z Epstein-Barr virus replication activator, 78
ZAP70, 78, 109
ZEBRA, 11, 78, 101
Zeta-chain (TCR) associated protein kinase 70kDa, 78